Scott
An aid to clinical surgery

EDITOR

H.A.F. Dudley
ChM, FRCS(Eng), FRCS(Edin), FRACS

Director, Academic
Surgical Unit, St Mary's Hospital; Professor of Surgery,
London University, London, UK; formerly Professor of
Surgery, Monash University and Consultant Surgeon, Alfred
Hospital, Melbourne, Australia

ASSOCIATE EDITOR

B.P. Waxman
BMedSc, MB, FRCS(Eng), FRACS

Senior Registrar, North Tees General Hospital,
Stockton-on-Tees, UK; formerly Research Fellow, Academic
Surgical Unit, St Mary's Hospital, London, UK, and Surgical
Registrar, Alfred Hospital, Melbourne, Australia

With the collaboration of

S.T.F. Chan
MB, FRACS
Senior Registrar, St Mary's Hospital

D. Hunt
MB, FRCS(Eng)
Senior Registrar (Orthopaedics), St Mary's Hospital

R.P. Jury
MB, FRCS(Eng), FRACS
Lately Research Fellow in Vascular Surgery, St Mary's
Hospital

C.R. Kapadia
MB, FRCS(Eng)
Lecturer in Surgery, St Mary's Hospital Medical School

S.E. Knight
MB, FRCS(Eng)
Consultant Surgeon, Wexham Park Hospital

V.R. Marshall
MD, FRACS
Associate Professor (Urology), Flinders Medical Centre, South
Australia

J.P. Masterton
MB, FRCS(Eng), FRACS,
Associate Professor, Monash University, Alfred Hospital,
Melbourne, Australia

A.N. Nicolaides
MS, FRCS(Eng),
Professor of Vascular Surgery, St Mary's Hospital

A.G. Radcliffe
BSc, MB, FRCS(Eng)
Lecturer in Surgery, St Mary's Hospital Medical School

THIRD EDITION

CHURCHILL LIVINGSTONE
EDINBURGH LONDON MELBOURNE AND NEW YORK 1984

CHURCHILL LIVINGSTONE
Medical Division of Longman Group Limited

Distributed in the United States of America by Churchill
Livingstone Inc., 1560 Broadway, New York, N.Y. 10036, and
by associated companies, branches and representatives
throughout the world.

First Edition 1971
Second Edition 1979
Third Edition 1984

ISBN 0 443 02684 X

British Library Cataloguing in Publication Data

Scott, Peter Robert
    An aid to clinical surgery. —3rd ed.
    1. Surgery
    I. Title   II. Dudley, Hugh   III. Waxman, B.P.
    617   RD31

Library of Congress Cataloging in Publication Data

Scott, Peter R.
    An aid to clinical surgery.

    Previous ed.: An aid to clinical surgery/rev. by H.A.F.
Dudley.
    Includes index.
    1. Surgery.   I. Dudley, Hugh Arnold Freeman.
II. Waxman, B.P.   III. Dudley, Hugh Arnold Freeman.
An aid to clinical surgery.   IV. Title.   [DNLM:
1. Surgery WO 100 S428a]
RD31.S363   1984   617'.9   83-15012

Printed in Singapore by Selector Printing Co (Pte) Ltd

Preface

This is an aid to clinical surgery rather than a comprehensive text though we believe that it contains nearly all that the student needs to know in factual terms to get through the standard surgical examinations. What we have included has been determined by our impressions of the student's common patterns of reading. He (or she) will probably buy a separate text on orthopaedics and on ear, nose and throat surgery. However he may or may not purchase one of the excellent small books on neurosurgery, urology or vascular surgery and is unlikely, unless he has a special interest, to equip himself with a special tome on cardiac surgery. Thus we have tried to include enough grounding in these latter subjects both to provide information that will enable the student to develop a clinical interest in these subjects and to help him pass his examinations. We have given a list at the end of the book of further reading which we hope the student will find interesting.

The purpose of the book is threefold. First, to give you, the student, enough basic vocabulary, principles and facts to make you feel at ease on surgical wards. Second we hope to equip you to pass your examinations, though it is of course impossible to write a set of notes or an aid which is exactly matched to all the surgical syllabuses that are found in different medical schools. Third, and to us most important, to provide the essentials with which to tackle the major task of analysing clinical problems. For this reason, though we have been not unjustifiably criticised for the number of lists we included in the previous editions, we have incorporated most of them into the present text. They provide a check against which you can match your own analysis rather than strings of words that should be learned by rote. Operative detail is included only where it is thought to be helpful in understanding an important surgical problem; otherwise we rely on you to consult the appropriate surgical operative texts which can be found in most libraries.

Nothing in clinical learning can substitute for the gradual acquisition of attitudes and relevant knowledge at the bedside. Books are resources to help in this process, not substitutes for it. We hope that you will use this one as a background to clinical experience and as a sounding board for what your clinical teachers tell you by word of mouth.

London, 1984

H.A.F.D.
B.P.W.

Contents

1. Pain   1
2. Body water and electrolyte problems   7
3. Metabolic response to injury   12
4. Shock   15
5. Some complications of surgery   20
6. Surgical wounds: healing and management   28
7. General management of injuries and fractures   31
8. Head injuries   37
9. Chest injuries and respiratory management in surgery   44
10. Abdominal injuries   51
11. Nerve and vessel injuries   55
12. Burns   59
13. Acute infections   65
14. Specific infections   69
15. Infections of specific sites   75
16. Scalp and intracranial conditions   84
17. Face, lip, tongue and mouth   93
18. Neck swellings   99
19. Thyroid   107

20. The breast   121
21. Intrathoracic conditions   131
22. Oesophagus and diaphragm   139
23. Peptic ulcer   148
24. Stomach   157
25. Biliary and pancreatic disorders   162
26. Intestinal obstruction   184
27. Inflammatory bowel disease   189
28. Acute appendicitis and other causes of acute abdominal pain   200
29. Large bowel tumours   206
30. Perianal conditions   215
31. Gastro-intestinal haemorrhage   222
32. External herniae   231
33. Testis and epididymis   241
34. Urinary tract disorders   248
35. Venous and related conditions of the lower limb   260
36. Arterial surgery and amputations   275
37. Skin conditions   283
Further Reading   292
Index   293

1

Pain

GENERAL FEATURES OF PAIN IN SURGICAL PATIENTS

Pain is among the commonest of all symptoms. Because surgeons deal predominantly with structural problems, that is things that affect peripheral structures, it is even more frequent as a presenting symptom for surgeons than it is for others.

The following observations are relevant both to surgeons and to others who deal with pain:

1. Pain is subjective—we cannot experience another person's pain, only judge it by reference to ourselves.
2. The individual's personality conditions the expression of pain. On the one hand the stoic who will recognise and admit to little; on the other hand the expressionist who will communicate every nuance and variable. Circumstances also alter cases—a loser is more likely to feel pain than a winner; the hungry more than the well fed; the anxious more than the man at ease.
3. Pain has to be expressed as communication either by language or by non verbal means. Such expression requires a common set of values and meanings between patient and doctor. Often this is difficult because adjectives such as 'burning', 'gripping', 'awful', 'terrible' have different meanings for doctor and for patient.

To get round the problem of communication it is well to say to the patient 'tell me about your pain' or 'how would you describe it?' and to watch the patient as he/she replies.

Mechanisms

Anyone dealing with pain must ask:

1. Can I conceive a mechanism which would explain *this* patient's pain in the clinical setting?
2. Is it possible for there to be a pathway along which pain of the type the patient has (or claims to have) can be transmitted?

There are five peripheral mechanisms:

1. Chemical irritation, including the products of bacteria—dropping acid on the hand, or release of bacteria into the peritoneal cavity are good examples. Exact chemical mediation unknown. Possibly release of prostaglandins is involved.
2. Ischaemia—probably rise in hydrogen ion concentration.
3. Inappropriate smooth muscle contraction—often called 'spasm'. Probably this pain is also ischaemic.
4. Tension and distension—there is a common mechanism of *stretch* but the first process usually takes place in solid organs (e.g., rapid distension of the liver capsule) and the second is the consequence of tension in relation to smooth muscle (e.g., the gall bladder).
5. Direct effects on peripheral nerves—direct stimulation by such things as a prick or cut, or by the infiltration of nerve axons say by malignant disease and by compression of a nerve root by bone.

The other mechanisms are *central*:

1. From the aberrant function of any pain conducting pathway or reception station (e.g. the thalamus) in the central nervous system.
2. From the malfunction of the psyche in which the patient perceives pain though there is not an organic cause.

Pathways

All pains generated peripherally are the consequence of nerve impulses passing along different fibres which have a ganglion station in the dorsal roots (Fig. 1.1). Skin and viscera have identical types of nerve pathways, though it is usual to call those arising from viscera *autonomic* or *visceral* afferents.

Within the spinal grey matter, pain fibres relay in the substantia gelatinosa and ascend in the spinothalamic and palaeospinothalamic tracts on the contralateral side. The ultimate fate of impulses in the thalamus is not well

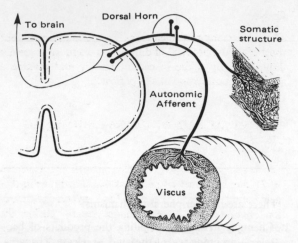

Fig. 1.1 Pain pathways from periphery

understood. It seems *unlikely* that pain is the result of a closed system of peripheral receptor—pathway—central analyser. It is more likely that pain is registered by the brain scanning a particular spatio-temporal pattern of impulses. Descending pathways probably discharging enkephalins may modulate transmission of pain impulses centrally so at least modifying the central perception of pain. A further factor which determines what the patient perceives is the activity of the central endorphin system in the midbrain. It is here that opiate receptors exist which are variably saturated by natural endorphins. Morphine and its analogues act here by filling empty receptor sites.

Reference

Pain is always (except in some mental illnesses) identified with a particular part of the body: in this sense all pain is 'referred' somewhere. Because the mental image of the body is largely of its surface (including the two extremes of the gastro-intenstinal tract), reference tends to be to a *surface*, though accuracy of localization (i.e. the ability of a patient to indicate one place rather than another) is more exact if the pain originates in a structure which *is* part of a surface (including *inner* surfaces such as parietal peritoneum or pleura).

The word 'reference' is also often used exclusively for what might better be called 'anatomically inappropriate reference'. Thus, pain produced by stimulation of the under surface of the diaphragm is appreciated over the shoulder. Though apparently inappropriate, this is embryologically appropriate. Exceptions can always be found to any rules, but the following are useful:

1. Pain of root or segment origin is referred usually to the surface dermatome of that segment.

2. Pain originating in a viscus is usually referred to the surface segment similarly corresponding, but is less well localized than pain originating in a segmental innervation or from a non-visceral structure such as a ligament.
3. Structures which have origin in the midline give rise to predominantly midline pain. Conversely, non-midline structures give rise to unilateral pain.
4. Pain which is segmental should never be ignored.

Patterns

Fully to delineate a pain it is necessary to ask Ryle's ten questions:

1. Site(s)
2. Radiation
3. Character
4. Severity
5. Duration
6. Frequency or periodism
7. Special types of description
8. Aggravating factors
9. Relieving factors
10. Associated problems

However, it is often adequate to build up a pain picture by defining *site, strength, duration* and *character*.

Irritation-produced pain is sharp, nagging, burning and usually continuous as long as the irritation lasts.

Ischaemic pain is of two types:
1. Produced in muscle by exercise—'angina' in the heart, 'intermittent claudication' in the legs. It is usually severe, gripping, crushing, ill localized (because it originates in deep-seated structures).
2. Ischaemia of nerve—continuous, severe, boring and intractable, e.g. the rest pain of severe ischaemia in the limbs.

Pain from inappropriate smooth muscle contraction is usually intermittent, though the periods may be many minutes in length. Slight to severe, gripping, lanceolating. Often called 'colic', but care must be taken to distinguish such intermittent pain from the continuous pain exacerbations seen frequently in distension of a hollow or solid viscus.

Tension or distension pain usually starts fairly suddenly, rises to a peak and persists with or without exacerbations until relieved by attention to the cause. Dull, aching, persistent, ill-localized pain unless a surface structure is involved, which is rare (but does occur, e.g. pain in infection of: the pulp space of the finger; the breast; and the ischio-rectal fossa).

Direct effects on nerves resembles ischaemia—continuous, boring, severe.

Central pain often does not correspond to a segment, descriptions tend to be bizarre, but remember the possibility of observer error on the patient's part.

Radiation is the description given to pain which starts in one place and then moves in a continuous fashion (initial pain usually persisting) to another. Causes possibly:

1. double reference—e.g. biliary tree represented in front and back of trunk.
2. spread of the pathological process across segments—e.g. radiation of pain into groin in renal colic.
3. involvement of adjacent structures—e.g. pancreas in biliary tract disease giving back-pain.

Not to be confused with two separate pains occurring in the course of some clinical circumstances, e.g. the development of right iliac fossa pain in appendicitis may appear to be but is *not* a radiation from the central pain which precedes it.

Associated features of pain. Vomiting is usually called 'reflex' and may be produced by any severe pain, but particularly by distension and muscle spasm. Salivation and nausea are lesser features of the same nature. Vasoconstriction and tachycardia may occur in severe pain. Fainting from pain is uncommon unless there is some additional factor such as blood loss or an added emotional situation.

Muscle spasm may be a consequence of the underlying cause of the pain (e.g. infection, irritation) or may occur reflexly to protect the source of the pain. '*Guarding*' is the term applied to any muscle contraction produced by additional stimulation. It can be further subdivided into 'voluntary' and 'involuntary' guarding. The first takes place when a threatened attack on a normally or abnormally sensitive site is perceived. This includes circumstances where the patients thinks the site should be painful, rather than when, in fact, it is so: hence the tense abdominal musculature of apprehensive patients. Involuntary guarding exists when a reflex is set up which invokes muscle spasm whether the patient wills it or not.

Rigidity is used to describe any muscle spasm permanently present in the conscious state.

ABDOMINAL PAIN

Nature

The appreciation of abdominal pain varies from patient to patient; what may be described as pain by some may be called 'wind', discomfort, heartburn or indigestion by others.

Cause

There are many possible causes for abdominal pain, but most often the problem of differential diagnosis is greatly diminished by taking a careful history and making a thorough examination of the patient.

ABDOMINAL PAIN OF EXTRA-ABDOMINAL ORIGIN

Pain that originates anatomically outwith the abdomen (p. 2) may be perceived as abdominal. Partly, as in thoracic conditions such as pleurisy and myocardial infarction, because the patient cannot clearly define the boundaries of his problem. Partly because segmental pain originating in the spine is referred along the line of the dermatome into the abdomen, as in vertebral column disease, tumour of the cord and tabes dorsalis.

Some more generalized conditions are associated with abdominal pain either because they produce disordered bowel contraction (lead poisoning), cause peptic ulceration (hyperparathyroidism) or because of an unknown mechanism (acute porphyria).

COMMON CAUSE

1. *The result of segmental stimulation that overlaps with the abdomen*
   a. Pleurisy
   b. Angina and myocardial infarction
   c. Vertebral column disease
   d. Spinal tumours
   e. Fractured ribs
   f. Herpes zoster
   g. Crisis of tabes dorsalis

2. *The result of a generalized disease*—mechanism postulated but unknown
   a. Acute porphyria
   b. Lead poisoning
   c. Crisis of haemolytic anaemia
   d. Hyperparathyroidism
   e. Sickle cell crises

3. *The result of abdominal wall disorder*—usually segmental, well-localized and accompanied by local signs
   a. Trauma
   b. 'Spontaneous' haematoma
   c. Rupture of muscles, e.g. rectus abdominis in pregnancy

4. *The consequence of peritoneal irritation*
   a. Rupture of a hollow viscus—peritonitis

b. Rupture of a solid organ—blood in the peritoneal cavity

5. *The outcome of hollow tube obstruction*
   a. Cystic or common bile duct obstruction
   b. Intestinal obstruction
   c. Renal obstruction

6. *From expanding lesions within a semi-rigid organ*
   a. Pancreatitis
   b. Malignant or inflammatory liver disease
   c. Infarction—gut or spleen

7. *Retroperitoneal causes*
   a. Ruptured abdominal aortic aneurysm
   b. Pancreatitis

Origins

GASTRO-INTESTINAL TRACT

The gastro-intestinal tract and its appendages are all, in embryological terms, midline structures. It is conventional, and for the most part correct, to say in consequence that pain originating in them and (an important qualification) unassociated with irritation of parietal structures such as the inner aspect of the peritoneum, will be referred to the midline. This is not an explanation—merely an expression of a general rule to which there are some exceptions, e.g. the occasional right-sided location of distension pain in biliary tract disease.

The gastro-intestinal tract is predominantly a hollow muscular tube; its appendages such as the liver (and more distantly, the spleen) are encapsulated and subject to distension either from the presence of excess blood or, as in the case of liver and pancreas, because of obstruction of the ducts that drain them. Two types of pain predominate: (1) distension pain consequent upon stretch of a hollow portion or of a capsule of a solid viscus, and (2) muscular contraction pain. The first is dull, dragging and continuous; the second the pain we all know to call colic—gripping, spasmodic, crescendo. Sometimes, as in so-called 'biliary colic' the two may be combined. Both are ill-localized and the patient will use the flat of his hand to indicate the site.

Localization

1. The foregut, which developed in the upper part of the abdomen, gives rise to predominantly epigastric and hypochondrial pain.
2. Midgut, to pain in the central abdomen and periumbilical region.
3. Hind gut, to suprapubic pain.

The predominantly central nature of 'gut ache' often helps to distinguish it from renal pain, which is well-localized to one or other side, and from segmental pain originating in the spine and spinal cord, which is usually band-like and, with rare exceptions, more severe to one or other side.

Additional helpful factors in most pain originating in the gastro-intestinal tract are an ill-localized nature, the type and the presence of associated features such as nausea and vomiting, though it must be admitted that the latter are not unique.

PERITONEAL PAIN

1. Direct stimulation. Where abdominal pain is well-localized ('precisely referred' may be a better phrase, see p. 2) it is good to think primarily of peritoneal irritation. The inner aspect of the abdomen has relatively accurate representation at the body surface so that when, for example, an inflamed anterior duodenal wall or a similarly inflamed appendix impinges against it, the patient can say 'I feel pain here' indicating the site with no more than one or two fingers. In addition, the precision of localization usually allows lateralization, though this may be false, as when pus tracking up from an inflamed pelvic appendix gives pain and tenderness in the *left* iliac fossa, or a long sigmoid loop containing an inflamed diverticulum lies pointing towards the *right* iliac fossa. Also, primarily intramural causes in the abdominal wall will have the same features, but can usually be distinguished by their context. Anatomically inappropriate localization or reference occurs when the subdiaphragmatic parietal peritoneum is irritated and pain is felt in the shoulder. Two maxims emerge: (a) acute *severe* shoulder pain in a patient with abdominal signs nearly always means blood, bowel content, exudate or gas in the peritoneal cavity (less severe pain on the right side may be a feature of biliary tract disease); (b) unexplained shoulder tip pain should direct attention to the abdomen as a possible cause, e.g. an acutely enlarging spleen with perisplenic irritation.

2. Stretch is also an effective mechanism in peritoneal pain. It operates when a hernial sac fills rapidly as a result of postural change, so stretching the neck and giving a dragging sensation well-localized to the site; common inguinal ruptures are thus *not* painless conditions and the patient's complaint should be treated with respect. Another much less common cause is sudden distension by ascites; surgeons have been foxed into thinking that a patient has diffuse peritoneal irritation because of generalized pain of this origin.

Establishing a diagnosis with particular reference to abdominal pain

SYMPTOMS

The following remarks—which are only guidelines—do not necessarily distinguish between acute and chronic pain.

1. Where is the pain?
   a. Flank—consider renal origin
   b. Beneath right costal margin—consider liver distension or gall bladder disease with peritoneal irritation
   c. Epigastric—consider peptic ulcer, oesophagitis from hiatus hernia, pancreatitis, epigastric hernia
   d. Xiphisternal—consider oesophagitis or peptic ulcer
   e. Suprapubic—consider pelvic causes

2. What kind of pain is it?
   a. Colicky pain—sharp intermittent gripping pains often indicate obstruction to a hollow organ, e.g. stone in common duct, stone in renal pelvis or bowel obstruction
   b. Crescendo pain in the abdomen may be the result of progressive distension
   c. Continuous or 'boring' pain may suggest penetration of a peptic ulcer, pancreatitis or malignant disease
   d. Throbbing pain suggests inflammation

3. Did the pain start suddenly or come on gradually?
   a. Sudden onset of severe pain suggests perforation, e.g. peptic ulcer or gall bladder
   b. Sudden onset after trauma may suggest fractured ribs, ruptured spleen or lacerated liver
   c. Gradual onset suggests obstruction or distension

4. Does the pain extend or radiate?
   a. Over the entire abdomen suggests perforation with peritonitis
   b. To the shoulder indicates diaphragmatic irritation, e.g. ruptured spleen or perforated peptic ulcer
   c. Beneath the right costal margin to between the shoulder blades suggests cholecystitis
   d. To the back suggests pancreatitis
   e. Down along the line of the ureter suggests ureteric calculus
   f. Into the vagina or perineum—pelvic causes

5. Is the pain getting better, worse or no change?
   Worsening pain, in severity and spread, indicates a progressive disorder, particularly if originally of sudden onset, with or without trauma.

   At this stage one often has a very good idea of the organ involved and various relevant questions can be asked.

Leading questions: for example, if suspect:
1. *Oesophageal lesion* (reflux oesophagitis, hiatus hernia): postural regurgitation, heart burn, dysphagia, haematemesis.

2. *Peptic ulcer*: previous exacerbations, perforations, haematemesis, medication, operations.
3. *Gall stones*: previous exacerbations, colour changes of skin, urine or faeces, which may indicate common duct obstruction. Attacks of fever may also suggest cholangitis.
4. *Liver disease*: contacts with hepatitis, alcoholism, etc.
5. *Pancreatitis*: alcohol intake, gall stone disease, weight loss, bulky stools, jaundice and diabetes.
6. *A urinary cause*: other urinary symptoms.
7. *An extra-abdominal cause*: enquire about such causes as myocardial, pulmonary or vertebral spinal disorders.

PAST HISTORY
1. Previous medication and X-rays may give clue to diagnosis.
2. Previous abdominal operations for peptic ulcer or gall bladder disease may suggest recurrent ulcer or stones.
3. Previous disease such as myocardial, pulmonary or haemolytic, may suggest a cause.
4. If there has been a hospital admission elsewhere *always* try and get the record.

SIGNS
1. *General,* particularly for:
   a. Estimation of degree of shock if an acute abdominal emergency
   b. Elimination of extra-abdominal causes, particularly lung, pleura and myocardium
2. *Local* (abdominal) particularly for site of:
   a. Local tenderness which indicates the site of an inflammatory process
   b. Presence or absence of peritonitis
   c. Presence of a mass which may be due to an aortic aneurysm, distended gall bladder, gastric tumour, enlarged liver in association with hepatitis or heart failure, or enlarged spleen in association with portal hypertension

SPECIAL TESTS
1. Urgent cases
If some intra-abdominal catastrophe is suspected then:
a. Plain X-ray of the chest and abdomen is advisable to visualize extra-luminal gas if perforated ulcer, fluid levels if bowel obstruction, radio-opaque calculi if acute cholecystitis
b. Serum amylase estimation if pancreatitis is suspected
c. Haemoglobin estimation and blood typing if suspect intra-abdominal haemorrhage
d. White cell count for evidence of leucocytosis in the presence of inflammation
e. Microscopy and culture of urine for red cells in association with renal calculi and for organisms in suspect pyelonephritis

2. Non-urgent cases

The investigation of abdominal pain as a presenting symptom should follow a sequence suggested by the history or physical findings. Such sequences will be found throughout this book, e.g. biliary disease p. 163. The advent of many methods of imaging (e.g. ultrasonography, CT) has greatly refined diagnosis and made the need for exploratory laparotomy that much the less. However, it is possible to 'study a patient to death' rather than get on to solve his problem, even if the evidence for cause is not cast-iron.

2

Body water and electrolyte problems

A thorough knowledge of the exchange of water and electrolytes both within the body and with the exterior is fundamental to good clinical care. Injury interferes with exchange or exaggerates it. This poses problems of maintenance or replacement, and thus quantitative knowledge is essential (important data for reference, but not memorization, are given in Tables 2.1 and 2.2).

ORGANIZATION AND DISTRIBUTION

Though water is distributed throughout the body, it can be divided into two sub-volumes separated by the cell membrane: intracellular fluid (ICF) and extracellular fluid (ECF) (Fig. 2.1). The ECF can be further divided into *intravascular* and *extravascular* (interstitial) components. In addition to these compartments, a certain amount of water is always present in the body cavities—gastrointestinal tract, CSF, aqueous humour. Such water has been processed through cells to reach these sites and is thus known as *transcellular* water. The instantaneous volume of transcellular water is usually small (about 0.5 l in an adult), but in certain sites, particularly the gastro-intestinal tract and kidney tubules, turnover is so rapid that many litres a day are processed. If the return pathway is blocked and production continues, then the ECF from which transcellular water is produced becomes depleted, e.g. small bowel obstruction.

Sodium and potassium are the major cations in body fluids and though their quantities within the body are roughly equal, sodium is restricted to the extracellular and potassium to the intracellular fluid. These ions are a major factor in determining both total body osmotic pressure and osmotic equality (isotonicity) across the cell membrane.

MOVEMENT OF WATER AND ELECTROLYTES ACROSS ANATOMICAL BOUNDARIES

The boundaries to the body fluid compartments are the cell membrane and the capillary membrane.

Though the *cell membrane* is freely permeable to both water and small ions, active transport mechanisms, which may be affected by hormones and other humoral factors, exist to maitain the differential in sodium and potassium concentrations within the ECF and ICF. Thus, changes in osmotic pressure (tonicity) within the ECF by solute confined to this compartment are equilibrated by movement of water to or from the ICF across the cell membrane.

The *capillary membrane* is freely permeable to water and small molecules. A decline in plasma osmotic pressure (e.g. hypoproteinaemia) or an increase in capillary hydrostatic pressure (e.g. venous obstruction) will favour

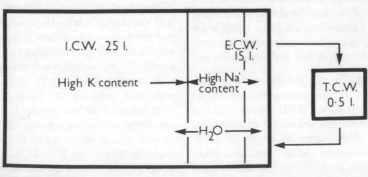

Fig. 2.1 Normal body fluid compartments

movement of fluid out of the vascular space into the interstitial (extravascular) space and thus oedema formation.

Turnover of water

There is an inevitable loss of water via the skin and lungs, water of *transpiration*, amounting to about 500 ml/day from each route in a temperate climate. This loss cannot be modified by the body's homeostatic mechanisms and is largely a consequence of:

1. Enviromental factors and the integrity of the skin envelope. The skin limits the transudation of water even though the external environment changes markedly in temperature and humidity. It is the rate of sensible perspiration (*sweating*) in man that is adjusted to deal with the problems of environmental change and that can result in ECF deficiency (see below.) Increased water of transpiration is associated with full-thickness destruction of the surface envelope, as occurs with full-thickness burns. Apart from an uncontrolled reduction in body water, consequent to insensible water escape, the latent heat of evaporation of water is such that considerable quantities of energy are required to vaporize the escaping water. Thus, cooling takes place unless increased supplies of energy are available. A patient with a deep burn of any extent must therefore expend more energy to stay normothermic.

2. The respiratory tract. A similar phenomenon occurs in the respiratory tract, and severe environmental temperature gradients may lead to an increased loss of water and heat, though the humidification mechanism tends to conserve heat.

If solute content remains the same, the insensible water loss would lead to a gradual increase in body tonicity. This is prevented in two ways:

1. *Water intake is maintaned*
2. *Kidney homeostasis.* The kidney excretes solute, an obligatory situation. However, it adjusts the rate of solute in water excretion to maintain constant body tonicity in the face of continued and fluctuating insensible losses. The kidney can alter the solute/water ratio; thus, if water loss exceeds intake this ratio rises; conversely, if water exceeds loss the reverse is true.

The control mechanism for the adjustment of urinary concentration is based on the osmoreceptor-posterior pituitary-antidiuretic hormone (ADH) system. Changes in the tonicity of plasma are sensed by hypothalamic osmoreceptors which then trigger the release of ADH. Increased tonicity increases ADH secretion while decreased tonicity lowers it. A minimal volume ('*volume obligatoire*') of approximately 400 ml is reached when intake is reduced or insensible losses increase (or both) in such a way that body tonicity rises stimulates maximal release of ADH. The exact *volume obligatoire*, i.e. the volume in which solute load can be excreted at maximum urinary concentration, is determined by:

a. The concentrating ability of the kidney; less in infancy and old age, as well as in diseases affecting the distal convoluted tubules.
b. As the solute load increases, urinary concentration falls and volume rises, presumably in part because the rate of flow through the counter-current multiplier is such that full diffusion cannot occur.Thus, increase in solute load from whatever cause, increase urinary volume in spite of maximal ADH secretion.

Water homeostasis is achieved in man with a turnover of approximately 2–2.5 l/day; of this, 1000 ml is expended as water of transpiration, the remaining 1–1.5 l being excreted by the kidneys apart from 200 ml in faeces. At this turnover, the urine is hypertonic to plasma.

Turnover of Sodium

Sodium is jealousy guarded by the body to maintain the ECF. The mechanism appears to reside in the renin-angiotensin regulation of renal sodium excretion. In temperate environments sodium losses, other than in the urine, are negligible, thus intake is directly proportional to output. Normal intake of sodium in the Western world is now between 150 and 200 mmol/day, but with sodium restriction, kidney output can fall to below 5 mmol/day. Sodium losses by the kidney are reduced in injury and situations of stress. Extra-renal sodium losses become significant with fistulae and excessive perspiration replaced by water only.

Turnover of potassium

1. RENAL LOSSES OF POTASSIUM

The turnover of potassium in a subject who is in sodium balance is of the order of 100 mmol/day, most of which is of exogenous origin. However, when sodium intake is restricted (i.e. electrolyte starvation, which is often associated with protein/energy starvation), potassium is maximally exchanged for sodium in the distal tubule; sodium excretion falling to minimal levels while that of potassium remains at 50–60 mmol/day. The potassium required for this process is removed from the plasma; however, the plasma concentration does not fall until urinary loss is in excess of 400 mmol, presumably by diffusion down the ICF–ECF concentration gradient, despite the activity of the sodium/potassium pump in the cell membrane. When the ECF potassium concentration falls, less potassium is available, and hydrogen ion excretion becomes the predominant method of renal sodium conservation.

2. EXTRA-RENAL LOSSES OF POTASSIUM

As with sodium, these amount to only a few mmol/day in sweat and faeces. Losses may be markedly increased in low small-bowel fistulae or large-bowel diarrhoea where mucus with a high potassium content is secreted.

Table 2.1 Normal chemical composition and fluid volumes for a man weighing 65 kg

		Litres
Total body water (TBW)		40.0
Intracellular fluid (ICF)		24.0
Extracellular fluid (ECF)		15.0
Plasma volume (PV)		3.0
Interstitial fluid (IF)		12.0
Transcellular water (CSF, pleural, peritoneal, intestinal)		0.5–1.0
Daily volume of:	Saliva	1.5
	Gastric juice	2.5
	Bile	0.5
	Pancreatic juice	0.7
	Succus entericus	3.0
Daily water losses in:	Expired air	0.4
	Faeces	0.1
	Skin (insensible)	0.3
	Urine (obligatory)	0.5
	Total	1.3
Daily losses in urine of:	Urea	25 g
	Nitrogen	12 g
	Sodium	150–200 mmol
	Potassium	100 mmol
Total body:	Protein	11.0 kg
	Fat	9.0 kg
	Carbohydrates	0.5 kg
	Minerals	4.5 kg

Table 2.2 Important ionic concentrations (mmol/l)

	ICF		ECF
(a) Na	10		135
K	150		4
Ca	2.5		2.5
Mg	7.5		1
Cl	10		100
PO$_4$	45		1
HCO$_3$	10		27
	Na	K	Cl
(b) Gastric aspirate	110	5	100
Intestinal aspirate	120	10	100

DISORDERS

Three major *deficiency* disorders are recognized. They may exist in pure form or intermingled.

1. Acute water lack
2. Acute extracellular (ECF) deficiency
3. Potassium deficiency

Each has its counterpart in *excesses*.

1. Water intoxication
2. ECF excess—congestive heart failure
3. Potassium excess

Acute water lack

Pathogenesis

When water intake is nil or losses exceed intake, loss continues by insensible routes. With maximal ADH secretion, the volume obligatoire is excreted by the kidneys. However, whole body tonicity rises because of continued extrarenal (insensible) losses. Gradually, the body becomes more hypertonic, eventaully enzyme systems fail, and there is hyperthermia and cell death.

Clinical features

Symptoms are thirst and anxiety; restlessness in the unconscious patient (the dangerous inference in this situation being that some other cause exists). Signs are minimal because the water loss equilibrates across the cell membrane (Fig. 2.2).

Laboratory investigations

Serum sodium concentrations may be slightly raised. Urea concentration is also raised. This is because with maximal antidiuresis the kidneys' ability to excrete a solute such as urea becomes less.

In the last stages of 'exsiccation' of this type, temperature regulation fails and the body heats up to +40°C.

Management

a. Do not let it happen
b. Pay careful attention to water balance, especially in the feeble or unconscious. Remember that water loss is increased with fever, mouth breathing and burns.
c. If acute water lack is present, rehydrate by mouth, stomach tube or vein, taking care not to swing into water intoxication
d. In complex circumstances, daily weight can be helpful

Water intoxication

Pathogenesis

Too much water input against too little output results in total solute dilution. This can occur when too much

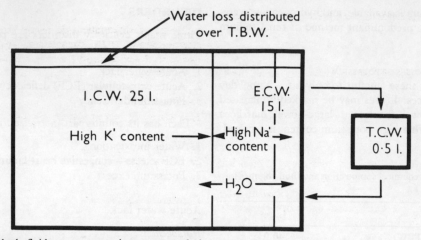

Fig. 2.2 Cange of body fluid compartments in acute water lack

solute-free water is infused during postoperative anti-diuresis. Symptoms are lethargy, mental disorientation, and coma. There is hypothermia.

Signs are few, as the excess water is distributed in both ICF and ECF. Oedema does *not* occur; this is a feature of sodium and water overload (see below).

Diagnosis is confirmed by finding a low serum sodium concentration (see 'sick cell syndrome').

Management
a. Water restriction
b. Rarely, hypertonic sodium chloride in small doses may be necessary
c. A diuresis may be induced by the use of a diuretic, but this removes as much sodium as water, and is less effective than allowing excess water to 'boil off' by insensible routes

Acute extracellular (ECF) deficiency

Pathogenesis
Diversion of transcellular water is the cause: excessive perspiration, gastrointestinal secretion, distal tubular urine. Because the loss is, to all intents and purposes, isotonic, water is not replaced from the ICF (Fig. 2.3). The ECF shrinks and shock supervenes, the cause of death being circulatory failure.

Clinical features
Sunken eyes, lax skin, dry tongue, oliguria, tachycardia, postural hypotension, low blood pressure, empty veins, and finally shock.

Management
a. Prevention by replacement of ECF losses as they occur.

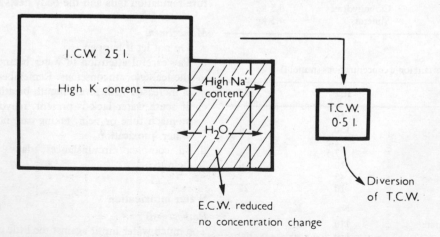

Fig. 2.3 Change of body fluid compartments in acute extracellular fluid depletion

b. Treatment replacement with saline or Hartmann's solution.

Control

By clinical restoration of circulation; skin tugor; haematocrit.

Acute ECF excess

Pathogenesis

Too much sodium and water in the face of diminished excretory capacity. Seen in congestive cardiac failure or in surgical circumstances after the injudicious infusion of saline in a patient whose renal excretory capacity is restricted, e.g. after injury (Fig. 2.4).

Clinical features

Dyspnoea: raised venous pressure, crepitation at the lung bases, oedema. The fluid chart may show a gradual increase in positive balance.

Management

Restriction of sodium and water intake. Use of diuretics, e.g. frusemide.

Potassium loss

Potassium continues to be lost by the kidney when sodium is conserved (as in starvation or after injury). A considerable deficit accumulates if this is allowed to continue over several days, serum concentration falling after 400 mmol has been lost. Hypokalaemia is further exaggerated by alkalosis, as occurs if there is concomitant gastro-intestinal loss of hydrogen ion, (e.g. pyloric stenosis). Potassium losses by extra-renal routes are rare; prolonged mucous diarrhoea can lead to hypokalaemia as mucus contains 10 times the plasma concentration of potassium.

Clinical features

Lethargy, disorientation, decreased striated and smooth muscle tonus with consequent ptosis, ileus, poor myocardial contractility, and potentially fatal cardiac arrhythmias.

Confirmation

Low serum K concentration, alkalosis, ECG changes.

Management

Stop loss. Replace K orally or cautiously intravenously.

Potassium excess

Pathogenesis

The kidney is responsible for potassium homeostasis; in acute renal failure, particularly when there is a large volume of dead tissue (including red cells) to provide a source of potassium, extracellular K rises. Starvation in this situation also leads to elevation of serum potassium concentration as protein is broken down. A doubling of the extracellular concentration of K is lethal; the situation is worsened by a low serum sodium concentration.

Clinical features

Non-specific features, similar to those with potassium deficiency, cardiac arrhythmias and cardiac arrest.

Confirmation

High serum K concentration, ECG abnormalities.

Management

a. No potassium intake
b. Reduce K concentration by infusion of glucose and insulin which pushes K into cells
c. Ion exchange resins
d. Haemodialysis in severe cases

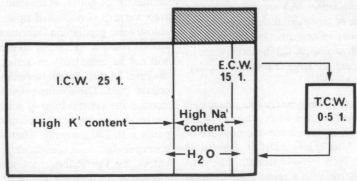

E.C.W. increased in volume
No change in concentration

I.C.W. 25 1.

High K' content

E.C.W. 15 1.

High Na' content

H_2O

T.C.W. 0·5 1.

Fig. 2.4 Change of body fluid compartments in sodium and water (ECF) excess

3

Metabolic response to injury

An understanding of the metabolic response to injury is desirable for the proper management of any severe illness. Just as wound healing is important to our knowledge of myocardial infarction as well as to the repair of an abdominal incision, so the changes typical of injury occur in a severe septic episode or a major medical crisis just as much as they follow trauma. However, they have been most intensively studied in relation to injury and they have their greatest importance in patient care in this setting.

GENERAL

Injury sets in train a complex neuro-humoral series of adjustments which, if interpreted teleologically, are designed to conserve body water and electrolytes in a situation where ability to obtain these may be reduced. Thus, the events seen are identical to those which take place when intake of water and electrolytes is withdrawn but in the case of injury they are driven by stimuli other than those involved in normal homeostasis.

SPECIFIC NEURO-ENDOCRINE RESPONSES

These are probably set off by pain but may be sustained by other things such as the products of injured tissue.

1. Secretion of catecholamines. An inevitable, almost immediate consequence of any painful situation. Begins within seconds, promotes vasoconstriction but is probably not of any great physiological significance except in circumstances where there are large changes in circulating blood volume (e.g. shock).

2. Secretion of antidiuretic hormone (ADH). Increased secretion of ADH normally occurs when intake of water is reduced because of an increased osmotic pressure of the total body water. After injury ADH is secreted in large amounts without such osmotic stimuli. The consequence is relative oliguria with a raised concentration of the urine, even though body water is normal. Because

the secretion of ADH is the result of the injury (mainly pain) the administration of water does not result in suppression of ADH secretion and a water diuresis. Instead, body water will expand and body tonicity fall. This can produce overhydration ('water intoxication'). The onset of ADH secretion is, like catecholamine secretion, within a few minutes of injury and lasts from 24 to 36 hours. During this time volume of urine secreted is the *volume obligatoire*—that necessary to excrete the solute load at the highest attainable concentration. Relative oliguria is thus the rule after injury—volumes down to about 0.4 ml/min. It is important to remember that this volume of highly concentrated urine will only be produced if glomerular filtration rate (GFR) is maintained. If GFR falls then urine volume will fall below 0.3 ml/min and more importantly, increasing the solute load will *not* increase urine volume. When GFR is normal the urine volume can be increased by increasing solute load, e.g. by the use of mannitol or urea. Sodium containing solutions have the same effect but this always results in the excretion of less sodium than is administered. However, the same solute loading effect can be obtained with frusemide which releases sodium from the proximal tubules.

3. Secretion of aldosterone and other adreno-cortical substances. There is a wave of increased adrenocortical secretion after injury, again starting within a few minutes and lasting about 36 hours. Cortisol levels in blood may double for 24 hours, as may aldosterone. As with ADH secretion this is not based upon the normal stimulus to aldosterone production—shrinkage in the extracellular space. Thus, if sodium is administered in this phase it will not be completely excreted, as would normally be the case. Instead, it will be retained, so expanding extracellular fluid. The sodium response is more sluggish than that for the conservation of water. On the first postoperative day 40–50 mmol sodium may be excreted as compared with 100 normally. Half this on the second postoperative day. As a consequence of reduction in sodium output by the kidney, potassium excretion tends to increase. This may also follow on the liberation of potassium from damaged cells.

In summary, the major changes seen after injury are:

1. *Reduced excretion of water*—because of ADH, *volume obligatoire* only is passed, say 500 ml/day.

2. *Reduced excretion of sodium*—50 mmol first day, less the next.

3. *Increased excretion of potassium*—up to 100 mmol/day for the first day. Thereafter the excretion is that in starvation which is approximately 50 mmol/day.

CHANGES IN ENERGY EXPENDITURE AND NITROGEN EXCRETION

For a long time it was thought that energy expenditure was markedly increased after injury. This was based upon the observation that nitrogen excretion rates seemed to be increased in some patients, so suggesting that tissue was being broken down. It is now known that such nitrogen excretion occurs in excess only when:

1. There is some labile nitrogen available as is usually the case in an individual on a normal protein intake who has a large pool of amino acids. When he is starved—the usual thing in relation to injury—some of the pool spills into the urine at a high rate producing a 'negative balance'.
2. When large areas of tissue are irrevocably damaged
3. In severe sepsis

Similarly increased energy expenditure is only seen:

1. When increased mechanical work is required—e.g. the work of breathing is markedly increased
2. When increased thermal work is needed—e.g. to evaporate water through a lost skin envelope as occurs in extensive burns, or when a fever is induced by infection

Apart from these situations there is little change in energy expenditure after injury. Should energy be supplied? The answer is roughly as follows:

1. If a patient is healthy and well nourished a few days starvation will make little difference to him. Exogenous energy can be withheld. The patient will metabolize his own fat and protein stores. After 24 hours nearly all energy is derived from fat stores and the respiratory quotient reflects this by falling to the vicinity of 0.7. In starving man there is a steady small attrition of protein for gluconeogenesis. This can be reduced to a minimum by administering this amount to conserve tissue protein.
2. In patients who have been severely depleted before coming under medical care, such as those with starvation from any cause or the effects of malignant disease, nourishment should always be provided before

and after injury because the additional stress of injury or acute illness seems to have a much more deleterious effect than in health. Furthermore, efforts should be made to get such patients into positive nitrogen balance before they have to undergo a surgical procedure.

ABERRATIONS OF THE METABOLIC RESPONSE

1. Renal
Conservation of water by the ADH mechanism and of sodium by the secretion of aldosterone only works if the kidneys are normal. Chronic renal damage from pyelonephritis or merely old age will render both endocrine mechanisms relatively ineffective. The patient will continue to pass large volumes of both water and sodium and therefore if adequate replacement is not undertaken, become depleted by the renal route.

2. Increased adrenocortical secretion
a. Diabetes. Cortisol is diabetogenic. If a patient is already not adequately handling carbohydrates, the extra effect of the increased circulating cortisol may drive him into frank, if temporary, diabetes mellitus. This is usually not a serious problem.
b. In severe stress states—massive infections, multiple injuries, extensive burns—the increased adrenocorticol secretion rates may be prolonged for many days: still stressed, still steroid secreting. The levels sustained may be high enough to prevent normal repair, sometimes of wounds and occasionally of the gastrointestinal tract. Vulnerable mucosal areas such as the stomach and duodenum may then ulcerate, or a previously present ulcer advance, producing so-called 'stress ulceration' (p. 148). Because of poor healing, this situation is difficult to treat.

NUTRITION

Man's normal energy requirements are 5000 kJ/m²/day (30 Cal/kg) accompanied by a minimum of 8 gN (50 g protein) a day. In addition to these *macronutrient* requirements a very wide variety of micronutrients are needed, amongst which are vitamins, minerals (e.g. calcium, magnesium, zinc, copper, manganese), essential fatty acids and almost certainly substances as yet unidentified.

After uncomplicated injury, energy and nitrogen requirements do not notably change, but the following circumstances often associated with injury do increase requirements.

1. Fever (10–13% rise in metabolic rate for every degree centigrade)

2. Physical demand—e.g. respiratory muscles
3. Severe sepsis even without high fever.

The last is often associated with increased amino acid wasting from muscle so that instead of drawing on fat stores as would the ordinary starving patient, there is selective muscle wasting which compounds the patient's problems.

Patients coming to surgery may be *depleted* by the effects of their disease. Their changes are those of starvation and sometimes electrolyte depletion (potassium most common). *After operation* normal feeding may not be possible because of a non-functioning gastro-intestinal tract.

Indications for supplementary or total feeding are:

1. Pre-operative repletion
2. Post-operative maintenance
3. Long term therapy for complicated intestinal diseases (e.g. Crohn's, short bowel)

Methods of feeding

If there is a normal gastro-intestinal tract then, if at all possible, it should be used. It may be necessary to get past an obstruction—e.g. dilating an oesophageal stricture or inserting a gastrostomy or jejunostomy. If *enteral* feeding is possible whole food mixed in a 'vitamizer' (homogenizer) can be employed as can various prepared packages. 'Elemental diets' are a particular example of the latter in which carbohydrate, amino acids and sometimes fat are provided so that digestion is not required and absorption is total.

When the gastro-intestinal tract is abnormal, *parenteral* nutrition is used. A plastic catheter is inserted into a large vein, usually the superior vena cava via the subclavian, and amino acid, carbohydrate and fat infused. An excess of Calories may be given to try to ensure weight gain, but it is usually difficult to get a patient to put on flesh and fat until he is completely well. Parenteral nutrition is not without hazard, both in terms of sepsis and the metabolic complications that may ensue. However, it can alter outcome in patients with cancer, intestinal fistulae and disturbed gastro-intestinal function.

4

Shock

Shock is a useful but imprecise term; useful because it describes a clinical appearance of circulatory collapse; imprecise as it neither gives information about aetiology nor guidance for a plan of treatment.

Shock may be defined in physiological terms as the body's *response* to a reduced *effective* circulating blood volume, but in everyday practice the word is used to describe the clinical state of affairs of *reduced peripheral blood flow* and resultant *peripheral tissue hypoxia*. It is these two mechanisms that explain most of the clinical manifestations of the shock syndromes: pallor; cold, clammy periphery; peripheral cyanosis; and mental confusion.

The method of production of reduced perfusion will vary from instance to instance, so when summoned to a patient said to be in shock, the first question to be asked is 'What is the cause?' Only so can a plan of treatment be arrived at.

The five major causes of 'shock' are:

1. Fainting and neural phenomena
2. Loss of circulating volume
3. 'Pump failure'
4. Massive sepsis
5. Metabolic and immunological disorders

The general principles of treatment are in three phases:

1. Immediate action
2. Assessment
3. Definitive treatment (see Chapter 7)

FAINTING AND NEURAL PHENOMENA

The fainting of emotional stress, also referred to as a 'vaso-vagal attack' because of the associated bradycardia, hypotension and hyperpnoea, has in the past been included under the heading of *shock*.

Certainly this is so to the layman who habitually describes as 'shocked' anyone who has had a fright. The term *neurogenic shock* is best not used, though peripheral tissue hypoxia in the brain is characteristic of fainting which has a neurogenic basis. What is important to remember is:

1. Other factors such as blood loss can, if the patient is upright, lead to the development of the physiological chain of events—adrenaline secretion, muscular vasodilatation, bradycardia and cerebral hypoxia—which leads to fainting. Thus, fainting may be a component of some particular circumstances of blood loss: perhaps the most frequently encountered in civilian practice is the patient who has a major gastro-intestinal haemorrhage and then either defaecates or vomits. The Valsalva effect so produced reduces venous return to the heart and precipitates a faint.
2. If, when a patient faints, he is prevented from falling, the cerebral hypoxia is self-perpetuating and may result in irreversible brain damage and/or a cardiac arrest. Death under light general anaesthesia in the dentist's chair and possibly some fatalities in elderly patients propped upright in bed in hospital may be assigned to this cause.

Management

Lay the patient flat, preferably with the legs elevated. Spontaneous recovery follows. Seek causes of bleeding.

Spinal shock

This is the clinical syndrome that may develop following damage of the spinal cord, and is discussed in detail in Chapter 7.

SHOCK FROM REDUCTION OF CIRCULATING VOLUME

There are three major causes of volume reduction:

1. **Whole blood loss** which may be either *external*, as from the body surface or the gastro-intestinal or genito-urinary tracts, or *internal* into damaged tissues (e.g. a

fracture haematoma or an infarcted organ) or a body cavity (e.g. intraperitoneal haemorrhage from a ruptured aortic aneurysm or ectopic pregnancy).

The effects of external or internal haemorrhage are the same, though the rate of loss may be slow and progressive into tissues where tension increases gradually.

2. Plasma loss occurs in burns as a consequence of leakage of protein and exudate through damaged capillaries. Dilute plasma is also lost into an area of inflammation or tissue damage, but the protein content of such loss is rarely important in considering fluid replacement, except in the case of fulminant pancreatitis.

3. Loss of extracellular fluid (ECF) is a consequence of three situations:

a. Deviation of normal exchange mechanisms (loss of *transcellular* water). Extracellular fluid is in a constant state of exchange across the gastro-intestinal tract and the nephron. Normally, though large quantities are moved every day in this manner, the net amount of extracellular water that is 'transcellular' (mainly in the lumen of the gut) at any instant is quite small. However, by interference with reabsorption the extracellular fluid can be continuously drained from its normal site. Such losses occur in vomiting, diarrhoea, fistulae and failure of tubular reabsorption of urine. In each instance the fluid lost varies in composition, but basically it is rich in sodium ions. Big losses are accompanied by shrinkage of plasma volume and the onset of shock (Fig. 2.3)

b. By increased loss of ECF along a normal pathway. The best single example of this situation is excessive sweating without replacement in a non-acclimatized individual. Sufficient dilute extracellular fluid may be leached out to produce a profound reduction in ECF and a shock state, but this is rare in temperate climates.

c. Disruption to the anatomical boundaries of fluid compartments (the 'third space phenomenon'). There are two kinds:

1. Loss of biochemical integrity of cell membrane, e.g. by hypoxia with leakage of sodium into the cell and thus a reduction in 'effective extracellular volume'. Probably uncommon.
2. When there is increased capillary permeability as in an inflamed area (see above).

Physiological adjustments to loss of circulatory volume

Two major physiological adjustments occur.

1. There is peripheral vasoconstriction which adapts the volume of the vascular tree to the reduced volume of blood it contains (it must be noted that a phrase beloved of many writers on shock—discrepancy between volume of blood and the capacity of the vascular tree—is a physical impossibility). The vasoconstriction is widespread, affecting the capacitance vessels on the venous side of the circulation as well as arterioles. In both instances as the vascular network shrinks the pressure tends to fall but initially, because of increased resistance to flow, it is maintained on the arterial side, with or without a mild increase in heart rate. Measurements of intravascular pressure are thus usefully made both on the arterial and venous side of the circulation, particularly the latter.

2. There is, by virtue of the altered pressure relations in the arteriole—capillary—venule loop, an ingress of extracellular water into the circulation which produces haemodilution. Initially, this is quite a rapid process and after a haemorrhage of 1.5–2.0 litres three quarters of the resulting haemodilution is over in 6–8 hours; this is of importance in the management of patients with suspected continued bleeding into, say, the gastro-intestinal tract. Repeated determinations over some hours indicating a progressively falling haemoglobin, haematocrit or red cell count (all rough indications of haemodilution) are more often than not indications of continued haemorrhage.

Reduction in circulating volume: correlation with physical findings

Computation of blood volume deficits is difficult and even direct measurement of blood volume is only accurate to about 5% (±300 ml in an average man). No single measurement should be relied on, rather a summation of the data in Tables 4.1 and 4.2.

In some circumstances it may be possible to correlate the clinical assessment with measured loss, e.g. blood during the course of an operation, or ECF from a fistula. Even if the measurement lacks refinement (as does simple swab weighing) it gives more useful information than an ill-educated guess. Historical evidence may also be useful though lay people and members of the medical and nursing profession all tend to exaggerate visible blood loss (except surgeons, who always underestimate the amount of blood they spill). Finally, semi-objective assessment may be possible by seeing the extent of injury and referring to previously established figures.

When an assessment of whole blood loss has been made a decision must be reached on the extent of additional 'third space' requirements.

Management of the loss

1. Replace volume appropriate to the loss with the type of fluid that is lost, e.g. ECF losses are replaced with

Table 4.1 Physical findings related to reduction in circulating volume. (Reproduced from Bailey H 1977 Emergency surgery, 10th edn, by permission of John Wright & Sons, Bristol.)

Clinical status	Vital signs	Intravascular deficit in adult
Patient well, not anxious	Pulse 70–80 BP 120 systolic Central venous pressure 5–10 cm water Urine volume at least 40–50 ml/hr	Less than 700 ml
Mild anxiety, restlessness, pallor, coldness, possibly sweating. Thirst. Fainting in upright position.	Pulse 90–100 BP 90–100 CVP 0–5 Urine volume less than 30 ml/hr	1–2 litres
Great anxiety, disorientation. Air hunger, icy extremities, fall in body temperature. Severe thirst.	Pulse 130+ BP 70 CVP −5 Urine volume nil	2–3.5 litres

Table 4.2 Points of differentiation between whole blood, plasma and ECF loss

	Whole blood	Plasma	ECF
Haematocrit	Normal initially; falls over some hours	Rises	Rises
Skin colour	Pallor	Usually unchanged	Usually unchanged
Tongue	Moist	Moist	Dry

Hartmann's solution. Crystalloids are the fluids of choice in the initial replacement of all types of fluid losses until blood or plasma are available.

Volume replacement is primarily more important than oxygen carrying capacity because if cardiac output is maintained, enough oxygen can still be delivered to the tissues down to a haemoglobin level of 8 g/dl. Care should be exercised in using large volumes of plasma or albumin, particularly when sepsis is present, as these forms of fluid replacement may be related to the cause of adult respiratory distress syndrome, so called 'shock lung'.

2. Stop the loss. Normally *replacement* precedes *stopping the loss* but occasionally replacement will be ineffective until the loss is stopped (e.g. massive arterial bleeding).

PUMP FAILURE (*syn* cardiogenic shock)

The causes are:

1. *Myocardial*: infarction, valvular damage or rupture and arrythmias.
2. *Pericardial*: cardiac tamponande or constrictive pericarditis
3. *Outflow obstruction*: pulmonary embolism causing pulmonary artery obstruction and dissecting aneurysm causing aortic obstruction may result in secondary pump failure

Cardiogenic shock is differentiated from low volume states by

a. no history and no signs of blood loss

b. raised rather than lowered venous pressure (jugular, venous or CVP)

c. evidence of a focal lesion on ECG.

Treatment

Cardiac tamponade and pulmonary embolism are emergencies requiring specific treatment. Other varieties of cardiogenic shock are managed by cardiologists with inotropic agents, transvenous pacing, correction of arrythmias, and occasionally intra-aortic balloon tamponade. The outlook in a surgical setting is usually gloomy.

MASSIVE SEPSIS (*syn* septic shock, bacteraemic shock, bacterial shock)

Definition. The term massive sepsis is preferred to septicaemia because the latter is, in fact, a bacteriological diagnosis which may be achieved only in retrospect if at all. Furthermore, there is some evidence that an acute local process may throw off not organisms but products of infection which cause the shock state.

Bacteria and toxins

1. Gram negative bacteria and endotoxins. The common pathogens are the aerobic *E. coli*, *Klebsiella*, *Pseudomonas* and *Proteus* species and the anaerobic *Bacteroides* species. Endotoxin is a liposaccaride released following the death of bacteria and is destroyed by the reticuloendothelial system (RES). Gram negative sepsis and endotoxemia are favoured by factors that impair host resistance and RES function, such as severe illness, diabetes, steroids and immunosuppressive therapy.

2. Gram positive bacteria and exotoxins. Exotoxins are secreted by living bacteria and are generally more toxic than endotoxins. Clostridial species secrete potent exotoxins which may cause massive local tissue destruction and also have cardiogenic and neurological effects. The more common Gram positive bacteria, staphylococci and streptococci, rarely cause massive sepsis. The 'toxic shock' syndrome is one exception. This occurs in women using vaginal tampons and has typical clinical features: high fever; erythematous rash followed by desquamation; and hypotension. The causative organism is a penicillin-resistant toxigenic *S. aureus*.

Surgical pathology

It is customary and desirable to distinguish two pathological forms of shock in massive sepsis—instances with and without a *focus*. In the latter the prognosis is worse than in the former and common portals of entry are the urinary tract, the portal tract and badly managed intravenous therapy. The pathophysiology of shock with sepsis is incompletely understood but the current view is that it is predominantly the result of intense arteriolar and possibly venular vasoconstriction, perhaps the consequence of catecholamine and catecholamine-like substances. The arteriolar vasoconstriction reduces or abolishes peripheral blood flow and the venous effects reduce the blood available for venous return. Thus, cardiac output falls, further aggravating the peripheral hypoxia. There is little evidence of a direct effect of bacterial toxins on the heart nor does selective hepatic vasoconstriction seem to have the same importance in man as it does in the dog and some other species.

Many other factors may contribute to the individual circumstances of a patient who presents with a presumed diagnosis of shock with sepsis. Acute ECF reduction, blood loss, respiratory insufficiency, metabolic acidosis and adrenocortical failure may complicate the picture and call for treatment in their own right.

Clinical features and diagnosis

Causes of blood volume reduction sufficient to account for the profound clinical disturbances are absent, but there may be a history of predisposing drug ingestion (e.g. steroids) or of a febrile illness. In favourable circumstances the diagnosis is made easy by the presence of obvious sepsis or of a portal of entry. On examination the patient is anxious, cyanosed, has an extremely sluggish capillary return, a cold periphery and tightly constricted veins. Arterial blood pressure and central venous pressure are both low.

Though blood cultures should be taken repeatedly in instances of shock thought to be associated with sepsis, they are more use for retrospective evaluation and the refinement of a chemotherapeutic regimen than for urgent diagnosis. By far the most important investigation is a peripheral blood smear. With rare exceptions this will show a leucocytosis and, of much greater importance, the neutrophils will usually contain toxic granulations and Döhle bodies. Both these are manifestations of severe infection and greatly strengthen the diagnosis.

Management

Treat sepsis by

1. systemic antibiotics, making a 'best guess' on the likely organisms.
2. draining any focal collection or removing dead infected tissue. Restore circulating volume if a deficit co-exists.

METABOLIC AND IMMUNOLOGICAL DISORDERS CAUSING SHOCK

1. Adreno-cortical insufficiency

This syndrome is rare, but perhaps not so rare as it used to be. *De novo* it may occur during the course of severe acute sepsis (e.g. the Fredrichsen-Waterhouse syndrome in relation to meningococcal septicaemia) or after a severe head injury but it is more common to encounter it after steroid drugs have been administered so suppressing endogenous cortical activity by depressing ACTH production. Thus, it may be seen when surgery is called for in a patient with ulcerative colitis or rheumatoid arthritis. Adreno-cortical suppression subsequent to steroid therapy may last up to 2 years, gradually declining in severity, but most instances of acute insufficiency occur within 18 months or take place while the patient is on a maintenance dose but is exposed to additional stress—an operation or infection. The clinical features are non-specific; the diagnosis is made only by a healthy sense of suspicion and the therapeutic trial of a large (200 mg) intravenous dose of hydrocortisone.

2. Insulin-induced hypoglycaemia

This occurs usually in young, 'brittle' insulin-dependent diabetics when the optimal ratio of circulating insulin to available glucose is exceeded. Mental confusion, profuse sweating and hypotension are rapidly followed by coma. In the surgical context this form of shock may be seen in a diabetic patient in the post-operative period or any patient receiving parenteral nutrition and insulin supplements. Treatment is an intravenous bolus injection of 50% glucose, having simultaneously taken a blood sample for glucose analysis to confirm the diagnosis.

3. Anaphylactic shock

This is the consequence of the release of vasoactive amines by mast cells following repeat exposure to an antigen. The common type of antigen is a drug, and penicillin and its derivatives are often implicated. An urticarial rash is quickly followed by the development of laryngeal oedema and stridor, compounded by severe brochospasm. Treatment with intradermal adrenaline should precede the use of an antihistamine, and is repeated until effective. Tracheostomy is rarely necessary.

5

Some complications of surgery

All operations are associated with a risk of complications which may be conveniently classified as general and local. General complications are those which may follow any operation, irrespective of its site. Local complications are those which are the consequence of the surgical procedure and may be related to a particular type of operation. The last are usually the problems of the specialist.

GENERAL COMPLICATIONS

Thrombotic and embolic events are thought to be the consequence of Virchow's triad—changes in the vessel wall, changes in the blood and stasis. Venous thromboembolism is dealt with on p. 267. Patients with known degenerative vascular disease (atherosclerosis) are more at risk for a post-operative arterial thrombosis, particularly cerebral or cardiac. The risk is difficult to quantify for the individual but obviously patients with symptomatic ischaemic heart disease or evidence of severe carotid stenosis (p. 279) should not undergo surgery unless

a. it is vital for their survival
b. the arterial lesion can be corrected first

RESPIRATORY

General anaesthesia and the effects of some operations (particularly chest and abdominal) produce a sequence of events that can lead to 'the post-operative chest'. Briefly, respiratory excursion and coughing are decreased (mostly by pain), tracheal cilial action is depressed, secretions accumulate, bronchial obstruction occurs and is followed by collapse-consolidation with subsequent bronchopneumonia. The best treatment is prevention by:

a. Avoiding operations on patients with known respiratory disease until the maximum improvement has taken place

b. arranging for good quality physiotherapy before and after operation
c. Using antibiotics during the perioperative period in patients who have purulent sputum and who must be operated upon. *Haemophilus influenzae* is the commonest organism and thus ampicillin an appropriate antibiotic
d. Ensuring adequate pain relief and mobility of the patient as soon after the operation as possible

Lesser degrees of respiratory problems can occur such as the tracheo-bronchitis that may follow operations on the thyroid.

Adult respiratory distress syndrome (*syn* shock lung; post-traumatic pulmonary insufficiency)

This still ill-understood condition follows very major operations or injuries and is nearly always associated with the development of systemic sepsis, usually of a severe variety. Fibrin, platelet and leucocyte micro-aggregates occur in the pulmonary capillaries. There is an interstitial exudate as a consequence of the microemboli, causing infarctions. The lung becomes progressively and patchily consolidated. There is also a tendency for the venous pressure to rise so that the clinical picture resembles pulmonary oedema.

CLINICAL FEATURES
The onset is insidious. The lung becomes stiff so that there is dyspnoea and tachypnoea; cyanosis ensues as arterial saturation falls, and then features of profound hypoxia—restlessness, anxiety and ultimately unconsciousness—may ensue. There is usually not much to be heard in the lungs—some signs of alveolar fluid and occasionally features of patchy consolidation. The chest X-ray is characteristic—small areas of patchy consolidation usually spreading outwards from the hilum. The whole process may take place within 24–48 hours, is made worse by any concomitant overinfusion of fluids and may lead to death from unrelenting respiratory failure. Treatment is:

a. Get rid of the cause—sepsis
b. Avoid overinfusion of liquids
c. Provide respiratory support with intermittent positive pressure ventilation (IPPV), often with positive end expiratory pressure (PEEP) which keeps the small airways open and possibly reduces interstitial oedema.

Aspiration of vomitus

The circumstances in which this may occur are:

a. Pre-operatively in 1. Intestinal obstruction
2. Haematemesis
3. Acute alcoholic intoxication
b. During induction of anaesthesia in any patient with a full stomach and particularly in intestinal obstruction or in pregnancy
c. After operation when an endotracheal tube is removed.

The effects are:

a. Complete respiratory obstruction leading to asphyxia and death
b. Bronchial obstruction with varying degrees of subsequent sepsis ranging from bronchopneumonia to lung abscess (often with anaerobic organisms such as bacteroides)
c. If the vomitus contains a large quantity of irritant acid, Mendelson's syndrome which is characterised by respiratory distress, bronchospasm and cyanosis with the development of pulmonary oedema.

PREVENTION

Aspiration can be prevented by:

a. Ensuring that the stomach is empty before anaesthesia is induced
b. Cricoid compression
c. Use of a nasogastric tube or gastrostomy postoperatively

TREATMENT

a. Immediate aspiration of nasopharynx
b. Endotracheal aspiration if necessary by the bronchoscope
c. Antibiotics against pulmonary sepsis
d. In Mendelson's syndrome, corticosteroids and bronchodilators

URINARY COMPLICATIONS

a. Retention of urine (see p. 256)
b. Urinary tract infections may occur
1. if an indwelling catheter has to be used over any significant length of time
2. in elderly females confined to bed

Strict aseptic precautions and mobility are safeguards, as is a high fluid intake. When infection occurs it should be managed by the simplest method possible to avoid the hazards of powerful antibiotics. Nitrofurantoin and co-trimoxazole are useful agents.

OTHER GENERAL COMPLICATIONS

Parotitis is now rare but follows serious illness when

a. Fluid and electrolyte balance is not well attended to, so that the patient gets a dry mouth
b. Mouth hygiene is deficient

The infected gland swells rapidly and pus forms quickly, adding to the systemic burden of illness.

Treatment is to correct the problems, administer antibiotics and drain the area early if there is any chance of pus being present.

Bed sores

These are wholly preventable but still occur in the elderly, the obese and the immobile, particularly when insufficient nursing care is given. The proximate aetiological factors are:

a. Prolonged pressure on a single point—buttock, sacrum, skin over the greater trochanter—which causes ischaemia
b. Shearing of the skin on the deep fascia which tears subcutaneous blood vessels and also produces an ischaemic lesion. There is sloughing of the skin and subcutaneous fat unless the causes are corrected, deep penetration down to bone occurs and there is often secondary infection with burrowing abscesses and a mixed bacterial growth.

Sores are prevented by ensuring constant movement so that pressure is not applied to a single place, by care in turning the patient and by rigorous skin hygiene. If they occur they are managed in the same way. Most are small and will heal—provided that the patient is able to mount a normal wound-healing response. Large ulcers may require skilled repair by a plastic surgeon.

Faecal impaction

Inability to evacuate the bowel after an operation is the consequence of:

a. inadequate pre-operative preparation
b. weakness
c. a bulky hard stool

The condition is usually seen in the elderly and bedridden but can occasionally occur in those who are frightened to defaecate–e.g. after surgical procedures on the anal verge. The presenting feature is 'spurious' diarrhoea which is the trickling down of liquid faeces through channels in an impacted solid collection in the rectum. Whenever diarrhoea occurs in post-operative patients a rectal examination is essential. The condition rarely responds to conservative measures (suppositories or washouts) and manual evacuation under sedation is usually required.

Pseudo-membranous enterocolitis

This is an uncommon complication which may follow the use of antibiotics, with the development of a fulminating bowel infection, usually due to resistant staphylococci but also clostridia particularly *Clostridium difficile*.

Surgical pathology
There is partial destruction of the bowel mucosa resulting in inadequate fluid resorption and dehydration. Casts may be passed with blood and mucus.

Clinical features
The diarrhoea usually appears 3–4 days after operation with associated abdominal distension, hypotension and shock.

Management

Prevention. Unnecessary use of antibiotics and particularly courses prolonged for more than a day or two should be avoided.

Therapy. Conservative management included intravenous replacement and supportive therapy, together with nasogastric suction and the use of the appropriate antibiotic. Unless there is reason to think otherwise, *Clostridium difficile* infection should be assumed and in this instance vancomycin is specific.

LOCAL COMPLICATIONS
WOUND INFECTION

This is the commonest complication in surgery. However the incidence varies from less than 1% (hernia and clean orthopaedic operations) to 20–30% in colonic surgery when this is unattended by suitable precautions.

Predisposing factors.

Pre-operative.
Infection at or near the site of the intended surgical wound as may occur with:

1. Skin infections—particularly those due to staphylococci from nasal, throat, or hand reservoirs
2. Wound contamination by infection from a diseased or perforated viscus such as may occur in perforated ulcer or appendicitis
3. Susceptible patients—particularly where malnutrition, hypoproteinaemia, avitaminosis, diabetes, carcinomatosis and prolonged steroid administration are present

Operative
1. Airborne infection from theatre environment, surgical and nursing staff where the organism is usually a staphylococcus. Though the incidence of this problem is now low, it is of great importance in relation to prosthetic implants
2. Contact infection from theatre staff, instruments, fluids (skin preparations, irrigating fluids) and dressings
3. Inadequate surgical technique—particularly when haematoma formation, incomplete obliteration of dead space, strangulating muscle layer sutures, or soiling of the wound by bowel contents is allowed to occur
4. Operations on heavily contaminated areas, e.g. large bowel, lower limbs of bed-ridden or diabetic patients

Post-operative
1. Continuation of preoperative factors
2. Self infection of the wound, particularly with staphylococci from the skin or nose, streptococci from the throat, or coliform organisms from the faeces
3. Cross-infection from the ward environment (surgical and nursing staff and patients) by airborne or contact routes. Particularly common in the presence of drainage tubes.

Bacteriology

Many wound infections are caused by a mixture of organisms.

1. *Staphylococci.* These have been in the past the commonest organism and often the coagulase-positive, penicillin-resistant staphylococci carried by the nose, face and hands of patients and attending staff can be incriminated. However, they have given way in frequency to intestinal organisms and opportunist pathogens.

2. *Coliform organisms. E. coli, Proteus* and *Pseudomonas* normally inhabit the bowel, and they may be the predominant organism in wound infections after operations on the intestinal tract.

3. *Haemolytic streptococci*. Beta-haemolytic streptococci, which are harboured in the nasopharynx in about 5% of the population, can result in wound infection by air-borne or contact routes, but this is now rare.

4. *Anaerobic organisms*. These were until recently thought to be a rare cause of wound infection. Specific infection with clostridia (tetanus and gas gangrene) are discussed in Chapter 14. *Bacteroides* infection is now known to be common following surgery of the large bowel (including the appendix) and these organisms may complicate vaginal and middle ear infections as part of a mixed picture.

Clinical features

The onset is usually within seven days after operation.

Symptoms
Malaise, anorexia, and pain, or discomfort at the operation site.

Signs
1. Local redness, tenderness, swelling, cellulitis, discharge, or frank abscess formation.
2. Elevated temperature and pulse rate

Treatment

PREVENTION
1. Pre-operative correction of any general problem
2. Pre-operative bowel cleansing before elective operations on the large bowel
3. Perioperative antibiotics (beginning before operation) are indicated

   a. When it is known or suspected that a contaminated or infected operative field will be entered, e.g. an inflamed appendix, operations which involve opening the gastro-intestinal tract
   b. When a prosthesis (e.g. arterial, cardiac, orthopaedic) is being inserted
   c. When there is known valvular heart disease (risk of sub-acute bacterial endocarditis)
   d. In debilitated patients and those on steroids
   e. In accidental wounds when there is any significant contamination

4. Sterile technique including instruments, skin preparations and drapes
5. Wound exclusion via plastic drapes, particularly when an infected abdomen is opened or when the bowel is to be cut, may have a place
6. Meticulous wound excision and toilet and washout of contaminated wounds

7. Careful wound closure, avoiding strangulating muscle sutures, haematoma formation and dead spaces, together with the use of wound drains and topical antibiotics before complete closure when contamination has occurred. Sepsis occurs predominantly in the subcutaneous tissue: if a contaminated wound is left open for 3 days and then closed (delayed primary closure—see p. 29), infection is much less likely
8. Post-operative wound dressings should be interfered with as infrequently as possible except when they become moist with discharge or exudate

TREATMENT
1. Isolate organisms whenever possible
2. Systemic antibiotics, specific to the infecting organism, are administered when cellulitis or septicaemia is present
3. When pus is present drainage is essential. This is performed by removing a skin stitch when a suture abscess is present, or by removing all stitches and opening up the wound for a larger collection
4. All wounds are then allowed to granulate and heal by a second intention. Wounds should not be tightly packed

RESIDUAL ABSCESS

After any operation sepsis may ensue deep to the wound but this is commonest in the abdomen and if the gut is opened. Further, after operation for sepsis a focus may persist. In both cases a residual abscess may form. Finally, an abscess may persist after drainage.

Predisposing factors

1. Inadequate drainage of an abscess cavity
2. Infection of a haematoma
3. Persistence of infective sources: in the abdomen such things as incomplete amputation of an appendix stump; in orthopaedics the presence of dead bone (a sequestrum); in any procedure a foreign body
4. Failure to carry out adequate treatment, e.g. complete peritoneal toilet in peritonitis

General features of residual abscesses

At a varying interval of 2–7 days, but occasionally much later, there are systemic features of sepsis—fever, malaise and a raised leucocyte count and ESR. Occasionally, organisms escaping into the circulation may give rise to rigors, and in severe cases septicaemia may complicate the local condition.

Locally, in accessible sites, there are the physical signs of inflammation—tenderness, heat, redness and swelling. Residual abscesses which are deep to wounds will usually 'point' to the surface via the wound, but others will have to be formally drained.

Principles of treatment

In nearly all instances drainage will be required but this must be undertaken

1. When spreading sepsis (including septicaemia) has been contained by antibiotic therapy. Conversely, drainage must be undertaken early if a focus is throwing off organisms into the circulation and so causing septicaemia
2. Without damaging other tissues or structures
3. Without spreading the infective process

Spontaneous discharge does not necessarily mean adequate drainage, and a surgical procedure may still be required.

Abdominal residual abscesses

Abdominal residual abscesses still occur with distressing frequency. In the classic sites—pelvic and subphrenic—they can usually be diagnosed (though the latter may cause difficulty) by conventional means (see below), but low-grade persistent sepsis in between leaves of the mesentery may pose much greater difficulty. New techniques—ultrasonography and labelled leucocytes that can be detected by scintiscanning—are helping to make the diagnosis earlier and to permit precise location. There is still an occasional indication for a laparotomy when sepsis is almost certainly present but cannot be precisely located.

Pelvic abscess

Pelvic abscess usually follows an operation for generalized peritonitis—perforated appendicitis, perforated ulcer, perforated diverticulitis. It can be the primary presentation of acute pelvic appendicitis. The organisms involved are enteric, with *Bacteroides* of importance.

CLINICAL FEATURES
Urgency of defaecation and mucus diarrhoea. Blood may appear with pus if the abscess has ruptured. Abdominal examination may show nothing or slight lower abdominal distension from coils of bowel lying in the abscess wall. On rectal examination there is a tender boggy mass which in the female may also be palpable on vaginal examination.

TREATMENT
Two groups:

1. *Pointing.* This is evidenced by fixation of the abscess, usually to the rectal wall, which becomes thickened and oedematous, and indicates that drainage through the rectum is required. Occasionally the abscess may point into the vagina or anterior abdominal wall and require incision and drainage at these sites.

2. *Not pointing.* As long as the patient's general condition remains satisfactory, conservative treatment is indicated. This includes the use of broad spectrum antibiotics and the maintenance of nutrition. Low-grade intestinal obstruction because of adhesions between loops of bowel and the wall of the abscess cavity may require gastric suction. The abscess may point and discharge spontaneously, require drainage, or resolve. Occasionally, deterioration will occur in the absence of localization of the abscess; then laparotomy and drainage will be indicated.

Subphrenic abscess

The subphrenic spaces are potential spaces only; they become real when distended by pus. Subphrenic abscess formation is an uncommon sequel to abdominal operations and occurs in less than 0.5% of cases.

SURGICAL ANATOMY
Terminology and classifications are conflicting. In practical terms there are only right and left subphrenic spaces, and the subhepatic space on the right.

CAUSE AND SURGICAL PATHOLOGY
The vast majority of subphrenic collections follow peritoneal contamination from either gastrointestinal operations or episodes of peritonitis associated with perforation of a hollow viscus. The condition starts as a cellulitis and is said to occur partly because the subphrenic spaces are in direct communication with the paracolic gutters to which pus gravitates, and partly because, once there is air beneath the diaphragm, the liver when it descends acts as a piston, sucking infected material upwards to the subphrenic space. An abscess develops and there is contiguous inflammation of the diaphragm and pleura, so leading to a 'sympathetic' pleural effusion. Gas often forms in the abscess cavity. If untreated the abscess may rupture into the general peritoneal cavity or into the chest. The latter situation may be associated with empyema, pyo-pneumothorax, bronchopleural fistula, suppurative pericarditis or mediastinal abscess formation.

CLINICAL FEATURES
A subphrenic abscess can occasionally be notoriously

difficult to diagnose. It is therefore important to remember that such a complication can occur, especially when conditions favourable to its formation are present.

Symptoms

1. *Onset.* In the more acute cases the features of a precipitating peritonitis may merge into those of a rapidly collecting abscess with continued pyrexia and general toxaemia.

   In delayed cases, the onset of suspicious symptoms may occur many days after apparent recovery from the predisposing condition. Later development is probably more likely to occur after intensive antibiotic therapy has been given for the original condition

2. *Anorexia and nausea* are usual
3. *Pain or ache* beneath or over the lower ribs should always raise suspicion; rarely is there shoulder pain
4. *Hiccoughs* are common

Signs

1. Patient may look unwell, pale or even wasted
2. Elevated temperature—the classical 'swinging' temperature is present in only 50% of cases, and in about 10% there is no elevation at all
3. Tachycardia is usual
4. Local tenderness beneath the rib margin may be present
5. Local redness is uncommon
6. Palpable liver edge on occasions
7. Palpable lump is rarely discernible
8. *Chest signs.* The classical sequence of percussion changes from above downwards of resonance (normal lung), dullness (pleural effusion), resonance (gas above abscess) and dullness (abscess) is rarely, if ever, detected. However, signs of consolidation or of pleural effusion may be present.

Special tests

1. Leucocytosis is usual
2. Blood sedimentation rate is elevated
3. X-rays, postero-anterior and lateral of the chest and screening the diaphragm, may demonstrate a pleural effusion, pulmonary consolidation, a raised, thickened, tented and immobile diaphragm, or an abscess cavity containing a fluid level
4. Barium meal is helpful on the left side to distinguish a stomach gas bubble from an abscess collection; it also may help in localisation of an abscess in the lesser sac
5. Radioisotopic scan of the liver-lung region may help to isolate an abscess which is distorting the liver surface on the right side
6. Ultrasonography has the same role as scintiscanning

7. Diagnostic aspiration is not recommended as a routine; the danger is that the pleural cavity may be infected if a trans-pleural route is inadvertently used
8. Labelled leucocyte scanning
9. CT scan

TREATMENT

In all cases when the diagnosis is certain pus should be evacuated and a large-bore drain tube placed in the cavity. Operation should be carried out under antibiotic cover on the assumption that enteric organisms are present. The routes used have varied considerably over the years, but most abscesses are now drained through anterior subcostal incisions.

When the diagnosis is not quite certain, continued observation is essential and rarely the patient's condition fails to improve; then either a diagnostic aspiration or a laparotomy *may* prove helpful in localizing the abscess.

WOUND DISRUPTION

Wounds break down because they are:

1. Septic
2. Pulled apart by distractive forces
3. Made in patients who cannot mount a normal healing response

The common wound disruption in general surgery is burst abdomen, the incidence of which remains at about 1% of all abdominal operations, and the mortality is about 10%. However, in that the causes are almost entirely technical, these figures are too high. Many surgeons now have recorded statistics with only one rupture in more than 1500 consecutive laparotomies. Apart from technical and general factors the common reason for an abdominal disruption is paroxysmal rise in intra-abdominal pressure from coughing or straining.

Surgical pathology

There are three types of burst abdomen:

1. *Superficial and revealed.* This occurs at about 2 weeks when the skin sutures are removed. There is separation of the skin and subcutaneous layers only, which is most often the result of wound haematoma or infection.

2. *Deep and concealed.* This occurs gradually, with separation of all layers of the abdominal wall with the exception of the skin. If not recognized while the patient is in hospital an incisional hernia always develops at a later date. Most often this type of dehiscence results from a combination of faulty technique and faulty healing.

3. *Complete and revealed.* This occurs at about the tenth day gradually or suddenly with the protrusion of a knuckle or loop of bowel or a portion of the omentum through a wound which is completely disrupted in the whole or part of its length.

Clinical features

Symptoms
1. There may be no warning of an impending wound dehiscence
2. Alternatively, there may be nausea, fever, and local pain or discomfort
3. Occasionally the patient describes a 'tearing' or 'ripping' sensation in the wound after a bout of coughing or straining

Signs
1. Sero-sanguinous or blood-stained discharge from the wound
2. Bowel or omentum protruding through the wound spontaneously or after removal of skin sutures

Treatment

Superficial and revealed
1. Evacuate blood clot
2. Treat wound infection if present
3. Allow wound to granulate and heal by secondary intention

Deep and concealed
1. If recognized while in hospital by presence of a 'tell-tale' sero-sanguinous discharge or the appearance of knuckle of bowel after removal of a few skin sutures—then urgent operation is required
2. If not recognised and the skin heals, then the subsequently developed incisional hernia is dealt with on its merits

Complete and revealed
Resuture with closely applied interrupted non-absorbable sutures passing through all layers of the anterior abdominal wall deep to the skin. The skin is best left unsutured. Any attempt to suture each layer separately is of no value, as the tissues are friable and oedematous.

ENTERIC FISTULA

This is any communication between the gastrointestinal tract and the body surface.

Predisposing factors

1. A disrupted intestinal anastomosis because of poor technique, avascularity or the persistence of some original disorder at the site of anastomosis (Crohn's disease, carcinoma, tuberculosis)
2. Intestinal obstruction distal to the site of anastomosis
3. Fistulating diseases such as Crohn's disease and diverticulitis
4. Injury to the bowel or its blood supply at surgery or subsequently, say, by a rigid intraperitoneal drainage tube

Clinical features

Either spontaneously or at a varying time after a surgical procedure there are features of systemic sepsis followed by the development of inflammation on the abdominal wall or in relation to a wound. Initially, pus may be discharged, but this is rapidly followed by intestinal content, the quantity of which varies according to the site of the fistula. Clinically fistulae are usually classified into:

1. High output
2. Low output

The first occurs predominantly in the upper gastro-intestinal tract, where even a fistula in the low ileum may produce many hundreds of millilitres of fluid a day. The second is characteristic of large-bowel fistulae or those which are not associated with complete division of the bowel or distal obstruction.

The *local effects* of fistulae are variable but if the site of discharge is at a point where there is much enzymatic activity in the effluent then rapid digestion and secondary septic infection of the abdominal wall takes place. Fistulae are not uncommonly multiple whatever their cause.

The *general effects* are loss of water and electrolyte (extracellular fluid volume deficiency) and malnutrition, the consequence both of failure of normal absorption, even if the patient can eat, and the increased catabolic rate associated with the severe local sepsis.

Treatment

Prevention. Clearly it is essential to avoid the predisposing factors, in particular poor surgical technique.

Treatment. Many fistulas will close spontaneously unless there is distal obstruction of the bowel, mucocutaneous union, or a persistently infective focus. Meantime the patient must be supported, and local treatment directed at protecting the skin around the fistula from digestion. If any of the factors which prevent closure are present, operation will be required once the fluid and electrolyte loss, malnutrition and sepsis have been corrected.

WOUND SINUS

A sinus is a track lined by granulation tissue which opens on to the skin.

Predisposing factors

In all cases there is persistent infection caused by:
1. Inadequately drained abscess
2. Residual dead tissue
3. Foreign material such as a ligature or swab
4. Chronic underlying disease such as tuberculosis, Crohn's disease or malignancy

Clinical features

Persistent discharge of material, other than gut content, from a wound beyond 1 month after operation.

Treatment

Prevention
1. Adequate drainage of an abscess so that healing takes place from its base
2. Removal of foreign bodies and avoidance of non-absorbable sutures in infected wounds

Treatment. The sinus is explored and any foreign material removed. An abscess cavity with an inadequately draining sinus must be opened widely so that it may heal from its base.

6

Surgical wounds: healing and management

The healing of wounds is fundamental to the practice of surgery, but its importance extends beyond this; a myocardial infarct, an area of acute inflammation in the lung, a gastric ulcer that is either healing or advancing are all examples of the same process.

Once tissues have been disrupted by injury, by the surgeon's knife or by some pathological process, a sequence of events sets in which follows a programme, i.e. one step must be completed or have reached a certain stage of completion before another will take over. Thus, if anything stops the programme by interfering with one step, all subsequent events are likely to be held up. This is helpful in understanding what clinical effects various pathological states may have.

Uncomplicated healing (say of an incised wound) may be divided into two phases:

1. Preparative

Blood clots, cellular debris, and perhaps external contaminants in the wound have to be cleared away. This is accomplished during that phase which corresponds to the acute exudative part of an acute infection. There is:

a. Capillary dilatation and increased premeability
b. Migration of polymorphonuclear leucocytes followed by macrophages

When uncomplicated, this phase is over at 36 hours and the visible oedema of the wound then subsides. Pain gets less at this point; if it does not, some pathological problem should be suspected.

2. Reparative

Repair takes place in all tissues by the invasion of the loose residual gel of exudate by capillaries which carry with them a perivascular cuff of active fibroblasts. The meshwork of young capillaries and dividing cells fills the wound interstices in 5–6 days and, as it does so, begins to lay down collagen, so that by 10 days there is a mass of ill-organized fibrils filling the wound (granulation tissue). Under the influence of tensile forces and other unknown factors these fibrils condense, cross-link and align themselves to provide a strong scar. This then begins to devascularize by about the twenty-first day, but final consolidation takes 3–6 months. The sequence of events is outlined in Table 6.1, which also enables one to work out the likely cause of impaired wound healing at any stage.

Tensile strength

For the first 3 days, the sound is held together merely by the stickiness of exudate and whatever means have been used to coapt it. From this point on it begins to attain some *intrinsic strength*, which in fascia by 21 days is 50% of its original strength. Thereafter, the gain in strength is slower but progressive to 6 months, by which time most wounds in connective tissue in normal people are almost as strong as the original tissue.

Contraction

During the whole of normal healing, the active zone of the wound contracts. This generalized shrinking is not the consequence of shortening of collagen fibrils but of an ill-understood condensation process. It is seen best in loose connective tissue such as abdominal wall or buttock, and is of surgical importance in that it reduces the area which requires epithelialization. In addition to this shrinkage, once collagen has been laid down it shortens. Where tissues surrounding the wound area are mobile, they are drawn toward the wound and become distorted. This leads to *contractures*—deformed areas of tissue produced by contracting scars.

The amount of collagen ultimately formed in a wound is roughly correlated with the following.

a. The size of the damaged area
b. The duration of the process (e.g. prolongation by infection usually increases the collagen formed)

Clearly these factors bear on wound management. The smaller the area and the more rapid and smooth the healing process, the better the end result will be.

Table 6.1 Programme of wound healing

Event	Time	Requirements	Aberrations
Tissue damage and bleeding	0–1 hours	Normal vascular responses to cut vessels	Bleeding diatheses (e.g. Von Willebrands disease)
Clotting	0–1 hours	Normal clotting factors	Clotting abnormality (e.g. haemophilia)
Clot stabilization	1–2 hours	Factor XIII	Factor XIII deficiency
Fibrinolysis	3–12hours	Normal fibrinolytic mechanisms	Excessive fibrinolysis; haem. Streptococci Uraemia—which stops fibrinolysis
Capillary dilatation and exudation	8–24 hours	Normal vascularity and membrane permeability	Ischaemia, glucocorticoids
Migration of white cells phagocytosis	8–24 hours	Normal leucocytes	Blood dyscrasia, e.g. leukaemia
Capillary-fibroblast migration and cell division	36 hours – 5 days	Active cells Adequate building blocks	X-irradiation Anti-mitotic agents Infection Malnutrition Zinc (Epithelium)
Collagen deposition	5–15 days	Source material Micro nutrients	Malnutrition Vit. C
Collagen cross linkage	10 days – 6 months	Tensile forces	Prolonged immobilization

In some situations in the skin, excessive, highly vascular collagen is laid down and constitutes a *keloid*. The reasons for this are not clear but it seems to be related partly to racial factors (common in Negroes) and partly to the site and depth of tissue damage.

Mechanisms of injury

A broad distinction can be drawn between low and high velocity wounds: the points of difference apply whether the wound is open—as in a missile or penetrating injury of any kind—or closed—as by the force of blunt injury, say from a motor vehicle.

In *low velocity injury*, only minor shock waves are set up along the path of injury. If there is a track, damage is only slight around it and damage away from the point of impact is minimal. By contrast, a *high velocity penetration injury* sets up shock waves around the track, followed by 'implosion' back into the cavity. Similarly, a high velocity blunt injury sends a shock wave through tissues that may disrupt distant structures (e.g soft viscera such as spleen, liver or brain). In blunt injury, rotational stresses are also often important. They may tear a mobile structure away from its underlying blood supply.

In closed injuries three important points must be noted:

1. By observation or inference, how much damage has taken place to deep structures?
2. How much blood loss is there?
3. In a limb particularly, are problems of compression going to develop as the part swells?

Management of the open wound

The *aim* is to secure a smooth, uninterrupted path to healing with minimal formation of fibrous tissue. The *chief hazard* is the ingress of infection—usually non-specific pyogenic but occasionally specific organisms such as clostridia. The way to avoid this hazard is:

1. To remove any organisms that have entered, plus those areas of lessened resistance that favor their growth. This is achieved by *excising* the wound (debridement)—removal of dead or doubtfully viable tissue, especially muscle, careful cleaning out of dirt and foreign bodies.
2. Attain haemostasis—blood is a good pabulum for organisms
3. Close the wound as soon as possible either by suture or by skin graft, but do not close it so soon that any organisms that may have been left in get good conditions for multiplication—warmth, the relative ischaemia that comes from increased tissue tension, and dampness
4. Immobilize the wound and/or patient to permit healing and prevent further damage

All this boils down, in practice, to:

1. In a relatively clean wound, *primary excision* and *primary closure*
2. In an early but heavily contaminated wound, primary excision, a period of 3–5 days delay during which organisms have less favorable circumstances to grow, followed by *delayed primary closure*

A primary closed wound and a delayed primary closed

wound heal the same way; the only difference is that during the preparative phase one is closed, the other open.

The disadvantage of leaving a wound open is the chance of added infection. This is reduced to a minimum by filling the wound with dry gauze and leaving it undisturbed. Such wounds are surprisingly pain free. For more details see p 32.

Wounds are occasionally not seen until they have already become infected, i.e. at +12 hours. It is then no use attempting excision. They should be *opened* to allow free drainage of the products of infection and removal of obvious dead tissue and foreign bodies. Infection can then run its course, and the wound—by this time containing granulation tissue—is closed secondarily either by:

1. Spontaneous contraction and epithelialization
2. Suture
3. Skin graft

Chemotherapy and wound management

Note that nothing has so far been said about chemotherapy, either in preventing infection or in controlling it once it has occurred. This is because it is secondary in importance to proper surgical management, though by no means without value.

The earlier high antibiotic concentrations can be achieved in the wounded tissues, the greater the likelihood of controlling infection. The best results are obtained when the tissues are already saturated with antibiotics before a wound is made; thus the surgeon begins antibiotics pre-operatively when the surgery is in an area containing bacteria, e.g. the gastro-intestinal tract.

In accidental injury the aim of prevention should be to establish high concentrations as early as possible. Should such treatment not succeed, it is little good going on giving the agent, and if it does succeed, there is no need to continue prolonged chemotherapy over successive days.

Recommended preventative regimens:

Gram positive organisms (e.g. staphylococci, beta-hemolytic streptococci, clostridia): penicillin G up to 5 Mu intramuscularly per day for 2 days

Gram negative organisms: Cephalosporin 0.5 g 4 times daily intramuscularly and metronidazole 500 mg 3 times daily, intravenously or rectally, for one day.

Ampicillin can no longer be recommended, as it is inactivated by beta-lactamase-producing *S. aureus* and *E. Coli.*

7

General management of injuries and fractures

PLAN OF ACTION

Management of the severely injured patient requires a list of priorities of treatment.

1. Immediate action

1. Check airway
2. Is patient breathing?
3. Intravenous line
4. Stop bleeding

2. Assessment

1. History
2. Examination
3. Special tests

3. Definitive treatment

IMMEDIATE ACTION

1. Ensure that the patient has an adequate airway, with intubation or tracheostomy if necessary
2. Check that the patient is breathing. Artificial respiration may be required. Immediate action may be indicated in chest injuries, for example insertion of an intercostal drain for a tension pneumothorax
3. Insertion of an intravenous line is of lower priority than the airway or breathing. There is little point in pouring fluids into a patient who is not breathing. Blood should be taken for cross-matching at this time. Volume replacement, usually in the form of normal saline, but occasionally plasma or plasma substitute, is primarily more important than oxygen-carrying capacity, because if cardiac output is maintained, enough oxygen can still be delivered to the tissues down to a haemoglobin level of 8 g/dl (See also p 16).

Normally *replacement* precedes *stopping the loss* but occasionally replacement will be ineffective until the loss is stopped (e.g. massive arterial bleeding).

4. Stop the external bleeding by direct pressure either with a gauze dressing and manual pressure or a pressure bandage. Application of artery forceps is time-consuming, unnecessary and often causes further damage.

ASSESSMENT

1. History

A full, relevant history is taken with particular attention to the following points:

a. Police, ambulance drivers or anyone present at the accident should be interviewed before they leave the accident department
b. The precise time of the accident (injury) should be recorded
c. The exact mechanism of the injury should be established

2. Examination

a. Examine all the injuries and look for injuries which may not be obvious, particularly:

Back injuries
Tendon or nerve injuries
Closed vascular injuries
Abdominal injury
More than one fracture in one limb

b. A full physical examination of all systems must be done, provided this does not interfere with urgent treatment.

3. Special tests

a. Full blood count, grouping and cross-match, and electrolytes and urea concentrations

b. X-ray. In addition to suspected fractures and chest X-ray, radiographs of deep lacerations, particularly of the hand, should be taken to exclude the presence of a foreign body. X-rays must not interfere with life saving treatment.

c. Specific tests for specific injuries (see appropriate chapters)

DEFINITIVE TREATMENT

GENERAL MEASURES

1. Pain relief. As soon as the patient has been assessed, analgesia should not be withheld. Intramuscular injections are poorly absorbed in shocked patients; intravenous injection of small doses, (e.g.5–7.5 mg morphine sulphate) of opiates diluted in saline given carefully is safe and effective.

2. Blood transfusion. Unless urgent transfusion of blood has been required, adequate replacement transfusion should follow full assessment of the extent of the injuries and estimation of blood loss, in particular taking account of amount of blood loss in association with fractures.

3. Catheterization of the bladder is the only way of monitoring accurately urinary output and thus the adequacy of volume replacement. Severely injured patients should be catheterized for at least the first 24 hours.

4. Anti-tetanus prophylaxis (see p 70)

5. Antibiotics. Most accidental wounds are contaminated and, particularly in the hand or in association with a fracture (compound fracture), prophylactic antibiotics are indicated. A combination of penicillin and a broad spectrum antibiotic is recommended

6. Care of the unconscious patient (see p. 40)

SPECIFIC INJURIES (see chapters on Head, Chest, Abdominal, Nerve and Vessel Injuries)

FRACTURES

Unless a fracture threatens the blood supply to the limb or is causing a severe vascular injury, it can usually wait until problems of head, chest and abdominal injury are dealt with.

Classification

1. Closed
2. Compound (a fracture associated with an open wound)

Both closed or open fractures may be either:

Simple, or
Comminuted (multiple fragments)

The healing of fractures

Normal healing requires:

1. Apposition of bony ends without other tissue in between
2. Adequate blood supply
3. Immobilization
4. Freedom from infection

The normal sequence of healing is:

1. Immediately after the injury haemorrhage occurs and a haematoma forms around the fracture site
2. Granulation tissue forms in the haematoma and osteogenic cells are mobilized
3. Provisional callus is laid down forming a bridge between the bone ends
4. Progressive remodelling of the provisional callus occurs leaving the fracture united by compact bone

Management of the open wound

OPERATION
1. The patient is given a general anaesthetic. Most cases will require a cuffed endotracheal tube and a gastric tube to prevent inhalation of stomach contents.
2. A tourniquet is not normally applied because it creates problems in the assessment of areas of doubtful viability; also the securing of bleeding points is made more difficult. In the presence of torrential haemorrhage a pneumatic tourniquet should, however, be applied and deflated later, after the haemorrhage has been controlled.
3. Clothing is removed, a sterile pad is placed on the wound, and the limb is scrubbed with soap and water. The area is then shaved and the wound washed out with 1% cetrimide solution. The limb is then elevated and the skin prepared with 0.5% chlorhexidine in 70% alcohol, and the wound prepared with 1% aqueous chlorhexidine solution. Sterile towels are clipped under and around the limb to isolate the wound area.
4. Wound excision (debridement)
   a. *Skin.* A minimum of skin should be excised, but this must include dead or doubtful skin and the ragged wound edges. The wound must be extended to expose the deeper tissues which are always involved in the injury.
   b. *Muscle and fascia.* Division of tight deep fascia

(fasciotomy) may improve the circulation to muscle which has been compressed by haematoma and oedema fluid. Necrotic muscle is excised and any foreign material removed.

c. *Vessels*. Small bleeding vessels are tied off with fine PGA (Dexon; Vicryl) ligatures. Major arteries are repaired if they are essential for limb survival.

d. *Nerves*. No attempt should be made to perform primary nerve suture, but divided ends are marked with coloured monofilament sutures.

e. *Tendons*. Tendon ends can be apposed if the wound is relatively uncontaminated.

f. *Bone*. If there is a compound fracture, completely detached fragments of bone are removed; foreign material is carefully cleaned from the bone ends and the fracture is reduced under direct vision. If the fracture is stable, external splintage with plaster of Paris is required. If the fracture is unstable, more complicated external or internal fixation may be employed.

5. Skin closure. The aim is to obtain primary wound closure. It is essential to suture the skin without tension, and this may necessitate the use of a relieving incision. When the skin cannot be sutured without tension, split-skin grafts should be carefully applied to the defect.

Primary wound closure is contraindicated when the wound is grossly contaminated or infected. In these circumstances the wound is filled loosely with dry gauze.

6. Immobilization. This is essential for healing. It should include the joints above and below the wound. A well padded plaster splint should be used and split from end to end to enable inevitable swelling to take place without compromising the circulation.

Principles of fracture treatment

1. Make a complete diagnosis in relation to:
   a. The patient—other injuries, other problems, shock.
   b. The injury—nature, bony displacement, involvement of joints surface, nerve and blood vessel injury, the extent of the wound if the fracture is compound. Obtain X-rays in two planes and special views as required.
2. Correct shock and establish an order of priorities of other injuries exist.
3. In compound fractures, early skin closure with adequate excision (debridement) of necrotic tissue is the aim of treatment, but skin tension must be avoided as it will result in skin necrosis as the swelling increases post-operatively.

4. Reduction. When a bone is broken, the periosteum is also torn but usually remains intact on one part of the bone as a 'hinge of soft tissue'. By understanding the deforming forces of the injury, the site of this hinge can be worked out.

Fractures can be reduced by:

Traction
Manipulation
Open reduction

Generally, with adequate traction most fractures will reduce. If not, manipulation is indicated. Initially the deforming force is increased, opening the bone ends on the soft tissue hinge, opposing the fragments and then closing the hinge.

When traction and manipulation fails, open reduction is indicated.

5. Immobilisation. This can also be achieved simply by traction or by splintage with, usually plaster of Paris or by internal fixation with plates, screws or nails. Internal fixation is sometimes the treatment of choice, for example, in fractured neck of femur in the elderly, where prolonged traction is accompanied by the problems of recumbency with pressure sores, pneumonia and deep vein thrombosis, and immobilization in plaster is clearly not possible.

In the immediate post-reduction period (particularly if immobilization includes a circumferential plaster) check repeatedly for circulatory inadequacy distal to the fracture, which is best demonstrated by pain on passive movements of toes or fingers.

Measures required to deal with this may vary from simply splitting a plaster to fasciotomy.

6. Rehabilitation. The surgeon's responsibility does not end with healing of the fracture. Rehabilitation starts from the time of operation. Active physiotherapy maintains muscle tone, improves circulation and reduces oedema and subsequent joint stiffness. It is continued after the fracture has united and the plaster has been removed. Occupational therapy is started to improve the patient's physical and mental well-being.

Complications of fractures

DELAYED WOUND HEALING IN COMPOUND FRACTURES
Healing may be delayed by persistent infection, sequestra or skin loss. Sufficient time must be allowed for control of infection and for dead bone to separate so that a healthy granulating surface is obtained.

To achieve this situation it is necessary to:

1. Provide free drainage of an infected wound by laying

it open and dressing it with non-adherent material until healthy granulation tissue is formed or skin healing occurs

2. Remove any obvious sequestra and leave the wound open to granulate as above

3. Continue immobilization for a longer period of time than usual as delayed union is inevitable

Once wound infection is controlled, skin closure must be obtained by delayed suturing or skin grafting.

Transfer of full-thickness free skin flaps, which may include bone or muscle, is now possible by taking the flap on its vascular pedicle and revascularizing the flap using microsurgical techniques.

DELAYED OR NON-UNION

If the fracture is mobile and there is little radiological evidence of callus formation at 3 months from the time of injury, bone grafting should be performed. If some signs of union are present, i.e. the fracture is almost immobile and there is X-ray evidence of obliteration of the fracture site by new bone, immobilization should be continued and clinical and radiological review carried out at monthly intervals. Sound union usually results, but if it is not present at 6 months bone grafting will be indicated.

MAL-UNION

If immobilization fails to hold the reduction, a fracture can unite with the bone ends incorrectly aligned.

JOINT STIFFNESS

This is usual after any limb fracture but is particularly marked after a compound fracture, especially one accompanied by infection. It is caused by adhesion of muscle and tendon to bone and fibrosis in the capsules and ligaments of associated joints. Prevention and treatment are by active exercises to the related muscles and joints.

ARTERIAL DAMAGE

Ischaemia results if circulation to the limb is impaired by arterial damage or a tight plaster, and this predominantly affects muscles and nerves. If untreated, Volkmann's ischaemic contracture occurs. Careful observation of pulses, capillary return and muscle function must be carried out regularly so that treatment can be instituted at the earliest possible moment before permanent necrosis of muscle and nerve tissue occurs. Treatment entails relieving compression on blood vessels by laying the plaster open down to skin. If this does not produce improvement within 1 hour the wound must be reopened and if necessary, the major limb arteries explored.

NERVE INJURY

If nerve section has been observed at the primary oper-

ation, nerve suture is undertaken after the bone has united and any wound infection controlled.

TETANUS AND GAS GANGRENE (see chapter 14)

SPECIFIC FRACTURES

Spinal fractures

Spinal fractures most commonly occur as a result of flexion injury in which one vertebral body is driven against another to produce a compression injury. At the same time there is often rotation, breaking the interarticular facet joints and so allowing dislocation with or without damage to the cord.

Less commonly, and nearly always in the cervical spine, an extension fracture or fracture dislocation may occur.

DIAGNOSIS

The spine should be specificially examined in any seriously injured patient.

Backache in relation to injury should always prompt an X-ray. Wedging or forward displacement may be seen.

Patients with injured spines must always be examined carefully for a neurological defect and moved with caution in a neutral position whether one is found or not. Ileus can complicate fractures of the lumbar vertebrae, presumably because there is retroperitoneal haematoma which stimulates the sympathetic chain. It usually resolves spontaneously.

TREATMENT

Compression fractures of a single lumbar vertebra are treated by initial bed rest followed by rapid mobilization. There is no place for immobilization in a plaster jacket, as used to be practised.

More complicated fractures and fracture dislocations require highly specialized treatment, particularly if there is also damage to the spinal cord. In the cervical spine this usually means *traction*; in the lumbar spine, immobilization on a spinal bed, which allows the patient to be moved without lifting.

Spinal shock

This is the clinical syndrome produced by damage to the spinal cord. It is a conduction defect which occurs particularly at the synapse. All functions which depend on conduction through the synapse, fail. In cases of mild damage, recovery occurs after 24 or 48 hours. If there is permanent damage to the cord, the stage of spinal shock lasts longer, approximately 3–6 weeks.

There is:

loss of voluntary movement
flaccidity
absence of reflexes
retention of urine

Mild cases may be differentiated from severe cases by:

a. Joint position sense. In mild cases, the posterior columns survive and this is present.
b. Change in sensory level. In severe cases, oedema of the cord around the lesion results in the sensory level moving proximally.
c. No recovery after 48 hours indicates a severe lesion

Severe lesions may be partial or complete.

Partial lesions
Recovery produces a spastic paralysis with extensor plantar responses and variable return of sensation.

Complete lesion
There is a spastic paralysis with a mass flexor reflex This is massive flexor response to minimal stimulation.

The bladder
The paralysis of spinal shock produces a atonic neurogenic bladder, and retention of urine. With recovery, if the level of the lesion is above the level of S2, spinal innervation to and from the bladder is intact, and an automatic bladder results, which empties every 2–4 hours.

Below S2, there is no sensation and no reflex arcs, except the intramural bladder reflexes are intact. The result is an autonomous bladder which tends to dribble spontaneously.

TREATMENT
Initially, the aim is to prevent complications and to preserve function.
  Specifically:

a. Prevention of pressure sores
b. Prevention of urinary infection through catheterization of the bladder
c. Prevention of constipation by the use of enemas
d. Physiotherapy to prevent hypostatic pneumonia and mobilization of joints to prevent contractures

Pelvic fractures and perineal injuries

Of all bony injuries, pelvic fractures are most likely to be the combined concern of orthopaedic and other surgeons. The reason is the concurrence of other injuries in different systems and particularly of damage to the bladder and urethra.

Pelvic fractures occur in their most severe form as the result of crushing injuries, when they assume particular importance because of the frequent involvement of viscera and the likelihood of associated damage to the bladder or uretha. They are thus in a 'no man's land' between general and traumatic surgery.

CLINICAL FEATURES
These can be considered under the following headings:

1. Due to pelvic fracture
a. Tenderness at site of an avulsion or impact of violence
b. Severe pain and inability to stand when pelvic ring disruption present
c. Shock, which is often marked when there is pelvic ring disruption especially if associated injuries are present

2. Due to urogenital injury
a. Extraperitoneal rupture of bladder or rupture of membranous urethra
  (i) Suprapubic pain
  (ii) Suprapubic tenderness
  (iii) Suprapubic mass, occasionally
  (iv) Inability to pass urine
  (v) Intense desire to micturate
  (vi) Extravasation of urine into anterior part of peritoneum or the anterior abdominal wall may occur, after days, with bladder rupture, but is uncommon after urethral rupture
  (vii) Blood at external urinary meatus
b. Intrapeperitoneal rupture of bladder
  (i) Severe suprapubic pain
  (ii) Abdominal distension, tenderness and later rigidity
  (iii) Inability to pass urine
  (iv) Fullness in recto-vesical pouch on rectal examination
  (v) Blood at external urinary meatus

3. Due to sciatic nerve injury
Anaesthesia and weakness of part of the leg when vertical type of pelvic ring disruption is present

SPECIAL TESTS
a. Plain X-ray of the pelvis for nature and extent of fractures
b. Cysto-urethrogram is performed if bladder or urethral rupture is suspected
c. Intravenous urogram to exclude renal trauma as cause of haematuria

TREATMENT
This entails the following:

1. Correction of shock

2. Catheterization. Do not do this without consulting an expert. In extraperitoneal rupture there is no hurry and the patient is best treated by suprapubic decompression and a later repair. The important things are to prevent further damage and sepsis.
3. Treatment of fractures. The fractures receive secondary consideration and nothing more is required other than bed rest for 3–4 weeks, until pain and discomfort have subsided. Skeletal traction to the leg on the affected side is necessary, particularly if there is sciatic nerve compression. This is usually maintained for about two months.

Occasionally, open reduction and internal fixation with a plate or screws is required. Alternatively, external fixation by means of a clamp which holds together pins inserted into the iliac crest can be used.

8

Head injuries

Head injuries are caused by motor car, industrial, sporting and home accidents in decreasing order of frequency. The best treatment of any condition is prevention. Motor vehicle accidents may be prevented by reducing blood alcohol and speed, improving road behaviour, road design and construction and improving vehicle design. Injuries in motor accidents may be prevented or minimized by wearing safety belts. Industrial accidents are reduced if safety helmets are worn.

CLASSIFICATION

Closed—non-penetrating

Injury to neurons occurs at the time (contusion, laceration) or later due to compression in a rigid skull by blood clot or oedema.

Open—penetration of the skull and/or the meninges

This may be direct, e.g. bullet, or by bony fragments. Meningitis is an ever-present risk.

SURGICAL ANATOMY

The tentorium cerebelli divides the cranial cavity into a supratentorial compartment containing the cerebral hemispheres and an infratentorial compartment containing the cerebellum, pons and medulla. The two compartments are continuous with each other through the tentorial hiatus (Fig. 16.1). Passing through this hiatus is the midbrain and its associated blood vessels. The important structures within the midbrain are the cerebral peduncles, the oculomotor nerves, the superior quadrigeminal bodies and the midbrain reticular formation. Lying immediately above and lateral to the tentorial hiatus is the uncus of the medial portion of the temporal lobe.

The reticular formation extends from the medulla to the thalamus and exerts a controlling influence on most cerebral activities. It can be subdivided into activating and inhibitory portions; the activating system lies predominantly in the midbrain and controls consciousness by its interactions with the cerebral cortex.

SURGICAL PATHOLOGY

Mechanisms

In *closed* injury the mechanism is nearly always *deceleration* or *acceleration*. The moving head comes into contact with a stationary object; the blow is usually tangential so that scalp and skull are arrested but the brain continues to move. Alternatively, the skull may be struck and accelerate, leaving the brain behind.

The initial (primary) damage is caused in three ways:

1. DIRECT IMPACT
Contusion of the brain occurs beneath the site of direct impact. At the same time there is an area of negative pressure on the surface of the brain opposite. This shearing force produces a 'contrecoup' injury.

2. BRAIN LACERATION
Lacerations are produced as the brain oscillates against sharp points of the skull, e.g. the sphenoid ridge; temporal lobe against middle fossa.

3. ROTARY-SHEARING FORCES
As the head pivots on the neck the line described by the brain after impact is an arc. This, together with the differing densities of regions of the brain, produces rotary forces. This is directed down the brain stem.

Direct impact, if severe enough, produces intracerebral haematoma. Less severe injuries produce oedema (with petechial haemorrhage) or only transient functional loss. Without structural damage, brain lacerations lead to the majority of acute subdural haematomas. Surrounding neuronal damage tends to be more severe.

Rotary forces damage long-fibre tracts, are transmitted down the brain stem and damage is proportional to severity (immediate death if respiratory centre is ruptured; unconsciousness if reticular formation is damaged).

Haemorrhage

Haemorrhage from any intracranial vessel may occur above or below the tentorium cerebelli and cause brain compression. Time is required for this to develop and it varies according to the number and calibre of the vessels, the pressure in the vessels and the *compartment* and *plane* in which haemorrhage occurs.

THE COMPARTMENT

Supratentorial haemorrhage. Intracranial haemorrhage and oedema acting as a space occupying lesion lead to secondary damage. If brain-stem function is intact after initial injury death may result from raised intracranial pressure. In most cases the space occupying lesion is supratentorial. Herniation of the uncus of the temporal lobe eventually causing haemorrhage in the brain stem. Initially it is function in the upper brain stem that is impaired (conjugate gaze). Superimposed on this cerebral hypoxia and hypercarbia increase oedema.

Effects of mid brain compression are:

1. Deterioration of the conscious state due to reticular formation compression.
2. Pupillary changes due to stretching of the oculomotor nerves. There is an initial transient constriction of the pupil on the affected side due to stimulation of the oculomotor nerve followed by dilation due to paralysis of the nerve. This is followed by similar changes on the opposite side as compression becomes more severe.
3. Hemiparesis due to compression of the cerebral peduncle. In two-thirds of cases the cerebral peduncle on the same side as the haematoma is directly compressed by the uncus giving rise to a contralateral hemiparesis. In one-third of cases the cerebral peduncle on the side opposite to the haematoma is pressed against the free edge of the tentorium giving rise to an ipsilateral hemiparesis. With continuing compression the following signs of damage to the pons occur:
4. Elevation of blood pressure
5. Slowing of the pulse
6. Irregular respiration

Infratentorial haemorrhage is less common. As the mid brain is not initially compressed, consciousness is not impaired.

THE PLANE

In each of the compartments haemorrhage can be classified according to the plane in which it occurs: viz. extradural, subdural, subarachnoid, intracerebral or intraventricular.

Extradural haemorrhage. This is commonly due to laceration of the middle meningeal artery in association with a fractured temporal bone as the result of a blow on the side of the head. Typically about 2 hours are required for clinical manifestations to appear, because though the haemorrhage occurs at arterial pressure, the dura (which is quite firmly adherent to the bone) must be stripped off the bone before a haematoma can form.

Extradural haemorrhage may also occur from the dural venous sinuses, when it may take 12 hours before compression effects are apparent.

Subdural haemorrhage. Less severe trauma produces a subdural haematoma over a period of about 10 days. The subdural space may be increased in elderly patients and thus the risk of bleeding from a venous sinus is present. In infants there is a soft surrounding skull. A further increase in the size of the haematoma occurs either because of osmotic forces or from rebleeding due to coughing, etc. The addition of leaking CSF produces the subdural effusion of infancy.

Chronic subdural haematoma occurs 3 weeks after an often forgotten incident. There is episodic drowsiness and confusion. Neurological defects are uncommon and papilloedema rare. Raised pressure leads to impaired conjugate gaze and dilatation of both pupils. Diagnosis is most easily made by CT scan and is easily missed in: alcoholics; epileptics; the elderly and patients with coagulopathy. A history of injury may not be obtained in infants.

Subdural hygroma. This is a condition in which yellow, high protein (400–1000 mg/dl) fluid accumulates in the subdural space extensively and bilaterally. It is commonly associated with severe head injuries.

Subarachnoid haemorrhage. This does not cause a space-occupying haematoma but gives symptoms and signs of meningismus, which include headache, photophobia, irritability and neck stiffness.

Intracerebral haemorrhage. This is associated with cerebral contusion.

Intraventricular haemorrhage. This is associated with very severe brain damage which is usually fatal.

MANAGEMENT

First aid

This must include:

1. Maintenance of an adequate airway, with artificial respiration if respiratory drive is reduced.

2. Oxygen if necessary
3. A light occlusive dressing to any compound head wound
4. First aid to associated injuries
5. Transport to appropriate medical care

Assessment in the emergency room

HISTORY

This must include an assessment of:

1. The nature of the injury
2. The patient's condition immediately following the injury
3. The time elapsed since the injury
4. The progress in the interim

EXAMINATION

1. Conscious state

The level of consciousness must be accurately assessed and recorded if deterioration due to intracranial haematoma is to be detected at an early stage. Changes in conscious level are likely to precede others. A system of record familiar to all involved in the patient's care must be used (e.g. Glasgow Coma Scale) and it is best to record over a range of 1–6 his response to given stimuli, viz:

a. Can give name; age; date; place
b. Eyes are open; can make purposeful movements and speech
c. Opens eyes, but speech and limb movement are only in response to command
d. Eyes closed, but aroused by pain to give appropriate movement
e. Does not respond to command; withdraws from painful stimulus appropriately
f. Deep coma; only response to pain is abnormal, i.e. extension of limb

2. Vital signs
a. Blood pressure
b. Pulse
c. Respiration
d. Temperature

3. Pupil reactions
Isolated cranial nerves lesions are likely to be due to initial injury

4. Fundi, other cranial nerves

5. Limbs
a. Power
b. Tone
c. Reflexes

d. Co-ordination (if condition permits)
e. Sensation (if condition permits)

6. Associated injuries
Of particular importance are injuries to the eye, ear and sinuses. Special care must be taken to exclude a cervical spine injury.

Penetrating injuries (there may be no period of unconsciousness) may injure bone and dura with subsequent meningitis. Such injuries must be evaluated (including skull X-ray) and the wound explored.

SPECIAL TESTS

1. Plain X-ray of skull and a lateral X-ray of the cervical spine (as soon as patient's condition permits)
2. CT scanning if facilities are available

From this information an assessment is made of the patient's condition and a decision taken about definitive treatment.

Definitive treatment

ALLOWED HOME

Patients are permitted to go home if they are conscious, mentally normal and have no skull fracture. They (and also a responsible relative if present) must be warned to return to hospital immediately if severe headache, vomiting, drowsiness or coma occurs. They should be reviewed either in outpatients or by their own doctor in a few days.

OBSERVED IN THE EMERGENCY ROOM

If there is mild impairment of the conscious state or mentality but no skull fracture, observation is essential. Ordinarily, patients are reassessed after 4 hours and a decision is then taken as to whether they have improved sufficiently to go home or whether admission is necessary.

TRANSFERRED TO THEATRE

Immediate operation is indicated if rapidly progressive deterioration of the clinical state occurs. Occasionally, severe scalp haemorrhage may require immediate operation for its control.

ADMITTED TO WARD

Admission is arranged if the patient is unconscious or stuporose, or when focal neurological signs (e.g. hemiparesis) or a skull fracture are present.

While the details of management will vary with the severity of the initial injury, the principles of management are: constant observation and care of the patient. Observation provides the information by which complications may be detected and treatment thus instituted.

Associated injuries are treated on their merits. The combination of a head injury with either or both of an abdominal injury and a long bone fracture may be particularly difficult.

The most important observation is of the level of consciousness (see above). Respiration and other variables are noted on a 'head injuries chart'. Signs of developing cerebral compression are:

1. Impaired upward conjugate gaze
2. Deterioration of conscious level
3. Changes in pupils (initial constriction and later dilatation). Direct damage to cranial nerves may occur at the time of impact so it is change that is important.
4. Appearance of haemparesis
5. Elevation of blood pressure
6. Slowing of pulse
7. Irregularity of respiration

The management of combined injuries can present conflicts in requirements, particularly with regard to the use of narcotics in the conscious patient. Narcotics are contra-indicated in the management of head injuries because they depress the conscious state and respiration and cause fixed constricted pupils. However, narcotics are important in the management of severe limb fractures and particularly in the management of chest injuries. In these circumstances no firm rule can be laid down and very close co-operation between the various surgeons concerned is required.

TRANSFER TO A NEUROSURGICAL UNIT

The necessity for transfer is clear when an intracranial haematoma is suspected. However the number with possible haematoma who ultimately require surgery is small. Nevertheless overall results improve with early and free transfer because of the expert opinion and treatment available at an experienced centre.

Other indications for transfer are:

a. Depressed fractures, CSF leaks, meningitis, epilepsy that is difficult to control
b. Those that do not show signs of recovery after 3 days
c. Deterioration. Although a CT scan can be performed, transfer may be harmful and the operation rate is low. Careful selection is required.

CARE OF THE UNCONSCIOUS PATIENT

This includes consideration of the following:

The airway (see also Chapter 9). In deeply comatose patients with impaired pharyngeal muscle tone and co-ordination, a plastic cuffed endotracheal tube is inserted and replaced by a cuffed plastic tracheostomy tube within 48 hours if the need persists. In less comatose patients an oral airway may suffice.

If endotracheal intubation or tracheostomy is performed, the inspired air must be adeuately humified to prevent encrustation of bronchial secretions. Regular suction of the bronchial tree must be undertaken with a soft sterile rubber or plastic catheter. The use of prophylactic antibiotics guided by sputum cultures is advisable.

Artificial respiration may be used before exploratory surgery. However it is most uncommon for a patient to survive following cessation of spontaneous respiration.

Fluids, electrolytes and nutrition. The patient is maintained in adequate fluid and electrolyte balance by intravenous, intragastric or oral fluids. In severely injured patients initial intravenous replacement is necessary. It is important in head-injured patients to avoid overhydration by excessive infusion. It is better to err on the side of underhydration in the initial 48 hours. It is important however to maintain an adequate haemoglobin in order that cerebral oxygenation is not impaired. Gastrointestinal absorption is usually absent for 2 or 3 days following severe head injury and a nasogastric tube is therefore required during this time to aspirate gastric secretions and later to provide nutrition.

Bladder. Retention of urine may occur, necessitating catheter drainage. Urine collection by either catheter or condom drainage is necessary to provide an accurate measure of fluid balance and to keep the bed and skin dry. If a catheter is used, prophylactic antibiotics must be administered and the urine examined frequently for evidence of infection.

Bowels. These are not initially a problem but troublesome constipation and faecal impaction will require treatment.

Back. The skin must be cared for by attentive nursing, frequent change of posture and by keeping the skin dry. Sheepskins are useful in this regard.

Temperature control. After severe head injury it is usual for hyperpyrexia to occur as a result of damage to central temperature regulating mechanisms situated mainly in the hypothalamus. It is important to control hyperpyrexia because not only may this cause death if left uncontrolled, but also it increases the patient's metabolic requirements generally and in particular raises the cerebral oxygen requirement. In addition, increase in temperature predisposes to cerebral oedema. It is therefore important to prevent increase in temperature and for the same reasons a moderate decrease in temperature is beneficial.

Reduction of temperature may be achieved with acetyl-salicylic acid (aspirin) orally or rectally (0·6 g, 4-hourly), promethazine (Phenergan 25 to 50 mg i.m. p.r.n.), or surface cooling with the aid of a wind tunnel, wet sheets and ice packs.

SPECIAL TESTS

These may be performed if the clinical pattern is not clear or when the patient fails to respond. The investigation chosen will depend on the time available, the condition of the patient and the type of complication suspected.

The investigations available are:

Plain X-ray of the skull. This is indicated in all patients with head injury sufficient to occasion admission. It may show a fracture, shift of a calcified pineal gland from the midline indicating the presence of a mass, an aerocele or some incidental problem.

Other tests aim to confirm or refute the presence of a space occupying lesion.

Computerized tomography (CT scan). This test is now available in most neurosurgical centres and has had a major influence on the management of intracranial haematomata. CT scan takes no longer than 10 minutes to perform; detects and localizes haematoma accurately; can be used to follow post-operative resolution of clot; but requires a co-operative or anaesthetized patient and is expensive.

Other special tests used less frequently following the introduction of CT scan are:

Echo-encephalography. This detects mid-line shift.

Carotid angiography. This takes 2 hours and localizes haematoma.

Pneumoncephalography and electro-encephalography are useful for investigating complications (e.g. epilepsy)

Exploratory burr holes may be made to exclude haematomas if time and resources preclude the above.

TREATMENT OF COMPLICATIONS

1. Intracranial haemorrhage

Death can be avoided by anticipation of complications. Other than maintenancy of an airway treatment of an intracranial haematoma is most likely to result in patient improvement. The chance of an intracranial haematoma are approximately as follows (it may not be remediable); coma (50%) focal signs (30%) fracture (10%) fit (8%) confused (6%) and not confused (1%)

Because CT scan detects haematoma very accurately, judgement is required in deciding which patients will benefit from surgery. It may however be necessary to evacuate an intracranial haematoma immediately.

Surgical treatment of haematoma is by burr holes, evacuation of the clot and securing haemostasis. *Craniectomy* (extension of the burr hole) or formal *craniotomy* may be necessary for adequate access.

Technique of burr holes. Either local or general

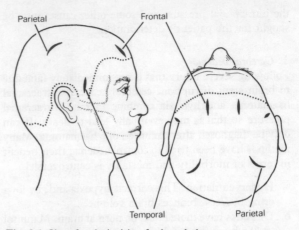

Fig. 8.1 Site of scalp incision for burr holes

anaesthesia may be used. The whole head is shaved and six burr hole sites marked out (Fig. 8.1).

The frontal incision lies in the line of the pupil and just behind the normal position of the hairline, angled obliquely forwards and laterally.

The temporal incision starts immediately above the zygomatic arch, one-third of the way forwards between the tragus of the ear and the external angular process of the eye.

The parietal incision is situated obliquely over the parietal eminence.

Each incision is 3–4 cm long and may be extended. The correct side to start is the one which pupil first dilates (note: it constricts first) or the side of a fracture or haematoma.

Steps in procedure. The skin incision is deepened to bone and the periosteum is scraped away on each side and a self-retaining retractor is inserted. Then a brace with a perforator is used to penetrate the skull until the tip of the perforator is just through the inner table; then a burr completes the hole in the skull.

If an extradural haematoma is seen, further bone is removed with rongeurs until sufficient exposure is provided to permit evacuation of the haematoma and the securing of haemostasis.

If no extradural haematoma is found the dura is opened using a sharp hook and a No. 15 blade scalpel. If a subdural haematoma is then found, further exposure is obtained as above and the haematoma is evacuated and haemostasis achieved. If no haematoma is present but the brain bulges, then further burr holes are made until a haematoma is found or is confidently excluded; in the latter situation cerebral oedema will be present.

If no haematoma is found and the brain is 'slack', that is it does not bulge and it pulsates gently with pulse waves and with respiration, then there is no elevation of the intracranial pressure and some other cause must be sought for the patient's deterioration.

2. Cerebral oedema

Following severe injury that is not immediately fatal due to brain stem disruption, cerebral oedema, intracranial haematoma and hypoxia combine to raise intracranial pressure so that is may eventually lead to death. If can only be diagnosed after exclusion of a haematoma. Many methods have been tried to control oedema; their benefit in terms of morbidity and mortality is controversial.

a. Hyperventilation. This corrects hypoxia and, by lowering of P_{CO_2}, reduces brain volume.
b. Diuretics have more effect on normal brain. Mannitol (0.25g/kg every 4–6 h) or urea can be used but electrolyte imbalance is easily produced
c. Steroids. Dexamethasone 4 mg i.m. 6-hourly.
d. Barbiturate-induced coma

3. Infection

Compound injuries of the vault are the result of direct trauma and are relatively uncommon in civilian life; commoner is compound injury of the base as a result of a fracture through an air sinus or the middle ear. When a CSF leak is obvious or suspected, sulphonamides (which cross the blood–brain barrier) are administered.

This may occur as a complication of compound fractures. It can be of the wound, the bone (osteomyelitis), the meninges (meningitis), or the brain (encephalitis). Treatment is ideally prophylactic with surgical closure of the defect in the coverings of the brain together with the administration of antibiotics. Treatment of established infection is by the administration of systemic, and if necessary, intrathecal antibiotics and closure of any site of continuing infection.

4. Skull fracture

Depressed fractures require removal of bone around the fracture followed by elevation in order to relieve raised intracranial pressure if they are large, or to relieve local cortical pressure and irritation (possibly leading to epilepsy) if they are small. Compound fractures associated with a scalp wound require primary closure of the sclap wound after debridement. The skin closure may require a rotation flap.

Compound fractures involving the paranasal sinuses or auditory passages with a dural laceration may lead to cerebrospinal fluid rhinorrhoea or otorrhoea. Both are initially treated expectantly but surgery will be required if the fluid loss persists for 2 weeks or more, if meningitis develops or if an aerocele is present.

5. Post-concussion syndrome

Temporary impairment of upper brain stem function by rotary forces is responsible for unconsciousness. Memory loss, confusion and disorientation are cerebral functions. Patients may awaken from coma completely demented due to severe neuronal damage. It is probable that a lesser degree of this is responsible for milder complaints described as 'post-concussion syndrome'. These may be very disabling but usually return to normality in 1–3 years. Residual brain-stem abnormalities reflect a greater initial injury. These include eye movements, speech, balance and co-ordination.

6. Personality disturbance

After severe head injury, that is, when the post-traumatic amnesia exceeds 1 week, personality disturbance and impairment of intellect are common. While improvement usually occurs with time, permanent changes may result.

7. Post-traumatic epilepsy

After mild head injuries there is an initial risk of 2% of developing epilepsy. If the post-traumatic amnesia exceeds 24 hours the risk increases to 10%. Following intracranial haematoma the risk is 30% and when cortical laceration has occurred the risk becomes 50%.

In all patients this risk diminishes with the passage of time (assuming no fits occur) and the risk becomes negligible after 5 years.

Prophylaxtic anticonvulsant therapy is required for patients with a depressed fracture and acute intracranial haematoma.

8. Brain death

Brain death is a controversial issue, particularly in regard to organ donation for transplantation. When brain death is established further artificial support is pointless. Permanent functional death of the brain stem constitutes brain death. The stringent criteria used aim to distinguish those who have a chance of even partial recovery from those who have no possibility of recovery.

Conditions for considering a diagnosis of brain death include:

a. *A working diagnosis*, e.g. intracerebral haemorrhage
b. *Coma* excluding: depressant drugs, neuromuscular blockers, hypothermia, metabolic crisis and endocrine crisis
c. *A requirement for artificial ventilation*

Tests to confirm brain death:

a. Pupils fixed
b. Absent corneal reflex
c. No eye movement to intra-aural instillation of cold water

d. No motor cranial nerve response

e. No gag reflex

f. No spontaneous respirations after discontinuing IPPV with P_{CO_2} 6.7 kPa (40 mmHg), i.e.

   (i) give pure O_2 for 10 min via ventilator

   (ii) give 5% CO_2 for 5 min via ventilator

   (iii) disconnect IPPV but supply 6 l/min O_2 for 10 min

The current code of practice for confirming the diagnosis of brain death is that two independent senior physicians make their examinations 30 minutes apart and at least 6 hours after the injury. Only then can consideration be given to withdrawing further treatment or proceding with organ donation.

9

Chest injuries and respiratory management in surgery

Trauma to the chest is a common occurrence particularly after road traffic accidents and it may be associated with potentially lethal pulmonary and cardiovascular injuries.

SURGICAL PATHOLOGY

1. Open injuries

Penetrating trauma of the chest wall by knife, gunshot, or other injuries is particularly liable to be complicated by the development of a sucking pneumothorax, intrathoracic visceral damage and infection.

2. Closed injuries

Direct blunt trauma to the chest wall due to crushing injuries and steering wheel injuries may cause rib fractures, a flail chest with paradoxical movement, rupture of the diaphragm, or serious cardiovascular complications: e.g. aortic rupture or myocardial contusion.

Deceleration violence, as can occur in aeroplane and motor car accidents is typically liable to cause rupture of the descending aorta just distal to the subclavian artery and rupture of the diaphragm.

Blast injuries are liable to be associated with intra-alveolar haemorrhage, pulmonary haematoma and hypoxia.

CLINICAL FEATURES

1. Recent history of violence

2. Symptoms of chest injuries

a. *Pain*—due to presence of fractures of the thoracic cage or pulmonary or cardiovascular complication.
b. *Dyspnoea*—due to fractures, pneumothorax, haemothorax, flail chest, ruptured diaphragm, ruptured trachea or main bronchus, or other serious visceral damage; rapidly increasing dyspnoea is typical of a tension pneumothorax.
c. *Haemoptysis*—due to lacerated lung with or without haemothorax, or pulmonary haematoma.

3. Signs of chest injury

a. *Shock*—may be due to: blood loss; tension pneumothorax or cardiac tamponade. It will be severe with associated visceral damage.
b. *Chest wall trauma*—will be evidenced by bruising, a sucking wound of the chest wall, paradoxical chest wall movement in association with a flail or stove in chest injury, or pain on 'springing' the chest wall when rib fractures are present.
c. *Surgical emphysema*—evidenced as a crackling sensation beneath the examining fingers, due to the presence of air in the subcutaneous tissues and caused by fractured ribs or a ruptured cervical trachea.
d. *Mediastinal emphysema with mediastinitis*—evidenced by pain on rocking the larynx and by a parapericardial clicking synchronous with the heart beat and is suggestive of a ruptured oesophagus or trachea.
e. *Tracheal deviation* is associated with displacement of the apex beat if there is pulmonary collapse (e.g. pneumothorax) or intrapleural collection (e.g. haemothorax). A tension pneumothorax will displace the trachea away from the affected side.
f. *Elevated jugular venous pressure*—occurs with cardiac tamponade due to haemopericardium.
g. *Lung fields*—hyper-resonance indicates pneumothorax and diminished or absent breath sounds indicate haemothorax, pneumothorax, or pulmonary collapse.

4. Special tests

a. *Chest X-rays*. These should invariable be performed and will demonstrate fractured ribs, pneumothorax, haemothorax, ruptured diaphragm, lung contusion and atelectasis. Injuries to the aorta and its major branches will be associated with haemorrhage and widening of the upper mediastinal shadow while a haemopericardium will show up as an enlarged heart shadow.

Chest X-ràys should *always* be taken *erect* unless the patient's condition totally precludes this (very rare). Supine X-rays provide limited information.

b. *Electrocardiogram.* This will be indicated when cardiac trauma is suspected.
c. *Aortography.* This should be performed when major artery damage is suspected, particularly when mediastinal widening is present on chest X-rays.
d. *Estimation of blood gases.* Regular estimation of arterial oxygen and carbon dioxide partial pressures is of considerable value in estimating the degree of respiratory insufficiency, particularly in those patients with paradoxical respiration and flail chest wall segments. Having excluded treatable conditions, e.g. pneumothorax, increasing hypoxia calls for added oxygen. Further deterioration requires endotracheal intubation and artificial ventilation.

An increasing PCO_2 (above 55 mmHg) is also an indication for ventilation.

MANAGEMENT

This will depend on the severity of the chest injury and the severity and extent of associated injuries.

In general there are four major considerations: the patient's respiration, his circulation, his progress, and any individual chest injuries.

Respiration

A clear airway and proper lung movements are essential for adequate respiration.

CLEAR AIRWAY
Sputum retention with bronchial obstruction and atelectasis is liable to occur when there is:

1. Unconsciousness (head injury)
2. Shock
3. Painful chest injury
4. Excessive production of secretions as in lung contusions, pulmonary oedema, massive pulmonary haematoma and in severe chest injuries

Treatment
This includes:

1. Adequate analgesia
2. Adequate sedation to relieve anxiety and apprehension
3. Posturing and physiotherapy
4. Antibiotics
5. Naso-pharyngeal suction
6. Naso-tracheal suction
7. Bronchoscopic suction
8. Tracheostomy

In mild or moderate chest injuries the use of anal-

gesics, sedation and physiotherapy may be all that is required, while in severe chest injuries endotracheal tube or tracheostomy suction may have to be included for effective clearance of airway obstruction.

PROPER LUNG MOVEMENTS
Inadequate lung movement may occur when there is:

1. A flail chest with paradoxical respiration
2. Severe head injury with brain stem damage
3. Blood or air in the pleural cavity

Treatment
This includes:

1. The urgent closure of a sucking chest wall wound
2. Removal of air from the pleural cavity by a chest drain, or blood from the pleural cavity by repeated aspirations, catheter drainage or operation
3. Tracheostomy and intermittent positive pressure respiration

Circulation

Restoration of blood and fluid losses is an essential requirement.

Blood transfusions will be indicated when major intra-thoracic visceral complications are present or when commonly associated upper abdominal injuries (rupture of spleen and liver) occur.

Regular assessment of progress

In moderate and severe chest injuries, repeated clinical and radiological assessment of the patient's progress is essential. In addition, repeated estimations of arterial oxygen and carbon dioxide partial pressures serve as valuable indices of respiratory function.

Individual chest injuries

OPEN CHEST INJURY
Closure of a sucking chest wall wound is an immediate requirement and may be performed temporarily with packing or sutures and later definitively.

Thoracotomy will be indicated if there is associated intra-thoracic visceral trauma, retained foreign bodies in the pleural cavity or if superadded infection should occur.

ISOLATED FRACTURED RIBS
This is the commonest injury to the thoracic cage which, because of the associated pain on breathing, may cause poor ventilation, sputum retention, atelectasis and pneumonia, particularly in the elderly.

Treatment

1. Relief of pain with analgesics, or local intercostal or paravertebral nerve block
2. Physiotherapy and encouragement to cough
3. Operation may be indicated for overlapping sternal fragments

FLAIL CHEST

An injury to the chest that results either in multiple ribs being fractured in two places or in the sternum being disrupted leads to an unstable or flail segment of the chest wall. With inspiration, the flail segment moves inward—paradoxical movement—so leading to hypoxia as gas moves from one lung to the other with movements of the mediastinum. Respiratory failure and lowered cardiac output result.

Treatment

1. Mild to moderate cases:
   a. Adequate analgesia
   b. Adequate sedation
   c. Posturing and physiotherapy
   d. Intranasal oxygen
   e. Respirator with mouthpiece
2. Severe cases: tracheostomy and intermittent positive pressure respiration is required for at least 10 days in addition to the simple measures above. The flail segment may rarely require surgical fixation.

In the absence of clinical evidence of respiratory insufficiency, regular blood gas estimations are of great value in determining the necessity for tracheostomy and assisted respiration.

PNEUMOTHORAX

This may occur as the result of:

1. Fractured ribs with lung puncture
2. Fractured ribs with valvular lung puncture, causing tension pneumothorax
3. Ruptured trachea or main bronchus, causing tension pneumothorax
4. Open chest wound, causing a sucking pneumothorax

Treatment

1. *Shallow pneumothorax* not inhibiting respiratory activity does not require any treatment unless a general anaesthetic or intermittent positive pressure respiration is indicated for some other purpose.
2. *Deep pneumothorax*, large enough to inhibit respiratory activity, requires the insertion of an intercostal catheter into the second intercostal space anteriorly in the mid-clavicular line and attaching the outlet to an underwater seal.
3. *Tension pneumothorax*. The tear in the parietal pleura may act as a valve. Air is sucked into the pleural cavity on inspiration but does not return to the bronchus on expiration. Rapidly increasing dyspnoea results, with increased intrathoracic pressure, impaired venous return and shock. Emergency treatment is insertion of a needle and/or intercostal drain into the cavity. If the lung fails to expand after catheter drainage then ruptured trachea or main bronchus should be suspected, particularly if there is blood-stained sputum. This diagnosis will be confirmed on bronchoscopy and will require thoracotomy and repair.

HAEMOTHORAX

This may occur from:

1. Parietal vessels (intercostal, internal mammary), when continued haemorrhage is likely.
2. Pulmonary vessels in association with lung trauma, when low pressure haemorrhage usually ceases spontaneously.
3. Diaphragmatic and sub-diaphragmatic trauma, when blood from a ruptured diaphragm and/or upper abdominal viscera is sucked into the pleural cavity.

Massive clotting of a haemothorax rarely occurs except in the presence of infection as with open chest injuries.

Treatment

1. *Minimal*—observe closely
2. *Moderate*—aspirate with syringe, needle, and two-way tap, completely and as frequently as is necessary
3. *Gross*—intercostal catheter and underwater drainage
4. *Continuing*—thoracotomy and secure haemostasis
5. *Clotted*—intrapleural fibrinolytic enzymes may be used but operation and decortication will be required at an early date
6. *Infected*—empyema formation will require thoracotomy and drainage

In all cases blood transfusions, antibiotics and analgesics will be given as indicated.

LUNG CONTUSION OR LACERATION

This is a cause of continued and profuse haemoptysis.

Treatment

1. The usual supportive measures, which include clearing the airways and tracheostomy
2. Any inadequately drained haemothorax is properly drained
3. A massive pulmonary haematoma is excised
4. Repair of a lacerated lung is rarely necessary

RUPTURED TRACHEA OR MAIN BRONCHUS

This is often missed but tends to occur with the more severe chest injuries.

It may present as:

1. *Acute tension pneumothorax*, with a persistent leak of air into the pleural cavity
2. *Chronic atelectasis* and recurrent lung infections when the leak seals off spontaneously

The diagnosis is usually made on bronchoscopy.

Treatment
1. *Acute*—thoracotomy and repair
2. *Chronic*—thoracotomy and pneumonectomy if lung inexpandable or bronchial secretions infected, or thoracotomy and bronchial anastomosis if lung expandable and bronchial secretions not infected

RUPTURED OESOPHAGUS
Rupture of the oesophagus is rare, but it may follow penetrating or crushing injury. It may also be torn from within by an oesophagoscope or a swallowed sword. Finally, nontraumatic rupture occurs in violent vomiting.

When due to a crushing injury there is most often a longitudinal tear associated with a tear in the posterior wall of the trachea which allows for tracheo-oesophageal fistula formation.

When due to an oesophagoscopy the tear is usually near the level of the cricoid cartilage and apparently the result of crushing of the posterior wall of the oesophagus between the instrument and the cervical spine, particularly when the latter is osteoarthritic.

A ruptured oesophagus presents as mediastinal emphysema and mediastinitis and when suspected the diagnosis is made on oesophagoscopy and oral water soluble X-ray contrast media (Gastrografin).

Treatment
1. Thoracotomy and repair
2. Intravenous replacement therapy or feeding jejunostomy
3. Tracheostomy and usual supportive measures if associated with a ruptured trachea

CARDIAC TRAUMA
Haemopericardium, cardiac contusion and laceration, cardiac rupture, pericardial rupture and injuries to the valvular mechanisms may occur after crushing, deceleration and blast injuries.

The diagnosis is often difficult but cardiac tamponade (i.e. inability of the chambers to fill) with a low arterial pressure, a high venous pressure, pulsus paradoxus and an enlarged cardiac silhouette will arouse suspicion.

Electrocardiography may show non-specific changes, QRS anomalies and various arrhythmias.

Treatment
In the presence of tamponade, pericardiocentesis or preferably thoracotomy is indicated.

RUPTURED THORACIC AORTA
This is usually rapidly fatal. Rupture occurs typically just distal to the origin of the left subclavian artery and usually follows a deceleration injury. If the patient survives it is because the wall of mediastinal pleura and aortic adventitia has contained a pulsating haematoma.

When the patient reaches hospital alive the diagnosis will be suspected if X-rays illustrate a widening of the upper mediastinum and tracheal displacement. Then an aortogram by way of the right brachial artery will reveal the defect.

Usually the flow of blood is not impeded but occasionally aortic obstruction occurs with a 'coarctation-like effect' with proximal hypertension, distal hypotension, and occasionally anuria and paraplegia.

Treatment
Left thoracotomy and suture or prosthetic replacement utilizing left ventricle to femoral artery by-pass.

RUPTURED THORACIC DUCT
This is a rare complication which may result from a severe crushing injury or hyperextension injury to the spine.

Dyspnoea due to chylothorax (usually rightsided) occurs and the diagnosis is established on paracentesis when white milky fluid containing fat droplets, cholesterol, lymphocytes and having a high protein content, is aspirated.

Treatment
1. Frequent aspiration or intercostal drain and suction.
2. Thoracotomy and ligature of the thoracic duct between the cisterna chyli and the site of injury will be indicated if conservative methods fail.

RUPTURED DIAPHRAGM
This may follow a penetrating, crushing or deceleration injury. Most ruptures occur in the left hemidiaphragm and most are centrally situated. Herniation of stomach, spleen, omentum, and small bowel may occur through the defect and often these structures are themselves traumatized by the injurious forces applied.

There are two phases of the condition:

Immediate consequences of rupture
1. Shock
2. Pain
3. Blood loss
4. Haemoperitoneum or haemothorax

Effects of migration of abdominal viscera into chest
1. Displacement of pulmonary, cardiac, mediastinal contents
2. Abdominal visceral obstruction or perforation

There are six signs of a ruptured diaphragm:

1. Diminished chest excursion
2. Impaired chest wall resonance
3. Absence of retraction of the intercostal spaces on diaphragmatic movement
4. Adventitious gastro-intestinal sounds in the chest
5. Cardiac displacement
6. Shock

Treatment
This includes:

1. Correction of shock
2. Laparotomy or thoracotomy
3. Reduction of abdominal contents
4. Repair of diaphragmatic rupture
5. Drainage of pleural cavity

RESPIRATORY SUPPORT IN SURGERY

Derangement of the mechanism of the chest wall, loss of surface for ventilation or merely muscular weakness may require:

1. Intubation so that secretion in the bronchial tree may be sucked out
2. Intermittent positive pressure ventilation until surface area is restored or mechanism improves, or both

The alternatives for IPPR are endotracheal intubation and tracheostomy. Both have advantages and disadvantages.

Endotracheal intubation is:
1. Easy to do
2. Does not create a wound
3. Provides a reasonable pathway for aspiration

but it also

1. May, if prolonged, lead to pressure necrosis of the vocal cord
2. Increases airways resistance
3. May be associated with severe tracheal infection

Tracheostomy
1. Reduces dead space more effectively than intubation
2. Allows a wide bore tube to be used and therefore results in low airways resistance
3. Is an effective portal for suction
4. Is often safer for long term intermittent positive pressure respiration

but it also

1. Creates a wound which often becomes infected
2. May be followed by tracheal stenosis

In both procedures proper humidification is essential.

Specific indications for either intubation or tracheostomy

The five 'R's:

RESPIRATORY OBSTRUCTION
Mechanical obstruction to the upper airway may occur with:

1. Ludwig's angina (mixed infection of the suboral space)
2. Angioneurotic oedema
3. Facial burns
4. Neck, mouth, and jaw injuries
5. Acute laryngo-tracheo-bronchitis
6. Laryngeal tumours
7. Laryngeal stenosis
8. Laryngeal diphtheria
9. Tracheo-bronchial injuries
10. Recurrent laryngeal nerve paralysis
11. Thyroid carcinoma
12. Foreign bodies

RETAINED SECRETIONS
Retention of secretions in the air passages may occur with:

1. Unconsciousness (head injury, cerebral tumour, cerebro-vascular accidents, cardiac arrest, drug over-dosage)
2. Painful chest injuries retarding coughing up of secretions
3. Overproduction of secretions as may occur in lung contusion and head injuries

Tracheostomy will be indicated when secretions cannot be removed by simpler measures such as the use of judicious sedation, adequate analgesia, assisted coughing, pharyngeal, endotracheal and bronchoscopic suction.

RESPIRATORY PARALYSIS
This results in inadequate ventilation with blood gas and pH disturbances and sputum retention. In addition those causes of respiratory paralysis associated with an inability to swallow (bulbar paralysis), allow for aspiration of pharyngeal secretions and vomitus.

Respiratory paralysis may be due to:

1. Poliomyelitis
2. Polyneuritis

3. Cord lesions
4. Tetanus
5. Myasthenia gravis
6. Flail chest

A cuffed tube should be used whenever assisted or controlled positive pressure respiration is necessary, or when aspiration of pharyngeal secretions or blood into the airways is a problem.

REDUCTION OF DEAD SPACE

Those with obstructive or restrictive lung disease in association with inadequate ventilation, especially after major trauma and major surgery, will benefit by a 30% reduction in the dead space with a tracheostomy.

RADICAL SURGERY

Tracheostomy will be necessary after:

1. Laryngectomy
2. Laryngo-pharyngectomy

Tracheostomy may be necessary after:

3. Total thyroidectomy
4. Bilateral block dissection of the neck
5. Excision of the jaw

Timing of tracheostomy

More lives are saved by leisurely prophylactic tracheostomies than by hurried emergency tracheostomies. Urgent situations are best dealt with by intubation or emergency laryngostomy.

1. URGENT

When respiratory insufficiency is obvious by virtue of cyanosis, stridor, chest retraction and retained secretions.

2. ELECTIVE

Tracheostomy will be performed when:

a. Anticipate patient will be unconscious for longer than 24 hours when removal of airway secretions by simple means becomes inadequate
b. Paradoxical respiration occurs in association with large flail segments of the chest wall. In these patients particularly, the decision to perform a tracheostomy should be made after repeated estimations of arterial or alveolar carbon dioxide partial pressures which are valuable indices of respiratory function in the absence of clinical features of respiratory insufficiency.
c. Retention of secretions is considered likely because of a combination of factors, viz. weakness, debility, chronic pulmonary disease, painful chest injuries

Method of tracheostomy

The operation should be performed under ideal conditions in an operating theatre.

The head is extended over a pillow. A local anaesthetic is used if an endotracheal general anaesthetic is contraindicated but it is better to have an endotracheal tube in place.

OPERATION

Through a transverse or vertical incision the operator 'burrows' his way down to the trachea keeping strictly in the midline. The trachea is best opened using an inverted U-shaped flap incision.

Management

MAINTAIN AIRWAY

This must include the following:

1. Effective and frequent atraumatic suction of the air passages through the endotracheal or tracheostomy tube. For this purpose a soft plastic single-end-hole catheter, fitted with a Y connection so that suction can be performed only during withdrawal, is recommended. Catheters with side holes allow for suction of air from above rather than secretions from below. The main bronchi are sucked out by turning the head from one side to the other.

2. Humidification of inhaled gases. This is essential to prevent drying and encrusting of the bronchial epithelium.

When there is an open tracheostomy, a heated nebulizer, utilizing oxygen or compressed medical air, at about 12 l/min, is used. When the tube is attached to a ventilator for assisted or controlled respiration then the humidification is provided by a cold nebulizer attached to the respirator.

3. Use of a mucolytic agent. Acetylcysteine 20% (Mucomyst) will liquefy and help to remove viscid or inspissated secretions when suction and humidification fail to prevent recurrent atelectasis. It can be administered by nebulization or intratracheal instillation but certain highly sensitive patients, particularly asthmatics, may experience varying degrees of bronchospasm at which time the medication should be discontinued.

4. Assisted coughing and physiotherapy to the chest

5. Avoidance of the tube impinging on the posterior wall of the trachea or being dragged out by the respiratory attachments necessitates repeated observation and suspension and support of heavy attachments.

6. Deflation of cuffed tubes for five minutes every hour if possible to prevent tracheal wall trauma.

7. Repeated clinical, radiological and, when necessary, blood gas estimations must be made to assess the efficiency of treatment.

PREVENT INFECTION

1. Aseptic suction technique; sterile tubes and catheters.
2. Frequent removal and cleaning of inner tube when a double metallic tube is being used and changing of single tubes every few days.
3. Antibiotics should be used only when pathogens are isolated. There is otherwise grave risk of super-infection.

Complications of tracheostomy

These include:

1. Encrustation, due to inadequate humidification and mucosal trauma
2. Haemorrhage from anterior jugular veins, thyroid isthmus and possibly the innominate artery
3. Tracheal ulceration and tracheo-oesophageal fistula
4. Tracheal stenosis at the site of the cuff, at the end of the tube, or at the site of tracheostomy
5. Infection of air passages and later atelectasis and pneumonia
6. Tube blockage or displacement
7. Surgical emphysema
8. Pneumothorax

10

Abdominal injuries

In civilian practice, 75% of abdominal trauma follows non-penetrating injuries, except in some communities with a tradition of using the hand gun and the knife to settle differences. Sometimes a force considered trivial may cause alarming visceral damage and even with an acute awareness of such a possibility, the diagnosis or elimination of intra-abdominal trauma can be extremely difficult, especially in the presence of a multiplicity of associated injuries.

CLASSIFICATION

1. **Non-penetrating (closed) injuries**
2. **Penetrating injuries**

SURGICAL PATHOLOGY

1. Non-penetrating injuries

In general the extent of damage depends on the speed, direction, and size of the force applied.

ABDOMINAL WALL
Contusions are common. Haematoma of the rectus sheath may occur with rupture of an epigastric vessel as the result of direct violence or sudden contraction of the rectus abdominis muscle.

INTRA-ABDOMINAL CONTENTS

Solid organs. The liver, spleen and kidneys are commonly affected by closed abdominal trauma because they are relatively fixed, large and comparatively exposed.

Haemorrhage is the outstanding feature and when severe, hypovolaemic shock will occur.

Hollow organs. The bowel, which is relatively mobile and able to move away from the path of a blow, is less likely to be damaged than solid organs, except at areas of relative fixation such as the duodenum, duodenojunal flexure, caecum, ascending colon and colonic flexures.

Peritonitis is the outstanding feature of hollow organ rupture and is due to bowel contents spilling out from tears, crushes or bursting defects in the bowel. The latter defect is uncommon but was occasionally seen as the result of underwater blasts from exploding depth charges in the vicinity of shipwrecked sailors during the major conflicts. Tearing of the mesentery is a particular feature of violent deceleration. A subserosal haematoma forms with subsequent rupture.

The mortality from hollow organ injuries is higher than that associated with injuries of solid organs because of the increased risk of infection. This risk is greatest with colonic trauma.

2. Penetrating injuries

The major effects depend on a combination of haemorrhage and shock when solid organs or major vessels are involved, and peritonitis and infection when bowel is perforated.

When a missile traverses soft tissue, the following may occur:

a. Low velocity missile (A stab or a missile up to 200 m/s). Structures traversed are lacerated.

b. Very high velocity missile (Over 200 and up to 1000 m/s).

The missile accelerates the medium through which it passes and moves it away from the path with such force that it continues to move once the missile has passed. As a result 'temporary cavitation' occurs which causes severe and widespread bruising, tearing, stretching and rupture of nearby viscera.

CLINICAL FEATURES

Non-penetrating injuries

HISTORY OF VIOLENCE
This may be insignificant. Road traffic accidents, falls, assaults and sporting injuries are commonest.

51

PREDISPOSING FACTORS

Adhesions and a flaccid abdominal wall (the unsuspecting or drugged) may increase the risk of intra-abdominal trauma.

PRESENTATION

There are two groups of patients:

1. Diagnosis certain

When haemorrhage from a solid organ or a major vessel occurs, or when peritonitis as the result of a perforated viscus is apparent, then little diagnostic acumen is necessary and operation is imperative. The outstanding features include:

a. Acute and persistent abdominal pain
b. Marked abdominal tenderness, rebound tenderness and rigidity indicating peritonitis due to blood, bile, or bowel content
c. Systemic evidence of continued internal haemorrhage despite resuscitation
d. Shoulder pain due to diaphragmatic irritation from blood or bowel content

(*Note.* Abdominal distension is a late sign and indicates paralytic ileus due to peritonitis or large retroperitoneal haematoma.)

2. Diagnosis uncertain

Abdominal signs may be masked early by shock, associated injuries, unconsciousness, or analgesics. Upper abdominal signs may, on the other hand, be exaggerated by the presence of fractured ribs. In such circumstances the diagnosis should be confirmed or confuted by peritoneal lavage. 500 ml of saline is run in through a sub-umbilical peritoneal dialysis catheter and then allowed to drain under gravity.

Return:

a. Crystal clear—no intraperitoneal injury
b. Blood or gut content—laparotomy essential
c. Slightly blood-stained—10% chance of injury. Reanalyse the clinical picture.

OTHER SPECIAL TESTS

These include:

a. Plain X-ray of the abdomen for pneumoperitoneum from hollow organ rupture and for fluid levels which indicate paralytic ileus
b. Abdominal paracentesis may be used if haemorrhage is suspected, but it is not recommended
c. Selective angiography in certain cases and under ideal circumstances may prove to be of great value, particularly when trauma to the liver is suspected

TREATMENT

1. Non-penetrating injuries

a. Diagnosis certain
  (i) Resuscitation
 (ii) Operation.

b. Diagnosis uncertain in spite of peritoneal lavage

Patients suspected of suffering from abdominal trauma must be considered as potentially serious problems; close and continuous observation is essential. This regimen must include the following:

  (i) Frequent recordings of pulse, blood pressure, temperature and respiration rates
 (ii) Frequent examination of the abdomen
(iii) Refraining from the use of analgesics such as morphine, pethidine or omnopon

Features which suggest the presence of intra-abdominal trauma include:

  (i) Persistent abdominal tenderness
 (ii) Persistent local abdominal muscle rigidity
(iii) Persistent elevation of pulse and temperature
 (iv) Persistent absence of bowel sounds
  (v) Development of paralytic ileus

The decision to operate in the difficult case must be made on a strong suspicion alone in the absence of frank signs or an absolute diagnosis, after careful and repeated observation.

2. Penetrating injuries

In low velocity injury (stabs) penetration may not mean visceral damage. Absolute indications for operation are

a. visceral or omental prolapse
b. continued bleeding—particularly dark venous blood probably coming from a portal radicle
c. faecal or other intestinal discharge
d. signs of spreading peritonitis
e. shock

All these being absent it is reasonable to observe the patient, making frequent abdominal examinations. Only about a quarter of stab wounds managed this way require exploration.

In high velocity injury exploration is mandatory. The principles of operation are:

a. Through laparotomy and assessment and treatment of associated injuries.
b. Wounds of entry (and exit, if present) must be excised and left open in the first instance at least.

SPECIAL CONSIDERATIONS

RUPTURED SPLEEN

This accounts for about 50% of visceral injuries following closed abdominal trauma.

A diseased spleen (malaria, leukaemia) is more likely to rupture than a healthy one.

About 25% of patients with splenic trauma remain well for days or even weeks before frank rupture occurs. In these cases subcapsular haematomata probably form and gradually increase in size before breaking through the capsule into the peritoneal cavity.

Clinical features

HISTORY OF VIOLENCE
This is often a crush to the left lower chest.

EVIDENCE OF INTERNAL HAEMORRHAGE
1. Signs of hypovolaemia: pallor; restlessness; tachycardia; hypotension
2. Signs of peritoneal irritation: pain; shoulder pain; guarding and rigidity
3. Signs of ileus: distension; absent bowel sounds
4. Signs of fluid—shifting dullness—rare

Special tests

1. Plain X-ray of the abdomen. This is performed to exclude haemothorax, fractured ribs or a ruptured hollow organ.
2. Kehr's sign is reliable if positive. Elevation of the foot of the bed causes pain to be experienced in the left shoulder.
3. Ballance's sign. Fixed dullness in left flank due to clotted blood about the spleen together with shifting dullness in the right flank due to unclotted blood in the peritoneal cavity is sometimes demonstrable.
4. Saegesser's sign. Pressure over the phrenic nerve in the left side of the neck is said to cause pain: not reliable.

Treatment

1. Resuscitation
2. Urgent laparotomy and splenectomy. Preservation of some or all of the spleen is now commonly practised, particularly in the child where there is a real risk of post-splenectomy acute infections with pneumococci and other related organisms. New compounds such as fibrillary collagen are more effective haemostatics and may be associated with effective cessation of bleeding in superficial tears. If splenectomy is done in the under-20 age group, anti-pneumococcal vaccination is mandatory.

RUPTURED LIVER

Trauma of the liver is common with penetrating abdominal injuries. After closed abdominal trauma, particularly sudden crushing injuries to the lower chest, the liver may be ruptured alone or together with other viscera. The right lobe is more commonly affected than the left.

The injuries vary from a simple capsular tear to gross irregular splitting throughout the whole organ. In some cases large fragments of liver may be completely detached.

The effects on the patient vary according to the amount of haemorrhage and the amount of bile leakage.

Clinical features

HISTORY OF VIOLENCE
Particularly crush injuries to the right lower chest.

EVIDENCE OF INTERNAL HAEMORRHAGE
As with ruptured spleen, but maximum pain, tenderness and rigidity are found on the right side of the abdomen.

Special tests

1. Kehr's sign. This is unreliable for liver rupture.
2. Plain X-ray of the chest and abdomen is performed to exclude haemothorax, fractured ribs, or a ruptured hollow organ.
3. Scintigraphy may show a filling defect.
4. Hepatic angiography. This is of considerable value in experienced hands particularly when major liver trauma is suspected and the patient is not in shock.

Treatment

Suspected minor liver trauma. Continuous and close observation if the patient is rapidly recovering from shock and abdominal signs are well localized or progressively improving.

Suspected major liver trauma. When shock persists despite repeated blood transfusion or when abdominal signs progressively worsen then laparotomy is an urgent requirement.

When severe liver trauma is present the first essential is to control haemorrhage. Deep 'through-and-through sutures' or packing of deep liver lacerations is often unsatisfactory and occlusion of the inferior vena cava above and below the liver together with compression of the portal vein and hepatic artery in the porta hepatis may be required through a thoraco-abdominal incision.

With haemorrhage controlled and after blood replacement has been achieved, the second essential is resection of non-viable liver fragments. This may rarely require a partial or complete hepatic lobectomy.

When minor liver trauma is present, small lacerations may be sutured, packed, or covered with omentum or the falciform ligament.

Occasionally haemobilia complicates liver trauma, usually a stab wound, and it is manifested by right upper abdominal pain, gastro-intestinal haemorrhage and transient jaundice. Selective hepatic arteriography may demonstrate the bleeding intrahepatic artery and treatment is by embolization or ligation of the feeding artery.

RUPTURED PANCREAS

This may follow closed abdominal trauma when the pancreas is compressed against the vertebral column and in its extreme form complete transection of the pancreas may occur. Injury may also occur with penetrating injuries at which time other organs are usually involved as well. Varying degrees of pancreatitis are liable to occur with oedema, haemorrhage, necrosis, infection and later pseudocyst formation.

Clinical features

There are two common methods of presentation:

1. *Solid organ rupture* with shock, severe abdominal pain, internal haemorrhage, spreading peritonitis and abdominal distension.
2. *Pseudo-cyst formation.* This develops at a variable period after the injury. The patient recovers but gradually develops an upper abdominal mass which may take months or years to become obvious.

Treatment

1. Laparotomy after resuscitation and remove necrotic pancreas, secure haemostasis and drain the lesser sac.
2. Pseudo-cyst formation (see Chapter 25)

RUPTURED KIDNEY

Trauma to the kidney may follow a heavy fall or a blow or crushing injury to the abdomen or loin. As a result there may ensue a subcapsular haematoma, parenchymal contusion, parenchymal rupture, complete split of the kidney or an avulsion of the kidney from its pedicle.

Clinical features

There is usually a history of violence
    There may be:
1. Pain in loin
2. Bruising in loin
3. Swelling in loin
4. Haematuria
5. Ureteric colic

Special tests

These will include:

1. Intravenous urogram (once the patient has recovered from shock) to assess renal function, to determine the presence or absence of extravasation and to demonstrate the presence of a normal opposite kidney
2. Retrograde pyelogram can be used as an alternative to an intravenous pyelogram when the latter is unsatisfactory because of overlying gas shadows or inadequate concentration of contrast in the presence of hypotension or renal artery damage
3. Renal arteriogram in selected cases and in ideal circumstances may be of great value in determining the nature and extent of renal trauma and may permit selective external ligation, conservative resection, or embolisation of a feeding vessel

Treatment

1. CONSERVATIVE MANAGEMENT
Is indicated when the clinical features and radiographic evidence indicate minor trauma, when there is no loin swelling and when haematuria subsides rapidly.

The patient is kept in bed until all symptoms and signs have abated.

A careful follow up is necessary and should include X-ray examination to detect complications which may develop later, such as infection, hydronephrosis, calculus formation or hypertension.

2. OPERATION
This will be indicated if there is:

a. Rapid deterioration with continuing shock despite transfusions
b. Continuous massive haematuria
c. Expanding loin swelling
d. Increasing pain, tenderness and rigidity suggesting haemoperitoneum

At operation, partial or total nephrectomy will usually be indicated. Rarely do the circumstances permit suture of lacerations with conservation of the kidney.

RUPTURE OF THE BLADDER AND DAMAGE TO THE URETHRA

See p. 35.

11

Nerve and vessel injuries

Blunt and penetrating injuries close to joints often involve damage to a combination of peripheral nerves and blood vessels because at these sites a neurovascular bundle forms to cross the joint. Of course, injuries of nerves and vessels may occur independently, and for simplicity they will be discussed separately in this chapter.

NERVE INJURIES

CLASSIFICATION

Nerve injuries may occur with open wounds, fractures or as a result of crushing or traction of the nerve.

Three stages of nerve injury are recognized:

1. *Neuropraxia*. The axons are intact but their ability to conduct has been lost, usually because of mild pressure or stretching
2. *Axonotmesis*. There is destruction or division of the axons in an intact neural sheath, a more severe injury
3. *Neurotmesis*. Complete division of the whole nerve sheath due to transection or tearing

ASSESSMENT

History

It is important to elucidate the mechanism and circumstances of the injury. Tidy injuries caused by broken glass or household utensils will frequently be associated with damage to deeper structures. Adequate tetanus prophylaxis should be assured for tetanus-prone wounds such as those occurring outside the home and with soil contamination. It is important to note the time from accident to examination, from the point of view of administering a general anaesthetic and also because prolonged periods of delay in treatment may influence the degree of closure carried out primarily in certain untidy wounds.

The patient's occupation should especially be noted, for this may influence the choice of operation.

Examination

Nerve injuries are frequently missed during the initial examination, often because the possibility of division is not thought of, because the injury is incomplete or the patient does not properly comprehend the instructions given by the examiner.

Tests of motor and sensory function are performed and where possible compared with the other side. To assess motor function it is simplest to place the patient's joint in the position of maximal contraction of the muscle to be tested and ask the patient to 'hold it there' against pressure exerted by the examiner. Remember that the patient will try to convince the examiner (and so himself) that his sensation is normal. Pin-prick is the only reliable test of sensation in these circumstances. In all penetrating wounds where nerves are at risk it must be assumed that the nerve is divided until proved otherwise, usually by direct vision at operative exploration.

Specific nerve injuries

1. Median nerve. This is most often damaged at the wrist, usually following a self-inflicted wound, as at the distal transverse crease the nerve is quite superficial. The motor function of the median nerve is tested by assessing the ability of the thenar muscles to maintain the thumb in a plane at right angles to the palm.

2. Ulnar nerve. This is susceptible on the medial aspect of the elbow and the wrist, and its deep branch following penetrating wounds of the palm. A reliable test, especially for distal injuries, is the ability to maintain abduction of the little finger. Integrity of the proximal nerve can be assessed at the same time by palpating the movement of the flexor carpi ulnaris tendon, on the medial aspect of the wrist, that contracts in synergy with abduction of the little finger.

Froment's sign is another similar test. It is elicited by asking the patient to grip a card in the cleft between index and thumb. In an ulnar nerve palsy, this is only possible by flexing the interphalangeal joint of the thumb.

55

3. Radial nerve. This is most commonly damaged in the upper arm as it runs around the radial groove of the humerus. The accompanying wrist drop and loss of extension of the thumb are characteristic. Lacerations in the forearm may cut the superficial, sensory branch of the radial nerve, which gives rise to a sensory deficit on the dorsum of the web space between the thumb and index finger.

4. Brachial plexus injuries.

Birth trauma. There are two main lesions:

a. Erb's palsy. The head is distracted from the shoulder, stretching the upper part of the plexus, causing a lesion at the upper trunk (C5 and C6). The external rotators of the shoulder, flexors of the elbow and the extensors of the wrist are paralysed. The arm is then held in internal rotation, extension and flexion of the wrist—the 'waiter's tip' position. There are sensory changes in the C5 and C6 dermatomes.

b. Klumpke's palsy. This is the result of forced abduction of the arm, disrupting the first thoracic root. The small muscles of the hand are paralysed and the sympathetic supply to the pupil, which runs with T1, is affected, producing a Horner's syndrome.

Adult injuries. In adults, these injuries are caused by pressure in the axilla (crutch or back of a chair) or high velocity impact and stretch injuries such as motor-bicycle accidents, when the whole of the plexus may be involved.

5. Spinal injuries (see p. 34)

6. Sciatic nerve. May be damaged by fractures of the pelvis or dislocations of the hip. It is also at risk from injections into the buttock and during operations on the hip. The common peroneal nerve is the major component of the sciatic nerve and foot-drop is the hallmark of any sciatic nerve lesion, with sensory changes on the sole of the foot.

The common peroneal nerve itself is vulnerable as it winds round the neck of the fibula. The clinical signs may be the same as for a high sciatic nerve lesion as only very severe injuries of the proximal sciatic nerve result in hamstring paralysis.

7. Femoral nerve. Injury is uncommon, but the usual cause is a penetrating injury of the groin. Paralysis of the quadriceps is produced, which can be missed clinically because the patient soon learns to lift the leg without flexing the knee by internally rotating the hip and using the tensor fascia lata to raise the leg.

8. Causalgia. Any incomplete nerve injury, particularly lower limb injury, can be followed by episodes of severe, burning pain which is very resistant to treatment. This is causalgia, the cause of which is unknown.

PRINCIPLES OF TREATMENT

Tidy injuries are closed primarily together with repair of divided deep structures and nerves can only be repaired initially in those circumstances where skin closure is assured, where further extension of the wound to mobilize these structures would not threaten the skin viability, and where there is no undue delay.

When a wound cannot be satisfactorily debrided (e.g. certain gunshot wounds) then neither should the wound be closed primarily nor the nerve repaired primarily. In this instance the wound is left open to granulate and closed at a later date, and repair of the nerve is delayed until skin cover is adequate.

Complete divisions must be repaired with an avascular field, adequate exposure of the nerve ends and magnification during repair.

The ends must be trimmed with a sharp blade until normal funiculi are identified, then the nerve ends precisely apposed while matching up corresponding funiculi, with very fine material. The related joints must be immobilized in such a position that all tension is taken off the repair.

Where there is loss of nerve substance, then this may be overcome to a certain extent by mobilization of nerve ends, posturing of related joints and, in the case of the ulnar nerve, by transposition of the nerve to the front of the elbow joint.

If the nerve ends still cannot be apposed easily, nerve grafting must be done using, usually, three or four equal lengths of suitable nerve such as sural nerve, interposed loosely between the cut ends and again anastomosed with very fine sutures under magnification.

Nerve injuries repaired by suture are completely immobilized for 4 weeks, then graduated mobilization is commenced.

VESSEL INJURIES

A vascular injury may be readily apparent with obvious ischaemia or haemorrhage; however severe arterial damage may be present with few initial symptoms or signs. Prompt diagnosis is vital to achieve satisfactory results.

In civilian trauma, vessel injuries are most likely to occur in young males involved in motor car accidents, whereas gun shot and stab wounds account for only a small number of cases outside the U.S.A. and some other violent communities.

CLASSIFICATION

1. *Contusions or crush injuries.* Probably the most common cause of vessel damage, as these are associated

with fractures and dislocations, the brachial and pop-liteal arteries being susceptible. External transmural compression of the artery produces a circumferential intimal tear, creating a 'valve' of infolded intima, with the formation of an intra-luminal thrombus and an intra-mural haematoma.

2. *Incisions and lacerations.* These are usually caused by glass or sharp objects and may or may not produce overt haemorrhage. A completely divided vessel may retract and constrict, with little bleeding, but a small lateral laceration may bleed profusely.

3. *Perforations.* High velocity missiles or sharp objects may perforate a vessel without external evidence of injury. The subsequent development of shock or a pulsating haematoma reveals the injury.

4. *Puncture wounds.* Percutaneous puncture of periph-eral arteries (in hospital for either arteriography or blood gas analysis) may result in a pulsating haema-toma (false aneurysm).

5. *Chemical injury.* Inadvertent intra-arterial injection of thiopentone or other agents will cause severe pain and intense vasospasm. A superficial ulnar artery at the elbow, a not uncommon anomaly, is often involved.

6. *Ruptured thoracic aorta* (see p. 47)

CLINICAL MANIFESTATIONS

Haemorrhage. External pulsating arterial bleeding or a persistent ooze of dark venous blood is obvious, but concealed haemorrhage may present as either shock or an expanding haematoma.

Ischaemia. The presence of a cold, pale, pulseless extremity distal to an open or closed wound means an arterial injury until proved otherwise at operation. Although skeletal muscle can tolerate ischaemia of 6–8 hours, time is a crucial factor in the salvage of an ischaemic limb.

False aneurysm. A false aneurysm may be formed by the outer layer of an encapsulated haematoma, following bleeding from a side hole in the artery. Usually proximal flow is not disrupted. An expansile and pulsating mass is palpable over the artery. At an early stage there is an *expanding haematoma* rather than a pulsating aneurysm.

Arterio-venous fistula. This may be acute, following synchronous laceration or ligation of artery and vena comitantes or delayed, when infected arterial haemato-mas erode into adjacent veins. A continuous thrill and murmur are usually present.

Venous injury and obstruction. Prominent distal veins and peripheral induration and oedema may indicate venous compression or obstruction.

PRINCIPLES OF TREATMENT

Severe associated injuries are common and should be treated appropriately.

Haemorrhage

External bleeding is best controlled by continuous press-ure or packing. Tourniquets and the blind application of artery clips are best avoided.

Operative repair of arterial injuries

The feasibility of repair is determined by the magnitude of the wound. For extensive wounds with gross contam-ination, as seen in military casualties, proximal arterial ligation and amputation may be life-saving.

The majority of civilian vascular injuries are, however, repairable as contamination and tissue damage is often minimal. The following principles therefore apply:

1. The artery is exposed by an *ample incision* in the long access of the vessel.

2. *Proximal and distal control* is achieved using slings then vascular clamps, and intravenous heparin given to prevent distal thrombosis

3. The injured area of the artery is dissected free and repaired according to the injury:

   a. *Simple laceration* is repaired by suture and when this is longitudinal a vein patch is incorporated to reduce narrowing of the artery

   b. *Partial or complete disruption* may be repaired by sutures, but more commonly contusion and retrac-tion of the artery necessitate excision and recon-struction with interposed autogenous vein graft. The use of prosthetic graft in trauma is avoided because of increased infection and thrombosis.

   c. *Intimal tear* The segment of artery involved is excised and either repaired by end-to-end anasto-mosis or interposed vein graft

   d. *Arterial spasm* alone is rarely responsible for vas-cular occlusion, except after chemical injury; then intra-arterial heparin and reserpine are infused

4. *Fasciotomy* is a useful adjunct to vascular reconstruc-tion to free swollen, ischaemic muscle compressed within fascial compartments

5. Fractures are stabilized by internal fixation *before* arterial reconstruction to avoid distraction forces on the repair

Operative repair of venous injury

The need for sequential venous and arterial reconstruc-tion is controversial, as the results following venous ligation alone are comparable. It would seem logical, however, to repair a damaged major vein to improve venous drainage of a revascularized limb. Venous reconstruction is mandatory during microsurgical repair of severed digits or limbs. The principles of venous repair are similar to those for arteries; however, thrombosis is a more common problem, and intravenous heparin is continued post-operatively.

12

Burns

In spite of many recent advances in care, an extensive burn remains one of the most dangerous and devastating of injuries. In physical terms, it involves the transfer of an excessive amount of heat energy to the body. The extent of injury will depend on the temperature, the magnitude and the period of exposure to the heat source. It will be modified by certain factors:

1. The insulating effect of clothing

2. The local blood supply
A good blood supply to an area, e.g. the face, will mitigate the effect of the burn because the blood will act as a heat exchange mechanism tending to reduce local damage.

3. The speed with which local external cooling can be applied
Cell damage occurs at temperatures at and above 44°C. Rapid cooling of a burn by application of cold in the form of ice or cold water may lessen that damage at the interface of damaged and viable tissue.

SURGICAL PATHOLOGY

Irrespective of the size of a burn, the pathological process is the same. There is damage or death of cells and the capillary bed of the skin is particularly susceptible. The latter leak, leading to loss of water, electrolytes and plasma proteins. The sequestrated fluid fills the interstitial space causing oedema, which can also be accompanied by blistering or actual surface loss of fluid. All such losses can amount to a very considerable volume in an *extensive burn* (defined as one covering more than 10% of total body surface area) and lead to shock if not dealt with by the appropriate fluid replacement.

As well as damage to the capillary network there is death or damage to all cells in the area of a burn, thus providing an admirable culture medium for bacteria, which multiply without interference. Burned tissue is like an ischaemic or gangrenous limb: there is a variable mass of dead tissue in which bacteria multiply freely and

from where showers of bacteria can invade the rest of the body across the interface of living and dead cells.

An understanding of the pathology of a burn as described above should lead to an understanding of the two major areas of endeavour in management: *shock* and the *burn wound and accompanying infection*. Both of these are influenced by:

1. The extent of the burn
2. The depth of the burn

1. The extent of the burn
The bigger the burn and the older the patient, the greater the likelihood of death. Other factors affecting the outcome are: pre-existing problems such as obesity, pulmonary disease and hypertension and how much of the burn is full-thickness.

The simplest way of estimating the extent of a burn for adults is by the Rule of Nines (Fig. 12.1). It should

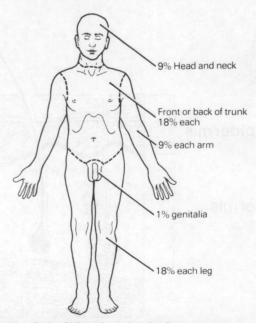

9% Head and neck

Front or back of trunk 18% each

9% each arm

1% genitalia

18% each leg

Fig. 12.1 Rule of Nines for estimating burn extent as a percentage of total body surface area

be emphasized that what might appear to be an easy method requires great care. Dirt, clothing and poor light can all prevent an accurate assessment. Early estimates done hurriedly tend to be inaccurate. Review and reassessment is essential. In children the Rule of Nines figures are a little inaccurate, in that the area of an infant's or a young child's head is comparatively greater compared with the rest of the body.

2. The depth of the burn

When examining a burned area, the question the clinician wants to know, and indeed the patient wants to know, is whether the area is going to recover. Is it partial-thickness burn damage or is the area going to require grafting because it is a full-thickness burn?

The skin consists of epidermis and dermis including hair follicles and sweat glands (Fig. 12.2). A *partial-thickness* burn ranges from one that spares some epidermis and all the dermis to one where there is involvement of all epithelial elements apart from some dermis from which re-epithelialization can occur. Re-epithelialization occurs best from surviving elements of epidermis but, if this is destroyed, it can occur from hair follicles and sweat glands. Provided infection does not cause further and total destruction of all epithelial tissue, skin grafting will not be necessary.

A *full-thickness* burn is one that destroys epidermis and dermis completely. Unless the area is grafted, healing can occur only by growth of scar tissue. A full-thickness burn which may extend to involve fat, muscle, tendon, nerve, major vessels and bone is the most dangerous, in terms of local restoration of function.

Differentiation of a partial-thickness burn from a full-thickness one clinically is not always easy even for an experienced clinician. However, certain clinical signs help in mapping out areas of partial and full-thickness damage. By doing this the treatment programme can be planned.

METHODS OF ASSESSMENT

1. Inspection
Partial-thickness burns are red, often blistered, and have a moist appearance. Full-thickness burns can be red, indicating entrapped red cells in damaged capillaries, but more often the surface is pale and parchment-like or has an appearance like marble. Blistering is rare in full-thickness burns and, if it is present, the blisters have usually ruptured and there are tags of loose dead skin hanging from the surface. In extreme examples, the tissue is charred and cracked. In such instances there is never any doubt.

2. Palpation
A partial-thickness burn is sensitive to touch, sometimes extremely so, whereas full-thickness areas are anaesthetic. Mapping the extent of each, using pinprick sensation, is useful. The red colour of partial-thickness burns disappears on pressure and there is blanching; this does not happen with full-thickness burns. The partial-thick-

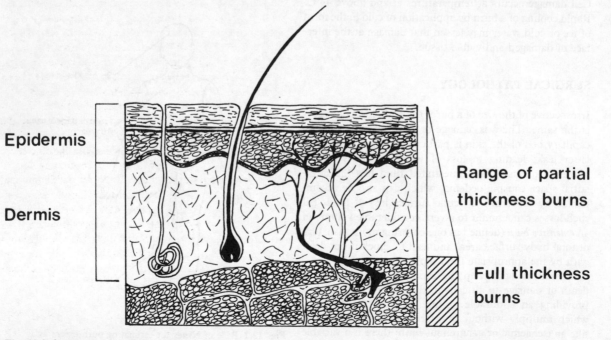

Epidermis

Dermis

Range of partial thickness burns

Full thickness burns

Fig. 12.2 Anatomy of the skin and depth of burns

ness burn has a resilient, soft feel about it; the coagulated skin of a full-thickness burn feels firm, like leather.

SHOCK

General aspects of the treatment of shock are discussed in Chapter 4, and need not be repeated here because the problem of hypovolaemic shock in a burn is not unique. Shock is likely to occur in a burn involving more than 10% of the body surface. The degree of shock is proportional to the total area burned and the depth. The hypovolaemic state is entirely due to loss of water, electrolytes and plasma proteins from widespread damage to the capillary bed. It is important to realize that losses occur into the interstitial space, into burn blisters and outwards from the burned surface, from which the fluid drips away, as well as being lost by evaporation. Oedema can be gross. For example, when the face is burned it swells to an inordinate degree, leading to inversion of eyelids and eversion of lips accompanied by a swollen tongue. The latter sometimes leads to partial upper airways obstruction, which is further aggravated by neck swelling.

A special circumstance may happen in burn shock that can also occur in crush syndrome. This is the phenomenon of haemoglobinuria and myoglobinuria. Perfusion of an area of damaged muscle and capillaries and their contained red cells washes the products of muscle and red cell destruction back into the circulation. This material is secreted in the glomerular filtrate and, as it flows down the loop of Henle, it is concentrated in the tubule, where it may cause blockage. Clinically, this possibility is suspected when a dark claret-coloured urine of small volume is produced and is a warning sign of the imminent risk of anuria.

Management of burn shock

A number of formulae exist which provide a guide to appropriate volume replacement in burn shock. These are helpful but usually depend on an accurate estimate of body weight and the area burned; both are not always attainable with any degree of accuracy and a practical alternative is to re-infuse the patient according to changes that occur in the usual parameters for assessing shock. Thus it is appropriate to measure pulse rate, blood pressure, central venous pressure, rate of urine output and haemoconcentration by haematocrit or haemoglobin. Other and more sophisticated measurements may occasionally be needed, such as mean arterial pressure via an intra-arterial cannula or pulmonary arterial wedge pressure via a Swan Ganz cannula.

GUIDELINES AND OBJECTIVES FOR FLUID REPLACEMENT
Shock is unlikely in burns covering less than 10% of the

body surface. Therefore, intravenous resuscitation is usually unnecessary. Over 10%, certain *guidelines* should be followed:

1. Burns of 10–20% require an intravenous infusion and may require urethral catheterization, particularly in elderly people who are more susceptible to changes in fluid dynamics.
2. Burns of between 20 and 30% require both an intravenous infusion and urethral catheterization, and it may be necessary to use a central venous cannula. The latter may be required in smaller burns because the arms are involved. Nevertheless an intravenous line can be inserted through burned tissue if necessary, either by puncture or cut down. Leg veins should be avoided at all costs because of the risk of early thrombo-phlebitis.
3. In burns of greater than 30%, insertion of a central venous line is mandatory in order to measure central venous pressure and provide access for adjuvant parenteral nutrition.

The objectives of treatment of shock should be to maintain:

a. a pulse rate of less than 120/min
b. a systolic blood pressure at or above 120 mmHg
c. a steady central venous pressure at between 0 and 5 cm of water
d. a urine flow rate of between 50 and 100 ml/h. In a burn of 50% this may mean infusion rates of the order of 1 litre or more per 2 hours in the first 24 hours.

The fluids to be used are a balanced or physiological salt solution (e.g. Hartmann's solution) and a plasma expander, preferably plasma itself or its equivalent, or one of the synthetic plasma expanders. In burns of less than 20%, plasma may not be required but in excess of this it is appropriate and practical to replace what may be quite substantial plasma losses to maintain intravascular osmotic pressure. The infusion is administered by giving crystalloid, alternating with colloid in equal volumes. Usually, maximum volume infusion rates are reached in the first 24 hours, after which the full picture of burn oedema will have developed and the situation will become more stable, except that there will still be continuing loss of water from the burn surface, both by exudation and evaporation. On about the third or fourth day postburn, oedema begins to lessen. At this time there is, in effect, an infusion of fluid back into the circulation from the interstitial space. When this occurs the intravenous infusion rate has to be reduced quite abruptly to avoid the risk of overloading which can lead to cardiac embarrassment, particularly in elderly people.

HAEMOGLOBINURIA
It occurs only in the very early post-burn period. The risk of tubular blockage is overcome by inducing a free urine flow at or above 50 ml/h. If this does not occur with

a fluid load then it may be necessary to give frusemide intravenously (initial dose 40 mg) or mannitol 20% in a bolus dose of 200 ml.

There are quite marked differences in management of shock from one centre to another. For example, some clinicians use whole blood while others may use plasma alone or balanced salt solution alone. Whatever method is used, the aim is to maintain adequate tissue perfusion, and the very best guide to this is urine output.

PAIN RELIEF

Consideration should be given to effective pain relief with morphine or its equivalent. In big burns this is achieved best by giving the drug intravenously. Analgesics should be avoided until effective resuscitation has been begun. The subcutaneous route is inappropriate because absorption is unpredictable in shock.

LOCAL MANAGEMENT OF THE BURN WOUND

A tetanus toxoid booster should be given to all who have been immunized already. Active immunization is begun on anyone previously unimmunized. In burns greater than 10% immediate passive immunization with human hyperimmune globulin should be considered in the unimmunized.

Small burns—less than 10%—because they do not require resuscitation can be dressed shortly after admission. The wound is cleaned with antiseptic solution and any loose skin tags snipped away. If possible intact blisters are left, as they protect the extremely painful underlying tissue. Silver sulphadiazine cream or its equivalent is applied to the burn and gauze dressings and bandages wrapped round it as appropriate. In certain circumstances it may be neither practicable or necessary to use antiseptic cream. For example, the face is best left alone and small burns require a sterile dressing only.

Big burns—greater than 10%—should be dealt with somewhat differently. First, if there are obvious circumferential full-thickness burns causing constriction of a limb or the chest, it may be necessary to incise these down to and including deep fascia to decompress the area. Because such an area is full-thickness it is insensitive and analgesia is desirable but not essential. The procedure can be carried out in the Emergency Department or in the ward. Apart from such treatment, the burn wound should be left alone until resuscitation is well under way and shock is controlled. This usually means a wait of 4–6 hours, and meantime it is essential to keep the patient warm and covered with clean or sterile sheets and blankets. An insulating 'space blanket' is very good for conserving heat.

Prophylactic systemic antibiotics are not recommended at the beginning of therapy, particularly when the patient is likely to be nursed in a clean environment such as most modern hospitals can provide. However, in less ideal circumstances, such as an open ward where staff are unused to burn care and techniques of preventing cross-infection, the patient should be given a course of prophylactic antibiotics for 10 days in the first place. One of the penicillins is appropriate. Irrespective of whether systemic antibiotics are used, the mainstay of infection control is a vigorous programme of burn wound antisepsis using some form of antiseptic washing which can include bathing, coupled with the application of an antibacterial cream such as silver sulphadiazine. A closed or open dressing technique can be used.

If the burn is all partial-thickness there is no need to progress beyond the stage of antisepsis and expectant treatment with baths and dressings until healing occurs. However, if there is a full-thickness burn it is expedient to attempt to excise the areas of full-thickness as soon as possible because such tissue remains a constant hazard for infection. Where extensive areas are involved with full-thickness, excision can rarely be done in one stage and a series of theatre visits will be necessary in order to achieve total wound excision and grafting. A conventional plan is to begin the programme of wound excision when the capillary lesion is well on the way to recovery. This will mean as soon after the fifth post-burn day as is convenient. It is usually found that around 10% of the body surface area can be excised and grafted in one session. Excision of areas greater than this can lead to unacceptably high blood loss. It is recommended that grafting is undertaken immediately after burn excision if at all possible. There are many variations in technique that are advocated and are acceptable. Broadly speaking, skin grafting is done using thin split skin autografts taken from whatever unburned or healed areas that are available, but preferably arms, legs or abdominal wall. Donor skin, not used immediately, can be stored for up to 2 weeks in an ordinary domestic refrigerator at +4°C. Techniques are available where allograft or xenograft skin can be used as temporary skin cover when there is a shortage of autograft material.

PROBLEMS OF MANAGEMENT IN BURNED PATIENTS

Burn scars

Even in the best of circumstances it is unusual in very extensive burns (>40%), where it is necessary to excise and graft large areas, for infection not to occur and for all grafts to take completely the first time. Were that to happen regularly, big burns would not present the major problem they do and the mortality would not be of the order of 15–20% in burns units which deal with a spec-

trum of small through large burns. Apart from any risk
to life there is an increased likelihood of development of
hypertrophic scars when grafts fail and regrafting has to
be done. It should be noted that in certain circumstances
even healed partial-thickness burns can lead to hypertrophic scars. Such scars are unsightly and, in addition,
they can lead to stiffness and disability through scar contracture, particularly when they are crossing joints.
Intensive efforts have to be made using physiotherapy,
splinting and compression bandaging to lessen the effects
of contractures and facilitate joint movement. Often
repeated and complex plastic surgical procedures are
necessary to improve matters. Much is demanded of the
patient and many have emotional problems requiring
understanding and support from their families and the
whole medical team. The distortion of body image that
occurs not only in a big burn but also in smaller ones
affecting hands or face can be devastating and long lasting. The aim of therapy should be to provide the support
necessary to overcome or mitigate this. Doctors, nurses,
social workers, physiotherapists, occupational therapists,
family, friends, clergy, other patients and employers all
play a part.

Chest problems

In the initial accident there may be burning of the upper
or lower respiratory tract. This may result from flames
sweeping across the face, fauces, pharynx and larynx, or
even extending lower down into the lungs. Apart from
flame, hot gases and noxious chemicals can be inhaled.
The latter occurs more often now because of the widespread use of plastics in furnishings and in industry.
When these become involved in fire, toxic gases can be
produced that cause significant alveolar damage when
inhaled. Such injuries are more likely when the burning
accident is in a confined space.

Respiratory tract injury should always be suspected
and looked for by examining the upper air passages. Stridor is an obvious sign that may demand immediate intubation. Damage to the lower respiratory tract is less easy
to pinpoint clinically and may go hand in hand with pre-
existing pulmonary disease or a problem of over-infusion
during the shock phase. The early development of a picture of pulmonary oedema is suspicious. Clinical examination, regular chest X-rays, monitoring of blood gases,
adjuvant oxygen therapy, antibiotics for added infection
and intubation with assisted respiration are all part of the
therapeutic regimen. Steroids and heparin are used but
their value is unproven. Tracheostomy can usually be
avoided provided recovery takes place in 7–10 days. If
there is a neck burn leading to compression of the trachea, intubation may be very difficult if left too late and
then one is committed to tracheostomy in less than ideal
circumstances. Tracheostomy can be done through
burned tissue but is best avoided.

Infection

By undertaking a vigorous programme using surface
cleaning and topical antibacterial agents, it is possible to
guide a patient through an illness without any clinically
apparent infection and without any need for systemic
antibiotics. Nevertheless, the risks of infection are ever
present.

Different environments create different sets of circumstances and the organisms causing burn wound sepsis
vary. In well-run burn units in temperate climates, streptococcal infection has virtually ceased to be a major problem. Characteristically, it occurs when patients are
admitted with neglected, infected burns that until then
have been treated at home. The organisms seen most are
staphylococci and the whole range of Gram negative
bacilli, headed by *Pseudomonas aeruginosa*, *Klebsiella*,
Proteus and coliforms. The burn wound can become col-
onized quickly and bacteria can migrate inwards remarkably rapidly from the surface. Infection is suspected
when there is fever, tachycardia, metabolic acidosis and
there are positive cultures from either the burn or the
blood stream. Hand in hand with burn wound infection
there is often pulmonary infection and invariably the
organisms isolated from sputum are the same as those
from the burns. Organisms cultured from urine are generally the same as from the burns. The need to monitor
urine output demands a urethral catheter with the inevitable hazard of infection. Intravenous cannulation sites
must be carefully watched for sepsis, and cannulae
should be changed and cultured on suspicion.

There is a characteristic progression of infection in the
big burn: for a number of weeks all is well and few cultures of the burn produce significant growth. Clinically,
there is no obvious infection. Then, after several visits
to the operating room, the chest radiograph begins to
cause concern. Blood gas measurements deteriorate and
Gram negative organisms appear in sputum and from
wound cultures. This is a danger period when, unless the
infection can be controlled, the prospect of survival is
gloomy.

Nutrition

Burns of greater than 20% invariably pose a problem of
nutrition and the very lack of adequate nutrition can
materially affect the outcome. Energy and nutrients in
excess of normal demands are required in order to offset
the deficit caused by heat loss, plasma loss and hyper-
metabolism. If infection is added, the combined metabolic demands may lead to energy expenditures of the
order of 5000–6000 kcal per day in an average adult.
It frequently happens that the burned patient is too sick,
apathetic and physically handicapped because of burns
to hands and face to be able to eat a diet that in any way
matches his energy needs. Not surprisingly, such

patients can and do lose weight. Only by the most vigorous counter measures can this be prevented.

Adequate oral feeding is the ideal but is seldom attained, particularly when the feeding regimen is interrupted by frequent visits to the operating theatre. Consequently, it is necessary to supplement oral food with either liquid tube feeds or intravenous food. The latter can now be given easily and in effective quantities via central venous cannulae. By a combination of oral or tube feeding and intravenous food, patients can and must be adequately nourished. As a corollary it is essential to recognize that these patients need to have an adequate haemoglobin level at all times. Frequent and ample blood transfusion is part of the total nutritional picture.

Stress ulceration (see Chapter 23)

Upper gastro-intestinal bleeding remains a difficult and serious problem in the big burn victim. If major bleeding occurs requiring transfusion, the mortality is in excess of 30%. The surgeon is faced with a dilemma. Conservative management, even with cimetidine, the histamine H_2 receptor antagonist, is not always effective. Operation may arrest the haemorrhage but may impose an insuperable burden on the patient's ability to respond to yet another injury. If the patient is elderly, the problem is insurmountable. There is evidence that antacids in high doses via a naso-gastric tube are an effective preventive.

THE AFTERMATH

Anyone dealing with a large number of burn victims will be impressed that after they have left hospital there are still many problems. The management of scars has been discussed. There are two others worthy of consideration:

1. Pruritis
2. Sweating

For as long as a year or more after burns have healed, either spontaneously or by grafting, the victim can be burdened by troublesome and almost continuous itching. This can be quite disturbing. He may wake at night scratching and find that delicate, recently-healed surfaces have been damaged and are bleeding. Treatment is not easy. Lanolin may help, as may 0.5% hydrocortisone ointment. A reliable hypnotic may be necessary to provide restful sleep.

In very extensive burns which have been grafted there has been a loss of large areas of sweat gland activity. Thermoregulation is deranged and in hot weather difficult to control. Sweat rates from unburned areas are high and, with females in particular, there is anxiety and

embarrassment about this. The victims feel they have unacceptable body odour. Reassurance is necessary to allay fears and anxiety over a problem that cannot be completely solved.

SCALDS, CHEMICAL BURNS, IRRADIATION

These three types of burn require separate brief mention.

Scalds

Scalds are mainly seen in paediatric practice. The lesion is from steam or a brief exposure to hot water. The injury is invariably a partial-thickness burn and not life threatening, unless it involves very large areas of the body. Treatment is as for other types of burn.

Chemical burns

These are caused by many different agents. Usually, the clinician first encounters the lesion when it is fully developed and treatment follows conventional lines. Washing in water helps to neutralize any chemical that remains. However, there are a number of chemicals that cause burns that are progressive—phosphorus is one and chromic acid another. Both of these should be dealt with by very early excision to prevent extension of the injury into deeper tissues.

Radiation burns

Radiation burns will be encountered only when there is the very occasional problem of patients accidentally exposed to an excess of local radiation as a therapeutic measure for treatment of malignant disease. Treatment is essentially one of protection of the area burned and application of antibiotic creams if there is infection. It is not the scope of this book to discuss the enormous problem of radiation burns in the event of a nuclear holocaust.

PREVENTION

A burn is a preventable illness. High risk groups can be identified. It affects the young, the socially deprived, the elderly, the ill-educated and the alcoholic, particularly those who smoke. Education and community awareness can make some impact on the problem. Finally, there is a group beyond our control in terms of prevention. These are those who see self-destruction by burning as a release from the burdens of life. For these people there seems to be no solution.

13

Acute infections

Infection is the invasion of the body by pathogenic microorganisms and the reaction of the tissues to their presence and to the toxins generated by them. Considering that man is surrounded by microorganisms, it is suprising that infections are not more frequent. Infection occurs when the fine balance between host resistance and the aggressiveness of the infecting agent breaks down. Acute and chronic bacterial infections should not be considered in isolation, in that the inflammatory response they engender occurs in a wide variety of conditions.

SURGICAL PATHOLOGY

Invasion of the body by a bacterial agent produces an inflammatory response which is variable and depends on the resistance of the host and the infecting organism. This response consists of a rapid exudation, similar to that produced in the early stages of any injury, called an *acute infection*. Once the early phase has taken place the infection may resolve, spread or become chronic.

1. Resolution

This is regression of the exudative phase, without any evidence of tissue damage. Many acute infections are aborted at this stage with or without the use of antibiotics.

2. Spread

Three forms can be distinguished.

a. Direct spread with local tissue death
b. By lymphatics
c. By blood stream

DIRECT SPREAD WITH LOCAL TISSUE DEATH
Direct spread into involved tissues leads to either local tissue death or further spread along tissue planes. *Local tissue death* takes place as a consequence of two factors:

1. *Direct toxic effects of organisms*—either their endo- or exotoxins
2. *Increased tissue tension*. The inflammatory response creates oedema regardless of the exciting agent. If the space in which the reaction takes place is limited, tension is inevitable. Such anatomically-bounded infection may occur in a variety of situations, e.g. in the pulp space of the finger, the breast or ischio-rectal fossa where fibrous septa separate fat pads; inside the skull where the bony cavity limits the expansion of tissue, and in bone itself where the rigidity of the tissue leads to a rapid rise of tension. Thrombosis of veins by the invading organisms will accelerate this process.

Local death of soft tissue results in two things.

1. The production of a solid area of infected dead tissue—a *slough*
2. The liquefaction of tissues and the products of infection—an *abscess*

When these events have taken place, the slough must first be cast off or removed or the abscess drained before healing will occur by granulation tissue formation—that is, by secondary intention.

In bone, similar processes occur. When bone dies, the resulting area of septic necrosis is known as a *sequestrum*, though this term is often reserved for a situation in which the dead bone has separated from the living. The complete picture of acute infection leading to tissue necrosis by a combination of tension and venous thrombosis is seen in the now rare condition of acute osteomyelitis. Here, a staphylococcal focus starts, usually in the metaphysis of a long bone and, unless aborted by early treatment, leads to bone death, subperiosteal abscess formation and ultimately the escape of pus to the surface. Because of tension in the lesion, organisms may be thrown off to give bacteraemia or pyaemia with metastatic foci, either in hard or soft tissues (see below).

Gangrene and its relation to infection. Tissues may die in either the presence or absence of bacteria. Aseptic necrosis is tissue death in the absence of bacteria, e.g. myocardial infarction. In the presence of bacteria, two events may occur—the dead tissue may harbour organisms which have little or no action on it, as occurs in a slough; or there may be wet gangrene in which proteolytic enzymes derived from the bacteria break down the tissues. These organisms tend to spread, so that wet gangrene may be associated with cellulitis in neighbouring tissues. Dry gangrene is necrosis with dessication of tissues.

Cellulitis is a spreading invasion of the connective tissue; characteristically, infection with haemolytic streptococci, where bacterial fibrinolysis breaks down the protective wall of fibrin and so allows spread of the organisms.

SPREAD BY LYMPHATICS

This is characteristic of organisms that do not cause coagulation of fibrin and thus is seen in streptococcal infections. The walls of the lymphatic vessels become inflamed and are often painful (lymphangitis). Embolization via lymphatics may also occur—though this mode of spread is more frequent with chronic infections, e.g., tuberculosis—the bacteria being trapped in regional lymph nodes setting up an inflammatory reaction that results in their enlargement with pain (lymphadenitis).

SPREAD BY THE BLOODSTREAM

Three forms of this are recognized:

a. *Bacteraemia*—the carriage of organisms by the bloodstream without specific symptoms being produced
b. *Pyaemia*—the carriage of clumps of organisms that can produce distant abscesses (metastatic abscesses)
c. *Septicaemia*—the multiplication of organisms in the blood (see p. 18)

CLINICAL FEATURES

The common local features are rubor, calor, and dolor. Fluctuation and pointing mean pus formation, but slough may be present without either. The presence of tension, judged by persistant pain, may necessitate decompression even in the absence of pus. The nature of the infecting organism may be recognized from its clinical appearance: haemolytic streptococcal lesions are associated with rapidly spreading lesions such as erysipelas (an intradermal infection) or lymphangitis, staphylococcal infection with local necrosis or with *Proteus* infection skin gangrene. But clinical appearances are not a good guide to therapy, which should always be designed to encompass all possibilities.

MANAGEMENT

Prevention

In wounds, prevention of infection is better than cure, and this is achieved by:

1. Proper handling of tissues.
2. Aseptic technique.
3. Appropriate chemotherapy.
4. Avoidance of gross contamination.
5. Care in handling infective materials.
6. Cleanly habits.

Principles of therapy

1. In the exudative phase, an infection may halt and resolve either as a consequence of host resistance or with the aid of chemotherapy. These measures may be aided by judicious immobilization. *Resolution is achieved by catching an infection early.*

Important features in determining outcome are:

a. Time of treatment in relation to onset
b. Host resistance
c. The vascularity of the tissues. This permits the development of an appropriate inflammatory response and the ingress of appropriate agents.
d. An effective chemotherapeutic agent

2. When treatment has failed in the exudative phase or the patient is not seen until tissue death has taken place, surgical intervention becomes necessary: slough must be removed, pus drained, or both. In infections under tension, it is important to reduce this to prevent further tissue death, e.g. in osteomyelitis, pulp-space infections or ischio-rectal abscesses.

When drainage has been undertaken, a cavity is left. Free escape of exudate must occur until the cavity has contracted and this may mean drainage for some time.

3. The defect in structures and function produced by an acute infection may require repair.

CHOICE OF CHEMOTHERAPEUTIC AGENTS

As it is nearly always impossible to know the exact nature of the organism and in particular its antibiotic sensitivity, treatment is begun based on

1. The likely organism on the grounds of clinical behaviour
2. Past experience with similar lesions

Often, particularly in serious infections that threaten the patient or tissue death, it is necessary to use two agents to fulfill the above conditions. Thus, in acute osteomyelitis the organism is almost certainly *Staphylo-*

coccus aureus, but it may be either penicillin sensitive or insensitive. Therefore until its sensitivity is known, either by analysis of a blood culture or some other source, it is desirable to use both pennicillin (which is cheap and highly effective and can be continued if the organism turns out to be sensitive) and another penicillin which is not susceptible to deactivating enzymes.

THERAPEUTIC SUMMARY
1. Treat early, aiming for resolution
2. Decompress, if necessary, on grounds of type of infection and tissue tension
3. Immobilize adequately
4. Choose chemotherapy by backing more than one infective horse
5. Remove pus and slough completely
6. Promote healing and rehabilitation

HOSPITAL-ACQUIRED INFECTIONS

These are clinical infections occurring in hospital patients that were not present at the time of admission. They occur in 5–15% of patients admitted to hospital, the incidence being higher in centres that treat the critically ill, and contribute to an increased morbidity and mortality.

Bacteriology

Gram negative bacilli are now the commonest cause of hospital-acquired infection, though *Staphylococcus aureus* remains on important pathogen particularly strains with multiple antibiotic resistance (multi-resistant *Staph. aureus*) The Gram negative organisms also have the capacity to develop resistance to many antimicrobial agents in common use, making them difficult to treat satisfactorily. In large part, this resistance is due to the acquisition of plasmids called resistance factors (R-factors). The R-factors consist of extrachromosomal DNA, which mediates antibiotic resistance by coding for enzymes that inactive the drug or by altering the permeability of the bacterial cell wall to the drug. Two properties of R-factors of major concern are: (a) resistance to several antibiotics is often linked to the same R-factor; and (b) transfer can occur across species lines from one Gram negative organism to another. Thus, under appropriate conditions, these properties make possible the dissemination of multiple antibiotic resistance among a wide variety of Gram negative pathogens. However the main reason for antibiotic-resistant bacteria is the use of antibiotics; by suppressing sensitive organisms, they allow colonization by resistant organisms,

often leading to overt clinical infections. In addition, infections may arise, especially in individuals with impaired host defences, caused by organisms (e.g. *Candida*) not normally regarded as pathogens (opportunistic infections).

Transmission is principally through a breakdown of asepsis and antisepsis; thus infection is contracted from contact with hospital staff, either from the hands or via respiratory droplets; via food, water, sinks, contaminated ventilation systems, catheters or respirators.

Common sites of infection

1. *Urinary tract*. Accounts for 40% of hospital-acquired infection, either secondary to instrumentation of urethra, bladder or kidneys or insertion of urethral catheter.

2. *Wound infections*; discussed in Chapter 5.

3. *Burns*. *Pseudomonas aeruginosa* is the most frequent organism. (see Chapter 12).

4. *Pneumonia*. Pulmonary infections are a leading cause of death in hospital-acquired infection. Infection with Gram negative bacilli and *S. aureus* both cause a necrotizing broncho-pneumonia. The organisms reach this site by inhalation or aspiration rather than by haemotogenous spread.

5. *Bloodstream*. Intravenous cannulae especially cannulae used for the infusion of hypertonic nutrient solutions, are particularly prone to infection and strict asepsis is of paramount importance. With peripheral cannulae, the risk of infection rises with the length of time they are left in a particular site.

Management

PREVENTION
1. Reduce the risk of patients acquiring infection. The basic principles remain the avoidance of transmission of infection between patients by hospital staff; identification and correction of potential sources of infection.
2. Isolate patients with nosocomial infection to prevent spread.
3. Protect patients by isolation of those more susceptible to infection e.g. patients with burns or depressed immunity.
4. Be restrictive with antibiotic policy. It is obvious that the indiscriminate prescription of a broad spectrum antibiotic without due consideration of diagnostic possibilities is dangerous and can lead to the emergence of multi-antibiotic resistant organisms. Thus it

is essential that antibiotics be used in full dosage only when necessary and only for the length of time required to eliminate the pathogen.

TREATMENT

1. Identify port of entry of organism. Drain wound infection if present; remove intravenous cannula.

2. Identify infecting organisms and its antibiotic sensitivity by blood culture, urine culture or culture of intravenous cannula tip.
3. Treat with appropriate antibiotic.
4. Discharge patient early, if possible, to prevent spread to staff or other patients.

14

Specific infections

These are so-called because, unlike the acute bacterial infections summarized in the previous chapter, each agent produces a number of clear-cut effects which allow the recognition of the clinico-pathological process. All are relatively rare though this varies with geography, but some knowledge of them is essential because, unrecognized, they can lead to disaster for the individual patient.

CLASSIFICATION

Two groups—acute and chronic—the second usually granuloma producing.

Table 14.1 Classification of specific infections

Acute	Chronic
Clostridial	Tuberculosis
Tetanus	Actinomycosis
Gas gangrene	Syphilis
Necrotizing fasciitis	Amoebiasis
Synergistic gangrene	
Anthrax	
Bacteroides	

ACUTE GROUP

CLOSTRIDIAL—TETANUS

Bacteriology

Tetanus is caused by *Clostridium tetani*, a ubiquitous, Gram positive, spore-bearing anaerobic bacillus that is commonly present in soil, particularly in agricultural areas, and faeces. Inadequately sterilized organic surgical materials (e.g. cotton or catgut) have in the past carried viable tetanus spores.

Cl. tetani is not an invasive organism, and it does not cause an acute inflammatory reaction. The clinical manifestations of tetanus are the result of the effects of its powerful exotoxin, which travels along nerve sheaths or via the bloodstream and becomes firmly bound to ante-

rior horn cells and neuromuscular junctions. Once bound, it is unaffected by circulating antitoxins. Tetanus is unusual in that it produces a poor antibody response; thus a patient can be affected on more than one occasion unless immunized.

Tetanus-prone wounds

The bacillus will only produce toxins under anaerobic conditions; in consequence, wounds likely to be affected are:

1. Deep and penetrating, associated with local tissue damage, foreign body implantation or soil contamination
2. Soil-contaminated, superficial and minor lacerations or abrasions
3. Crushing injuries of fingers and toes, especially those associated with fractures
4. Surgical, particularly when a second operation is performed; the operative trauma may activate dormant tetanus spores
5. Deliberately contaminated raw surfaces; the umbilicus of a neonate 'dressed' with earth containing spores—a tradition in certain communities

In about a fifth of cases of tetanus, no obvious source of infection is apparent.

Clinical features

1. *The wound.* This may be trivial or even impossible to detect. There are no signs of inflammation unless infection by another organism is also present.
2. The course of the disease can be considered under three headings.

   a. *The incubation period.* Tetanus usually develops within 14 days of inoculation; it may, however, be fulminant and develop after a few days of injury or lie dormant in an old wound for over 12 months, becoming activated by trauma. There appears to be a rough relationship between the incubation period and the distance from the CNS; head early, limbs later.

b. *Phase of tonic spasm.* The diagnosis is made in this phase of exaggerated muscle tone (hypertonicity). The patient complains of stiffness or cramps of the limbs, back, abdomen, neck, jaw (trismus) and facial muscles (risus sardonicus). Hypertonicity isolated to the injured limb (localized tetanus) is unusual. Examination reveals a hypertonic and alert patient with hyperactive reflexes.

c. *Phase of clonic spasm.* In more severe cases, progression from the tonic phase occurs over 24–72 hours with episodes of sudden, severe and painful increases in muscle tone. Though initially confined to the injured limb, these episodes quickly become generalized and increase in duration and frequency; then arching of the back (opisthotonus), hyperextension of the head and hips and flexion of the knees and elbows appear simultaneously. These clonic spasms resemble those associated with strychnine poisoning and epilepsy, differing in that the patient is completely alert and that there is incomplete relaxation between spasms. Two life-threatening situations may arise:

(i) *Laryngeal and pharyngeal spasm.* This occurs suddenly, lasting only a few seconds, but, when the spasm is prolonged, respiratory obstruction and death may follow.

(ii) *Respiratory fixation.* Hypertonicity of the intercostal muscles and diaphragm results in impaired respiration and causes respiratory fixation. This is aggravated by frequent clonic spasms, when impaired ventilation predisposes the patient to atelectasis, stasis and infection.

Differential diagnosis

The diagnosis is entirely clinical, only strychnine poisoning, certain North Australian fish poisons or phenothiazine idiosyncrasy presenting a similar picture.

Management

PREVENTION

1. Active immunization with tetanus toxoid is recommended as standard practice. Full immunization is obtained with 0.5 ml of the phosphate absorbed toxoid intramuscularly in three injections, the first two separated by an interval of 6 weeks and the third 6–12 months later. Immunity is maintained by booster doses every 5–10 years.

2. Presence of tetanus-prone wound.

a. If previously immunized, give tetanus booster.

b. If not previously immunized, give 250–500 units of human antitoxin. In addition to antitoxin, active immunization should be started.

c. Any wound should be meticulously debrided and pus drained freely. Antibiotics should be administered if infection is present.

CURATIVE TREATMENT

All patients should be managed in a unit experienced and equipped to cope with the variable patterns of the disease. The patient should be isolated from sudden stimuli and should be spared unnecessary movement and excitement.

1. *The wound.* The same meticulous debridement is necessary. There is no place for amputation or wide excision.

2. *Antibiotics.* While penicillin is bactericidal to *Cl. tetani*, it is of limited value, as it is ineffective in reaching organisms in an avascular or devitalized wound and has no effect on the toxin.

3. *Antitoxin.* 'Free' toxin should be fixed by giving 3000–6000 units of human immune globulin intramuscularly. This dose maintains adequate levels of circulating antitoxin for 3 weeks after which it may be repeated. The antitoxin has no effect on toxin already fixed to the CNS.

4. *Nutrition.* Should be maintained, preferably via the gastrointestinal tract (naso-gastric or gastrostomy feeding). Intravenous feeding should rarely be necessary.

5. *Intravenous infusion.* May be necessary for the administration of drugs in a severe case.

6. *Tracheostomy.* Is indicated for airway obstruction or when total paralysing therapy is indicated.

7. *Antispasmodic therapy.* Various drugs are available and their dosages are dependent on the patient's age, weight, and general condition. Drugs commonly used are:

a. In *mild spasms*: barbiturates (e.g. Amytal), chlorpromazine, and diazepam (Valium) orally

b. In *severe tonic spasms* (interfering with rest and respiration): barbiturates or chlorpromazine intravenously

c. In *clonic spasm*: mephenesin (Myanesin) or related drugs, or diazepam intravenously

8. *Intermittent positive respiration and muscle paralysis.* Indicated if spasms continue to affect respiration or complications occur from drugs used (e.g. hae-

maturia, haemoglobinuria or vein thrombosis). Therapy entails paralysis of the patient, establishment of a tracheostomy and positive pressure respiration. The management of prolonged artificial respiration should only be undertaken in a recognized respiratory centre.

CLOSTRIDIAL—GAS GANGRENE

Bacteriology

Gas gangrene is an acute and devastatingly rapidly-spreading infection caused by a mixture of gas-forming organisms on the *Clostridia* group in which the predominant ones are *Cl. welchii*, *Cl. septicum*, *Cl. oedematiens* and *Cl. sporogenes*. All are Gram positive anaerobes which are inhabitants of soil and the bowel of man.

Like *Cl. tetani*, this group of organisms produces disease by virtue of powerful exotoxins but, unlike *Cl. tetani*, the effect is predominantly at the wound of entry.

Some of the organisms ferment sugar (saccharolytic) and others destroy protein (proteolytic) with the liberation of carbon dioxide, hydrogen sulphide, ammonia and hydrogen—a mixture of which results in the formation of the characteristic, foul-smelling gas.

Gas-gangrene-prone wounds

The mere presence of toxigenic species of *Clostridia* in a wound does not necessarily lead to gangrene; the physical conditions of the wound and the general virulence of the organisms determine the outcome. The anaerobic conditions required for the growth of tetanus organisms pertain also for the gas-forming *Clostridia*. They are particularly prone to grow in deep penetrating wounds which are associated with much tissue-damage, ischaemia, haematoma formation and soil contamination. In current surgical practice, the wounds most at risk are amputations of the lower limbs in bed-ridden diabetic patients.

Surgical pathology

Unlike *Cl. tetani*, there are dramatic changes at the wound of entry. The organisms proliferate and spread rapidly, aided by the destruction caused by the powerful exotoxin. Spread in the subcutaneous tissues results in the formation of a dry, hot and oedematous cellulitis, containing gas bubbles (clostridial cellulitis). This is followed by destruction of blood vessels and haemolysis of liberated blood, which causes the area to assume a brick-red colour. Later, proteolytic organisms destroy muscles, liberate further gases and the tissues assume an olive-green colour (localized myonecrosis), the process eventually spreading to involve other muscle groups (spreading myonecrosis).

Clinical features

1. The *incubation period* is short, usually 24–72 hours.
2. The *wound* is never trivial; it soon becomes unusually painful and swollen, with the development of brick-red and olive-green colour changes and a 'sickly-sweet' smelling discharge containing gas bubbles. As the infection progresses, the skin becomes gangrenous, and black friable muscle is exposed in the depths of the wound. Palpable crepitus beneath the skin can be elicited and visualized in tissue planes on radiographs.
3. The *patient* has marked toxaemia associated with tachycardia and pyrexia. Death may occur from circulatory failure or extensive gangrene.

Differential diagnosis

The diagnosis should always be made on clinical grounds alone and without delay for bacteriological confirmation. Wound infections due to other gas-forming organisms such as some anaerobic streptococci, coliforms and *Proteus* organisms occur more slowly and are not associated with putrefaction or the production of the characteristic discharge.

Management

PREVENTION

Gas gangrene, unlike tetanus, cannot be prevented by the production of active immunity. Moreover, the effectiveness of passive immunization with polyvalent antitoxin at the time of wounding has never been proven. Prophylaxis is dependent on two measures.

1. Wound debridement
Meticulous attention must be paid to all gas-gangrene-prone wounds. All dead skin, subcutaneous fat, fascia, muscle, loose bone fragments and foreign bodies must be removed so that the wound becomes macroscopically clean.

In the presence of gross and widespread crushing of tissues where heavy contamination has occurred, or when suppuration is already present, the wound must be left open and allowed to heal by second intention. However, when the wound appears to be clean and not heavily contaminated, primary closure followed by careful observation is permissible; but if doubt exists about the potential infectivity of the wound, then it should be left open and re-assessed about 5 days later, when delayed primary closure may be possible.

2. Antibiotics

Large and frequent doses of penicillin are given by injection for all gas-gangrene-prone wounds.

CURATIVE TREATMENT

Once gas gangrene has been established, the following treatment is instigated.

1. *The wound*. Wide and ruthless debridement is essential, with removal of all dead and doubtfully-viable tissues and the laying open widely of all pockets of pus or potential cavities. When more than one group of muscles of a limb is involved, serious consideration must be given to amputation; it will certainly be indicated if all muscle groups are involved. Whatever is done, the wound must be packed lightly and left open.

2. *Antibiotics*. Large and frequent doses of penicillin parenterally are essential.

3. *Antitoxin*. Polyvalent antitoxin containing antibodies against *Cl. welchii*, *Cl. septicum*, and *Cl. oedematiens* (9000 units intramuscularly) is sometimes given but its effectiveness is very doubtful.

4. *Supportive therapy*. This includes

   a. Correction of shock and peripheral failure with intravenous therapy
   b. Correction of anaemia with blood transfusions
   c. Correction of metabolic acidosis
   d. Hyperbaric oxygen. With increase in the amount of oxygen available in the tissues, the production of *Clostridia* toxins, particularly in the alpha-toxin of *Cl. welchii*, is inhibited.

      Intermittent exposure of patients with gas gangrene to oxygen at 3 atmospheres absolute causes dramatic benefit in the first 48 hours of therapy. Patients, severely toxic with clostridial myonecrosis, benefit from $2-2\frac{1}{2}$ hours of hyperbaric oxygen therapy before debridement, provided it is not associated with any complications such as oxygen convulsions or disorientation. Hyperbaric oxygen together with wound debridement and antibiotics has now become standard practice in centres equipped with hyperbaric chambers.
   e. Relief of pain with analgesia
   f. Sedation only if absolutely necessary

The overall mortality rate from gas gangrene is about 25% and most deaths are due to late diagnosis, inadequate excision of devitalized tissue and multi-organ failure.

NECROTIZING FASCIITIS

Necrotizing fasciitis is an invasive infection of fascia due to a mixed infection with microaerophillic streptococci or staphylococci or both, as well as Gram negative bacilli.

Clinical features

The process begins in a localized area such as a puncture wound or leg ulcer and spreads along relatively ischaemic fascial planes. Vessels penetrating between skin and deeper structures thrombose, leading to skin death. The skin becomes anaesthetic, and crepitus may be present. The patient is pyrexial and has a tachycardia. Surgical findings are of dull-grey necrotic fascia and subcutaneous tissue which contain thrombosed veins.

Differential diagnosis

Is between ischaemic and clostridial gangrene.

Management

a. *Antibiotics*. Penicillin in large doses parenterally, once material has been taken for smear and culture.
b. Thorough *debridement*. The wound should be left open for secondary closure.
c. Restoration of tissue perfusion with blood
d. Correction of other disorders, e.g. diabetes mellitus

SYNERGISTIC GANGRENE

First described by Melaney. This condition is caused by a mixed infection with *Staphylococcus aureus* and a microaerophilic non-haemolytic streptococcus.

Clinical features

The condition usually starts around puncture sites or wounds and spreads as a painful, increasing area of pale red cellulitis with a purplish central area that finally ulcerates.

Management

a. Radical excision of the ulcerated area with secondary closure
b. Antibiotic therapy. Penicillin in large doses parenterally. This may have to be changed once sensitivity of the staphylococcus is obtained.

ANTHRAX

Bacteriology

B. anthracis (a Gram positive rod) inhabits domestic cattle, goats and wild animals. Infection is nearly always cutaneous through a small skin scratch or septic spot. There is a very acute local and general reaction. The local reaction is haemorrhagic necrosis; the resulting black lesion is known as a *malignant pustule*. Progression ultimately leads to septicaemia.

Prevention

Careful handling of animal products such as skins and hides.

Management

Early recognition is vital. If this is done, chemotherapy aborts the condition. Penicillin and tetracycline should be given in combination, because a few strains of *B. anthracis* are penicillin-insensitive.

BACTEROIDES INFECTIONS

Bacteriology

A large number of *Bacteroides* species are found in the gut and genital tract. They are either obligatory or facultative anaerobes and, though of relatively low aggressiveness in isolation, are synergistic with aerobes and produce more aggressive mixed infections. Their occurrence as pathogens has been underestimated because of the special techniques required to culture them. To ensure that they are not missed, specimens should be handled anaerobically and placed in Stuart's transport medium for transfer to the laboratory. A special request for anaerobic incubation must also be made.

Surgical pathology

The organisms are largely opportunistic, gaining access to and growing in damaged and devitalized tissues in close contact with the gastrointestinal or genital tracts. They are a common feature of chronic middle ear infection (and therefore otitic brain abscesses), intraperitoneal abscess, abdominal wound infection, some chronic skin infections and septic incomplete abortion. The infection produced is a progressive cellulitis with the formation of foul-smelling pus and slough.

Management

The site is drained or a wound laid open. Bacteroides are nearly always sensitive to metronidazole, the tetracycline group of antibiotics and to clindamycin or lincomycin. Metronidazole is currently regarded as the treatment of choice.

CHRONIC GROUP

TUBERCULOSIS

Once a common surgical disease but now rare in the Western world.

Bacteriology

Two forms: human and bovine. The organism is a rod which stains characteristically with the Ziehl Nielsen method. Culture, which takes 6 weeks, is the method of identifying the disease.

Surgical pathology

The effects of tubercle bacilli depend largely on host resistance. A large dose in an undernourished patient without natural 'herd resistance' may produce a relatively severe subacute infection which is relentless and causes death. A small dose in a healthy individual with a naturally high level of resistance or one that has been raised artificially by BCG administration produces a more chronic infection with which the body may either come into equilibrium or even eliminate.

The lesions produced are granulomas. They destroy the tissue in which they form, leading to the formation of necrotic 'caseous' material and pus (cold abscess) which is 'sterile' unless a secondary infection supervenes. Healing is by fibrosis with or without calcification. Common sites are:

a. Lymph nodes of the neck, mediastinum, and abdomen. In the first site, abscesses and sinuses occur, and necrotic material has to be removed.
b. Serous surfaces: joints, peritoneum and pleura
c. Viscera: e.g. Kidney, gut

Management

All surgical tuberculosis is initially managed conservatively with antituberculous agents unless there is an emergency (e.g. spinal cord compression, intestinal obstruction). Surgery is used to:

a. Obtain tissue for diagnosis, either by histological examination or culture
b. Evacuate pus and necrotic tissue
c. Stabilize or reconstruct
d. Deal with complications

ACTINOMYCOSIS

Actinomycetes is a fungus which grows in conditions of relative oxygen lack. It gains access through a breach in the mucosa of the gastro-intestinal tract anywhere from teeth to anus but is most common in the neck and right iliac fossa, the latter secondary to appendicitis.

Pathology

A woody cellulitis is followed by pus formation contain-ing the yellow sulphur granules which are clumps of fungus.

Management

Always conservative, with large doses of penicillin over a period of many weeks.

SYPHILIS

This condition is almost entirely the province of vener-eologists. It should be kept in mind in circumstances of unusual genital, anal and oral ulcers and in exanthemata. Gumma, the third stage, is now virtually unknown.

AMOEBIASIS (see p. 198)

15

Infections of specific sites

ABDOMEN AND CHEST

CLASSIFICATION

Infections of the abdominal wall

Omphalitis

Wound infection (see p. 22)

Persistent discharging sinus (see p. 27)

Infection of the parietes

Peritonitis

Empyema

Residual abscess, pelvic abscess and subphrenic abscess (see Chapter 5)

INFECTION OF THE ABDOMINAL WALL

Infection of the skin of the abdominal wall is essentially similar to superficial infections occurring elsewhere on the body (see p. 65).

Omphalitis

This is an infection of the umbilicus. Predisposing factors are:

In neonates contamination of the umbilical stump. In adults poor hygiene

BACTERIOLOGY

Usually a mixed staphylococcal and streptococcal infection.

CLINICAL FEATURES

Redness, heat, swelling, tenderness and pus. There may be cellulitis spreading from the naval.

MANAGEMENT

Prevention
1. Avoidance of contamination of the umbilical cord when it is severed and during healing
2. Cleanliness

Treatment
1. Drainage of pus
2. Antibiotics systemically in neonates to prevent possible complications

COMPLICATIONS

Usually confined to neonates

1. Septicaemia
2. Portal pyaemia and liver abscess by spreading along patent umbilical vein
3. Portal vein thrombosis and portal hypertension

INFECTION OF THE PARIETES

PERITONITIS

Classification

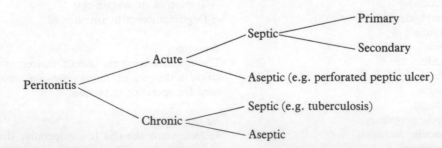

75

Peritonitis is inflammation of a portion or all of the parietal and visceral surfaces of the abdominal cavity. Primary peritonitis caused by the haematogenous spread of a single type of bacterium is exceedingly rare, being seen in patients with cirrhosis and ascites or nephrosis. 'Peritonitis' when used by surgeons today is taken to mean acute septic or aseptic secondary peritonitis and it is this condition that will be described.

Surgical pathology

LOCAL

Regardless of cause there are two immediate local responses: inflammation and ileus.

Inflammation of the peritoneal membrane leads to increased transudation of fluid into the abdominal cavity, depleting the ECF. After a few hours, exudation supervenes, the fluid in the abdominal cavity becoming turbid, containing leucocytes, protein, fibrin, cellular debris and blood. Even when the irritant is initially sterile, bacterial contamination ensues after 12 hours. Bacteriological culture invariably shows a mixed growth of aerobic (e.g. *E. coli*, *Proteus*), and anaerobic (e.g. *B. fragilis*) organisms.

Ileus. The gut responds to peritonitis by initial hypermotility, quickly followed by paralytic ileus. Fluid accumulates in the bowel as a consequence of increased secretion and decreased resorption. This further depletes the ECF.

GENERAL

The hypovolaemia caused by ECF sequestration results in a diminished cardiac output and reduced perfusion of peripheral tissues. In addition, abdominal distention and pain reduce ventilation and consequently the availability of oxygen. The metabolic rate increases in response to stress, with a corresponding increase in peripheral oxygen demand; thus a shift to anaerobic metabolism ensues with a metabolic acidosis.

Common causes of acute peritonitis

These are discussed individually in their appropriate chapters, and will only be listed here.
—Acute appendicitis
—Mesenteric lymphadenitis
—Acute cholecystitis
—Acute salpingitis
—Acute diverticulitis
—Perforated peptic ulcer
—Acute pancreatitis
—Abdominal trauma
—Ruptured ectopic pregnancy
—Mesenteric vascular occlusion
—Gall bladder perforation

Clinical Features

These depend on the precipitating causes.

Symptoms
Abdominal pain, nausea and vomiting.

Signs
Fever, abdominal tenderness, and rigidity. Bowel sounds may be hyperactive initially, becoming silent later. Without treatment, there is rapid progression leading to abdominal distention, hypotension, shock with, ultimately, respiratory, renal and cardiac failure.

Laboratory findings

Leucocytosis, haemoconcentration. Serum electrolytes vary. The urea concentration may be elevated. There is often a picture of metabolic acidosis with a compensatory respiratory alkalosis. Plain X-ray of the abdomen may show distention of both large and small bowel with fluid levels. Free air may be seen under the diaphragm when perforation of a hollow viscus has occurred.

Differential diagnosis

GENERAL
—Uraemia produces abdominal distention, especially in the elderly
—Diabetes mellitus often presents as an acute abdomen in children

THORACIC
—Inferior myocardial infarction
—Basal pneumonia with diaphragmatic pleurisy
—Ruptured oesophagus

RETROPERITONEAL
—Renal calculi
—Pyelonephritis
—Tabes dorsalis
—Osteoarthritis of the vertebrae

PELVIC
—Ruptured ovarian follicle
—Torsion of an ovarian cyst
—Degeneration of uterine fibroid

TREATMENT
The initial assessment should concentrate on resuscitation of the patient, finding the cause of sepsis and the need for operative correction.

PRE-OPERATIVE
1. *Intravenous therapy*. It is imperative that ECF losses be made good. These are best replaced by Hartmann's

solution, with an electrolyte composition similar to plasma.

2. *Central venous pressure monitoring* is essential in the critically ill and the elderly, where cardiac impairment may be exacerbated by large fluid loads.

3. *Nasogastric suction*, to empty the stomach and prevent further vomiting.

4. *Urinary catheter*, allows assessment of urinary flow and fluid replacement.

5. *Antibiotics* should be commenced as soon as diagnosis is made. An aminoglycoside and an anti-anaerobic agent should be used, e.g. gentamicin and metronidazole.

6. *Analgesic*. Morphine in small doses should be administered intravenously, preferably as a continuous infusion or as a bolus hourly.

7. *Laboratory investigations*
   a. Full blood count
   b. Group and cross-match blood
   c. Serum electrolyte concentration
   d. Serum amylase
   e. Blood gases, especially in the elderly
   f. ECG also in the elderly

OPERATIVE

The operative management will depend on the cause of the peritonitis. General points of note are:

1. *Peritoneal toilet and lavage*. All necrotic material and contaminated fluid should be removed. Lavage with saline and a broad spectrum antibiotic (e.g. tetracycline) reduces post-operative complications.

2. *Intestinal decompression*. Distended bowel should be decompressed retrogradely via a naso gastric tube. A gastrostomy may be fashioned for post-operative decompression of the stomach, as prolonged ileus is a frequent complication of peritonitis.

3. *Drains*. Drains should only be placed for the egress of purulent or necrotic debris or blood.

4. *Wound closure*. The deep muscle layers should be closed with monofilament nylon or polypropylene sutures. Delayed primary closure of the subcutaneous layers and skin is prudent.

POSTOPERATIVE

1. *Intravenous replacement therapy* to maintain intravascular volume and the hydration of the patient, monitored by central venous pressure measurement and urinary output. This is continued until it is judged safe for oral intake to be resumed, i.e. the return of bowel sounds, passage of flatus or faeces and reduced gastric aspirates.

2. *Nasogastric or gastrostomy drainage* continuously until drainage becomes minimal. At this point the nasogastric tube may be removed or the gastrostomy spigoted and fluids may be cautiously started by mouth.

3. *Antibiotics* commenced pre-operatively are continued unless cultures of the peritoneal aspirate at the time of operation show that the causative organism is resistant to these, in which case they are changed to appropriate ones.

4. *Analgesia*. Morphine given continuously intravenously is the most comfortable and safest way to administer analgesia. If this method is not available, small doses at frequent intervals may be administered intramuscularly or intravenously.

Prognosis

The prognosis depends on the cause, the age of the patient, and the duration between onset of the disease and its correction. In early peritonitis the prognosis is good.

EMPYEMA

An empyema is an acute or chronic suppurative pleural exudate, which may be caused by a multitude of organisms.

Surgical pathology

The initial inflammation of the pleura leads to an exudation of fluid into the pleural cavity. Though the exudate may at first be sterile, if the inflammation was caused by an adjacent lung lesion it is soon invaded by bacteria.

SPREAD

This is by:

—Direct extension of pneumonia
—Lymphatic from infections of the lungs, mediastinum, chest wall or diaphragm
—Haematogenous
—Direct innoculation by direct trauma or surgical incision of a lung abscess
—Ruptured thoracic viscera, e.g. oesophagus
—Extension of subdiaphragmatic process, e.g. subphrenic, hepatic or perinephric abscesses

Bacteriology

This depends largely on the source of the infection. The organisms most frequently encountered are:

1. *Staphylococcus aureus*, most common organism in all age groups. Spread is directly from staphylococcal pneumonia.

2. *Streptococcus pyogenes*, a frequent complication of streptococcal pneumonia; it is characterized by thick green pus that becomes loculated early.

3. *Bacteroides*, seen as a complication in women with pelvic inflammatory disease and in elderly debilitated men. It is also seen in pleural rupture of a subphrenic abscess, when it is often associated with other enteric organisms. It is characterized by the massive accumulation of thick, foul-smelling pus that rapidly returns after evacuation.

4. *Klebsiella pneumoniae* principally affects debilitated, elderly, chronically ill or alcoholic patients.

Complications

1. Invasion of the chest wall and osteomyelitis of the ribs or costal cartilages
2. Brochopleural and bronchial fistulae. These require urgent closure, because of the danger of flooding of the opposite lung with pus.
3. Mediastinal abscess
4. Septicaemia
5. Metastatic abscess

Clinical findings

Symptoms. Chest pain, shortness of breath, weakness and haemoptysis.

Signs. Fever and the signs of a pleural effusion are usually present.

Special tests

—Anaemia and leucocytosis
—Chest X-ray. There is opacification of part of the pleural space, occasionally with a fluid level. A pneumonic infiltrate may be seen, though this is usually obscured by the effusion.

Treatment

LOCAL

Antibiotics. Prompt diagnosis and treatment are essential. Sputum, pleural fluid and blood cultures should be obtained and antibiotic treatment instituted on the basis of clinical findings and smears.

Drainage of pleural space. Early, closed, underwater-seal drainage of the empyema is necessary to avoid chronicity. If the chest X-ray suggests loculation, this should be broken down through a limited thoracotomy, with removal of all necrotic material and the resection of a short segment of rib. The empyema cavity is usually isolated from the remaining pleura within a week, the underwater seal becoming unnecessary. The tube can then be cut, and slowly withdrawn as the cavity becomes obliterated.

GENERAL

Anemia should be corrected with blood transfusion. The patient should be fed a high energy, high protein diet supplemented with vitamins.

Prognosis

The mortality rate for patients developing empyema in association with pneumonia is about 10%, rising to 25–55% in postoperative patients.

HAND INFECTIONS

Though hand infections are not now associated with the serious consequences which were common in the pre-antibiotic era, they are still frequently encountered and responsible for the loss of many man hours in industry.

Hand infection commonly follows the ever-increasing number of hand injuries. Such infection is often attributable to inadequate treatment and serious disability may result from impaired tendon and joint function.

CLASSIFICATION

Subcutaneous

1. Acute paronychia
2. Pulp space infection
3. Web space infection

Deep

4. Thenar space infection
5. Middle palmar space infection
6. Suppurative tenosynovitis
7. Non-specific tenosynovitis
8. Wound infection

Miscellaneous

9. Osteomyelitis
10. Septic arthritis
11. Foreign Bodies

SURGICAL PATHOLOGY

Bacteriology

Organisms usually enter the hand from minor cuts, abrasions, pricks, or burns. In some cases no source of entry is found. The organisms usually involved are:

Acute infections
1. *Staphylococcus aureus*
2. Haemolytic streptocci
3. *Escherichia coli*
4. *Protcus*

Chronic infections
1. *Staphylococcus aureus*
2. Tuberculosis
3. Candidiasis

INDIVIDUAL INFECTIONS

Acute paronychia

Infection starts as a cellulitis of the nail fold, and within a few hours a subcuticular abscess forms. When this is not controlled, rapid spread follows to involve the entire nail fold, usually in association with subungual extensions (Fig. 15.1A).

Pulp space infection (felon)

Infection is most common in the distal pulp space following a penetrating injury. An initial phase of cellulitis involving most of the pulp is quickly followed by the collection of pus, because of the honeycomb between the fibrous bands intersecting the space between phalanx, tendon sheath and the skin (Fig. 15.1B). There is rapid necrosis of the pulp tissues and of a varying amount of overlying skin, due to the action of necrotizing staphylococcal exotoxins. Untreated, the infection leads to further skin necrosis, and possibly osteomyelitis of the distal phalanx, or suppurative arthritis. In the case of more proximal segments an important danger is involvement

of the tenosynovium which often leads to disastrous effects on flexor tendon function.

Web space infection

Infection may follow a penetrating injury in the region of the web space and is quite common in manual labourers or hairdressers. Pus collection occurs in the subcutaneous compartment of the web beyond the distal palmar crease and is limited on each side by vertical septa of the palmar aponeurosis passing to the intermetacarpal ligaments. Untreated, the infection may spread to involve the deep palmar spaces.

Thenar space infection

This space is bounded in front by the flexor tendons, behind by the fascia covering the transverse head of adductor pollicis, medially by the intermediate palmar septum and laterally by the fascia covering the muscles of the thenar eminence (Fig. 15.2). True collections in this space are rare, and many which are so-called are simply abscesses deep or superficial to the palmar aponeurosis or extensive collections in the first two space.

Middle palmar space infection

This space lies between the medial palmar septum medially and the intermediate septum laterally and is bounded in front by the flexor tendons and behind by the third, fourth and fifth metacarpal bones and the fascia covering the intervening interossei (Fig. 15.2). Subcutaneous abscesses of the palm may occasionally extend to involve this space.

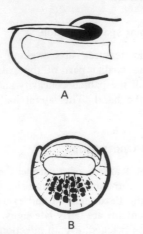

Fig. 15.1 A. Subungual extension of acute paronychia B. Pulp space infection

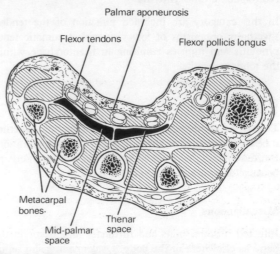

Fig. 15.2 Thenar and mid-palmar spaces

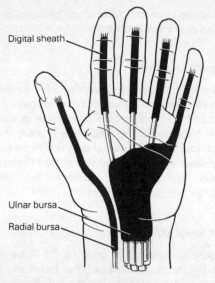

Digital sheath

Ulnar bursa

Radial bursa

Fig. 15.3 Flexor tendon sheaths

Suppurative tenosynovitis

Though infection of a tendon sheath is uncommon, when it occurs prompt diagnosis is imperative if there is to be any hope of salvaging flexor tendon function. Suppurative tenosynovitis may develop as the result of a penetrating injury, as an extension of one of the aforementioned infections or following the operative repair of an injury involving the flexor sheath. The infection is confined to the tendon sheath and, if untreated, it will result in extensive destruction of the synovial membrane, tendon adhesions and even sequestration of the flexor tendons in advanced infections (Fig. 15.3).

Non-specific tenosynovitis

In this category are included infection of the tendon sheath by organisms of low virulence, traumatic tenosynovitis and injuries resulting in haemorrhage within the tendon sheath.

Wound infection

This is the commonest form of hand infection, whether it be an infection of an abrasion or of a sutured laceration. It often follows the primary repair of lacerations, perhaps because of errors in surgical technique.

Miscellaneous

Infected blisters, boils and furuncles may occur in the hand as elsewhere in the body. Osteomyelitis and septic arthritis also occur, either as a result of one of the above infections or as a primary infection.

CLINICAL FEATURES

Acute paronychia

The nail fold becomes red and swollen, and later a sub-cuticular collection of pus appears with or without a subungual extension.

Pulp space infection

Infection of this space is suggested by the onset of severe throbbing pain following a penetrating injury of the involved segment, in association with a diffusely swollen and very tender pulp. Maximal tenderness overlies the centre of abscess formation. In the early stages the pulp is tense and reddened, but with impending skin necrosis the pulp develops a mauve or blue colour. In an untreated case osteomyelitis or spread to the tendon sheath may result.

Web space infection

This infection is characterized by the onset of pain and tenderness in the area, together with obvious distension of the web space, usually following a penetrating injury. Considerable swelling of the dorsum of the hand may be associated.

Thenar space infection

The important features are severe pain and extensive swelling centred on the thenar eminence and the corresponding region of the dorsum of the hand, but without obliteration of the palmar cavity, which distinguishes this infection from one in the middle palmar space. The distension of the thenar space tends to force the thumb into palmar abduction.

Middle palmar space infection

Characteristic features are swelling and tenderness involving the medial part of the palm, flattening or obliteration of the palmar concavity and swelling of the dorsum of the hand. The lateral half of the hand is spared.

Suppurative tenosynovitis

The classical features of a swollen, reddened finger, affecting all segments, with exquisite tenderness along the line of the flexor tendon and excruciating pain on passive movement, are fairly late signs. If this advanced stage has been reached, even if infection controlled, considerable tendon dysfunction is likely to result.

Pain on passive movement of the fingers is the best sign of developing tenosynovitis.

Non-specific tenosynovitis

One occasionally encounters patients who have some of the local features of a suppurative tenosynovitis, such as pain on finger flexion and localized tenderness along the flexor sheath, but little local swelling, cellulitis or systemic disturbances. These are cases of non-specific tenosynovitis due to trauma to the synovium, as may occur in process workers carrying out long periods of rapid and repetitive hand movements. Suppuration does not occur and recovery takes place fairly quickly with rest to the affected part.

A similar condition is De Quervain's disease, which is tenovaginitis of the long extensor of the thumb. There is pain on thumb movement and tenderness over the tendon on the postero-lateral aspect of the distal third of the forearm. Most patients recover with rest, but a few require incision of the sheath.

Wound infection

There is obviously an infected wound with or without suppuration. In addition there may be the signs of infection of one of the above spaces indicating spread of infection.

Miscellaneous

1. OSTEOMYELITIS

Acute osteomyelitis may accompany any of the above infections, in which case the features are those of the infection with radiographic changes of bone destruction. If the infection has become chronic there may be sequestration of bone and sinus formation. Tuberculous infection of the metacarpals or phalanges is common (tuberculous dactylitis). There is pain with swelling and the development of a 'cold abscess'. There is constitutional 'ill health' and radiographs show bony destruction.

2. SEPTIC ARTHRITIS

A painful, red, swollen joint with or without evidence of infection elsewhere is indicative of a septic arthritis. There is usually associated constitutional disturbance and a fever. It is particularly likely to complicate rheumatoid arthritis.

PRINCIPLES OF TREATMENT

There are four fundamentals of treatment:

1. Drainage. When pus has formed, simple incision suffices to drain unilocular collections in the palm, the web spaces and the proximal segments of the fingers; but for the honeycombed collections of pus in the pulp space adequate drainage can only be assured by incision and meticulous debridement of all necrotic tissue.

Incisions must be transversely placed parallel to the skin creases, centred over the area of maximal tenderness and swelling, but when there is a draining sinus or an area of skin necrosis, this should be included in the incision. In finger collections, any longitudinal extension of the drainage incision must be made in the mid-lateral axis of the finger to minimize the incidence of longitudinal scar contracture and tenderness.

When local anaesthesia is used the injection should never be introduced through or in the vicinity of areas of cellulitis. Distal digital pulp infection may safely be drained under a digital block but infections extending on to the palm will require a general anaesthetic or an infra-clavicular brachial plexus block. There is no place for ethyl chloride freeze anaesthesia in the treatment of hand infections, because the duration of anaesthesia so produced is too short to allow deliberate removal of necrotic tissue.

2. Antibiotics. Where cellulitis has not progressed to pus formation some early infections can be reversed by the prompt administration of antibiotics. This applies particularly to early paronychiae and certain beta haemolytic streptococcal infections.

Antibiotic therapy should begin before surgery, the initial choice usually being an empirical one based on the fact that *Staphylococcus aureus* is the most likely pathogen. When the infection is acquired in a hospital, as in the case of nursing staff, a penicillinase-resistant penicillin, e.g. cloxacillin, should be used. At the time of drainage, pus is sent for culture and sensitivity tests. The initial choice of antibotics may need revision within 24 hours if the area of cellulitis is extending or pain is not relieved, particularly when the results of the culture and sensitivity tests indicate that a more effective antibiotic should be chosen.

3. Immobilization. Post-operatively the area involved and related joints should be immobilized with an appropriate plaster of Paris splint and supporting sling. If the infection is severe the patient should be confined to bed with the limb elevated by suspension from a vertical stand. Immobilized joints should be placed in the position of function of slight dorsiflexion of the wrist with the metacarpo-phalangeal joints at 90° of flexion and interphalangeal joints fully extended.

4. Rehabilitation. Once infection has been controlled and healing is progressing, graduated finger movements are started to minimize stiffness which may result from tendon and joint adhesions. These are always a likely complication of hand infections.

SPECIAL CONSIDERATIONS IN TREATMENT

1. Acute paronychia. Once pus has collected, management depends on the extent and direction of spread. In very early cases elevation of the fold with a small pair of scissors breaks into the abscess and establishes drainage, which is maintained with a small double layer of tulle gras.

In most late cases, some subungual extension has occurred (Fig. 15.1A) and more efficient drainage is obtained by a vertical incision alongside the nail. The proximal half of the nail must be excised together with its prolongation beneath the nail fold (Fig. 15.4A)

2. Pulp space infection.

A common error in drainage of these infections is simply to incise the pulp—this releases a bead or two of pus only but takes no account of the slough, which will prolong the infection if it is not excised.

In early cases, before pus has pointed, a lateral incision is used (Fig. 15.4B). This is deepened across the pulp space, in front of the terminal phalanx, breaking down the fibrous septa which connect the skin to the terminal phalanx, allowing the entire space to be cleared out. In late cases, when suppuration has progressed to produce skin necrosis and sinus formation or if pus is clearly pointing in the centre of the pulp, drainage is carried out at this point by excising a circle of skin 2 mm in diameter (Fig. 15.4C).

When the slough has been excised, the cavity is loosely filled with a narrow strip of tape moistened with acriflavine emulsion or glycerin. No wound should be packed so as to plug the escape of discharge. A bandage is lightly applied and the dressing is renewed daily for 3 to 4 days by which time granulations will have begun to obliterate the cavity. Healing should be completed in about 10 days. It is helpful to dust the abscess cavity with a little antibiotic powder prior to redressing.

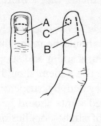

Fig. 15.4 Incisions for draining pulp space infections A. For subungual extension B. For early pulp space infection C. For late pulp space infection pointing in the centre

3. Web space infection.

A transverse skin incision is made over the point of maximal tenderness or fluctuation, then artery or sinus forceps are opened in a longitudinal direction (to avoid damage to the digital nerves and vessels), through the subcutaneous tissue to enter the abscess cavity and allow drainage (Fig. 15.5A). A small glove drain, about 1 cm wide, should be retained to hold the edges apart and maintain drainage for 48 hours, when it can be removed.

4. Thenar and middle palmar space infection.

These are drained through skin incisions as indicated (Fig. 15.5B). The abscess is then entered by opening artery forceps in the line of the digital nerves and going either medial or lateral to the common flexor sheath.

5. Suppurative tenosynovitis.

In early cases where tendon sequestration has not occurred, the sheath is drained by short transverse incisions down to, and including, the fibrous, flexor sheath, opposite the distal and proximal finger segments (Fig. 15.5C). It is also helpful to irrigate the sheath with an antibiotic solution introduced through fine polythene tubing at the points of incision. In the case of the little finger the infection may extend to involve the common flexor sheath at the wrist and may require more extensive palmar drainage, including drainage of the ulnar bursa proximal to the flexor retinaculum.

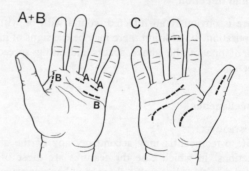

Fig. 15.5 Incisions for draining infections of the hand A. For web space infections B. For thenar and mid-palmar space infections C. For early suppurative flexor tenosynovitis

6. Non-specific tenosynovitis.

The affected finger is immobilized for 7–10 days in the position of function, and antibiotic therapy is prescribed.

7. Wound infections.

All sutures are removed, necrotic material is debrided and, if necessary, the wound may need to be extended to allow drainage of a collection which is beyond the limits of the wound.

8. Osteomyelitis.

If associated with pulp space or other infection, adequate drainage must be achieved with incision and debridement of necrotic material when that space is drained. A primary osteomyelitis of a bone of the hand should be treated by incision over the swelling and drilling of the underlying bone. Pus must be cultured to identify the causative organism, including culture for tuberculosis.

9. Septic arthritis.

Similarly, infection involving a joint must be treated by drainage of the joint, culture of pus and antibiotics. The hand must be rested until the infection is controlled, but careful rehabilitation is essential if permanent stiffness is to be avoided.

FOREIGN BODIES

The presence of a foreign body in the hand must always be considered in hand injuries. They may present a difficult problem. The diagnosis may be difficult, the functional consequences if untreated may be significant and surgical removal can be technically very demanding. The commonest causes of foreign bodies are:

1. Fragments of glass or metal in lacerations
2. Penetration by a nail or needle which breaks

Diagnosis

A foreign body may be present in any puncture wound of the hand. X-rays should always be taken, preferably in two planes, and with an opaque marker at the entry site.

Management

Open wounds should be explored and carefully excised until all foreign material is removed. Exploration for a fragment of needle following a puncture wound should be undertaken in an operating theatre with full aseptic conditions, tourniquet control and the image intensifier (or X-ray facilities) available.

16

Scalp and intracranial conditions

SCALP

SURGICAL ANATOMY

The scalp is superficial to and freely mobile upon the pericranium (periosteum of the skull) and consists of four tissue layers:

1. *Skin*
2. *Subcutaneous connective tissue* which makes the scalp stiff and unyielding, and within which the blood vessels ramify.
3. *Aponeurotic layer or galea* to which are attached the frontal and occipital muscles.
4. *Loose areolar tissue*

The arterial blood supply is from terminal branches of the external carotid artery and the ophthalmic artery a branch of internal carotid. Scalp lacerations bleed profusely because the walls of these arteries are tethered by connective tissue of the subcutaneous layer which reduces spasm and contraction, and the muscles which are attached to the deeper galeal layer play little part in limiting scalp haemorrhage.

Venous drainage is via venae commitantes of the arteries but drainage of the frontal area occurs via emmissary and diploid veins which traverse the skull, communicate with the cavernous sinus and are relevant to the intracranial spread of infection.

CLASSIFICATION

1. Laceration
2. Haematoma
3. Infection
4. Tumours

Laceration

Minor lacerations of the scalp form a major part of the suturing load of most casualty departments. More extens-ive wounds may involve an underlying skull fracture or defect of scalp tissues.

The thickness of the scalp and the overlying hair provide a cushion for the skull and brain and blunt trauma commonly causes a stellate laceration involving all layers of the scalp. Haemorrhage from scalp lacerations is often brisk and may be so profuse to cause shock even in the absence of any other injury.

TREATENT
1. *Stop the bleeding*. Digital pressure with the fingertips placed at the edge of the laceration is the best first-aid measure until clotting occurs. Avoid grasping the bleeding artery with artery forceps, but instead use a series of artery forceps, grasp the galea and swing the forceps back over the wound edge. This man-oeuvre controls the bleeding very effectively and is useful both for elective scalp incisions and for dealing with extensive lacerations.
2. *Closure*. Through-and-through sutures of silk or, preferably, monofilament material, picking up all layers, will not only control bleeding but will be sufficient for apposition of the skin edges. Elective incisions are closed in two layers—galea and skin. Healing is rapid because of the rich blood supply.
3. *Repair of scalp defects*. As for any laceration the hair-bearing skin is shaved up to 2 cms from the edge, and for large defects with loss of scalp tissue the scalp is extensively mobilised, deep to the galea, in the areolar layer. Large defects are closed by either a reversed S-plasty or a rotation flap, and split-skin grafting is rarely necessary.
4. *Antibiotics*. The rich blood supply restricts the need for antibiotics to circumstances where there is a combination of scalp laceration and skull fracture—i.e. an open fracture.

Haematoma

Whether as the result of the obstetricians' forceps (cephalohaematoma) or because of an unsuspected low doorway, haematomas of the scalp are common. Predictably, the haemorrhage after blunt trauma is within the subcutaneous layer and its spread is restricted by the dense connective tissue, producing the characteristic egg shape. Subaponeurotic haematomata may develop after penetrating injuries or neurosurgical procedures. Spread of blood is limited by the bony origins of the muscles that attach to the galea, the frontal bone and occiput. A black eye, or ecchymosis of the periorbital skin, is therefore a not uncommon sequel to penetrating scalp wounds.

Treatment is conservative in that scalp haematomata resolve quickly because of rich venous and lymphatic drainage.

Infection

Because of a rich blood supply, infection of the scalp and scalp wound infection are both uncommon. Retrograde spread via emissary veins from a distant source in the skull (osteomyelitis) or brain (cerebral abscess) may present as a subaponeurotic abscess with localized tenderness and pitting oedema (Pott's puffy tumour).

Conversely the rare occurrence of scalp infection, especially in the frontal region, may theoretically cause cerebral abscess or cavernous sinus thrombosis.

Tumours

All tumours of skin (p. 285) may occur on the scalp. The more common and specific scalp tumours are:

1. *Epidermoid cyst* (*wen*). These are often multiple, arise in the skin layer and may be excised with ease under local anaesthesia. Recurrence at that site or elsewhere on the scalp is not uncommon.
2. *Cock's peculiar tumour*. An infected and ulcerating epidermoid cyst, which may resemble a squamous cell carcinoma.
3. *Cylindroma* (*turban tumour*). The growth presents as an extensive turban-shaped swelling and histologically the stroma forms peculiar transparent cylinders. It behaves like a basal cell carcinoma and, despite the same name, should not be confused with the invasive adenocystic carcinoma of the salivary glands (p. 104).

INTRACRANIAL CONDITIONS

The majority of a neurosurgeon's workload involves dealing with head injuries (Chapter 8), brain tumours, intracranial aneurysms and to a lesser extent intracranial abscesses. In this chapter the pathophysiological effects of these intracranial space-occupying conditions and the general principles of their management will be outlined before discussing each condition.

RAISED INTRACRANIAL PRESSURE

Pathophysiology

The cranium is the only body cavity that is wholly rigid and inelastic, and any rise of intracranial pressure (ICP) causes compression of the brain. Changes of ICP reflect changes of intracranial contents which are the sum of brain volume, cerebrospinal fluid (CSF) volume and intracranial blood volume.

1. *Brain volume*. This increases with brain oedema, which is a result of:

   a. Vasogenic factors that increase ECF accumulation secondary to changes of endothelial permeability, e.g. tumour or abscess
   b. Cell damaging factors, such as hypoxia that increases intracellular sodium and water.

   Any lesion within the brain increases brain volume by its own mass.
2. *CSF volume and circulation*. Cerebrospinal fluid is formed in the choroid plexus of the lateral ventricles, passes through the foramen of Monro to the third ventricle, along the aqueduct of Sylvius to the fourth ventricle, then via the foramena of Luschka and median foramen of Magendie to the cisterna magna and the spinal subarachnoid space. It recirculates through the cisterna ambiens, around the mid-brain at the level of the falx cerebri (Fig. 16.1), to the subarachnoid space of the cerebral hemispheres and is absorbed by the arachnoid villi of the superior sagittal sinus into the venous circulation. Obstruction at any one of these very narrow passages will cause increased pressure and obstructive hydrocephalus.
3. *Intracranial blood volume*. Cerebral vasodilatation due to hypercapnia and hypoxia and increased central venous pressure both cause marked increases of blood volume in the brain. Respiratory obstruction is therefore a potent cause of raised ICP.

A space-occupying lesion may increase ICP by:

1. Increasing brain volume, by its very presence
2. Altering endothelial permeability
3. Obstructing CSF flow
4. Increasing cerebral blood flow

The brain has an intrinsic elastance or stiffness which allows it to absorb increases in volume and pressure, but when normal compensatory mechanisms are exhausted any small changes in ICP will cause major clinical effects (Fig. 16.1).

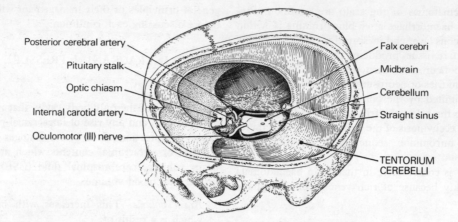

Posterior cerebral artery

Pituitary stalk

Optic chiasm

Internal carotid artery

Oculomotor (III) nerve

Falx cerebri

Midbrain

Cerebellum

Straight sinus

TENTORIUM CEREBELLI

Fig. 16.1 Tentorial hiatus. Cerebral hemispheres have been removed to display the anatomical relations at the free edge of the tentorium cerebelli. The subarachnoid cisterna ambiens (in black) lies at the side of the midbrain

Clinical features

The common clinical features of raised ICP are:

1. *Headache.* Typically occurs in the morning and is aggravated by coughing, sneezing and stooping.
2. *Vomiting.* Again occurs in the morning, and is common in children with posterior fossa tumours.
3. *Mental disturbance.* Responsiveness can be equated with brain function. Coma is therefore equivalent to 'brain failure'. Increased ICP causes a deterioration of brain function culminating in coma. Clinical assessment of responsiveness, coma and brain death is discussed in Chapter 8.
4. *Papilloedema.* The optic nerve is an extension of the brain with all its meningeal coverings. Raised CSF pressure in the subarachnoid space causes congestion of the central retinal vein with oedema and haemorrhages.

LOCALIZING SYMPTOMS AND SIGNS

The neurosurgeon has no equivalent to the general surgeon's exploratory laparotomy as he cannot open the skull and pass a hand around the brain feeling and looking for a lesion. He is therefore dependent on a detailed knowledge of neuroanatomy and, from the history and examination, attempts to locate the site of the lesion and choose the best investigation.

Supra- and infratentorial lesions

The tentorium cerebelli (Fig. 16.1) is the important divider in the cranium. Lesions above and below the ten-

torium produce different clinical syndromes, require different investigations and cause different complications. Space-occupying lesions may therefore be classified anatomically as being:

1. Supra- or infra-tentorial
2. Lateral or central
3. Right or left

LATERAL SUPRATENTORIAL LESIONS

These lesions cause:

1. *Epilepsy,* which is usually focal and often heralds a tumour but is more common with abscess than haematoma
2. *Dysphasia* (temporal lobe)
3. *Parietal spastical disorders,* with incorrect perception of self with disregard for left or right side
4. *Anosmia* (frontal)
5. *Homonomous hemianopia* (occipital)
6. *Hemiplegia* (pre-frontal)

CENTRAL SUPRATENTORIAL LESIONS

1. *Pressure symptoms*: lesions of the roof of the third ventricle obstruct the foramen of Monro causing increased ICP
2. *Hemiplegia and dementia,* when invading the corpus callosum
3. *Bitemporal hemianopia* (*chiasmal compression*), for sellar and parasellar lesions (Fig. 16.1)
4. *Cavernous sinus syndrome,* with proptosis, diplopia and ptosis (third, fourth and sixth cranial nerves) and facial pain (fifth), also from sellar and parasellar lesions (Fig. 16.1)

INFRATENTORIAL LESIONS

More commonly seen in children (e.g. with cerebellar medulloblastoma) and in general causes more problems of raised ICP from CSF block due to the proximity of the fourth ventricle.

Central lesions cause predominantly pressure symptoms and *lateral lesions* cause ataxia, nystagmus, dysphonia and cranial nerve palsies of seventh, eight and the bulbar nerves (ninth to twelfth).

Brain shift and herniation

Supratentorial masses push brain through the hiatus causing transtentorial herniation (temporal coning) and infratentorial masses push brain through the foramen magnum causing foraminal impaction (tonsillar coning). 'Coning' is an illustrative term to describe the cone shape of the plug of herniated brain.

TENTORIAL HERNIATION

The clinical features are:

1. Decerebrate rigidity (mid-brain compression)
2. Bradycardia and hypertension (brain stem buckling)
3. Ptosis and mydriasis (third nerve stretched)
4. Homonomous hemianopia (thrombosis of the posterior cerebral artery and occipital infarct)
5. Hemiplegia (compression of cerebral peduncles).

FORAMINAL IMPACTION

The clinical features are:

1. Irregular respirations and apnea, so-called Cheyne–Stokes respiration (medullary compression)
2. Loss of gag and cough reflexes (bulbar cranial nerve compression)
3. Nuchal rigidity and opisthotonos (dural irritation)

INVESTIGATIONS

1. *Plain X-ray skull.* Certain features may indicate underlying disease:

   a. *Raised ICP* indicated by thin dorsal sellae, erosion of posterior clinoids or widening of sutures (in children).
   b. *Intracranial calcification.* The pineal, choroid plexus and falx cerebri are commonly calcified in normal adults. Suprasellar calcification is seen in craniopharyngioma. Displacement of the pineal from the midline may be present.

2. *Lumbar puncture.* Included as a warning. Although this test is easily performed, the potential risks to a patient with raised ICP of brain shift and herniation are hardly worth the meagre information obtained.

3. *Electroencephalogram (EEG).* This investigation is of limited value, requires an expert technician to perform the test and a high degree of skill to interpret the results. Most useful when lateral supratentorial lesions are suspected, particularly abscess.

4. *Isotope scan.* Gamma-emitting isotopes of technetium are injected intravenous and the head scanned with a gamma camera. Uptake of isotope is related to vascularity. Meningiomas and metastases have a dense uptake and abscess, infarct and haematoma may be satisfactorily demonstrated. Measurements of cerebral circulation may also be performed. Isotope scanning is a useful screening test to show mass lesions but negative scans are quite unreliable.

5. *CT scan.* Computerized tomography uses a series of narrow beams of X-rays to obtain a density picture of the brain in horizontal slices, the density equation being computerized. Greater clarity of vascular structures can be obtained by intravenous injection of contrast (contrast enhancement). A range of densities can be determined by altering the 'window' of the X-ray beam. Needless to say CT scanning has revolutionized the investigations of the brain and is the investigative cornerstone of all neurosurgical units.

   The only limitation is that the patient must remain still for several minutes and children or restless patients may need sedation or general anaesthesia.

6. *Contrast radiology*

   a. *Carotid angiography.* Displacement of vessels, especially midline shift of pericallosal vessels, and tumour circulation are well demonstrated.
   b. *Ventriculography.* This requires a burr hole and injection of air into the lateral ventricle, and is useful in defining the pathological anatomy of CSF circulation in patients with raised ICP. By-products are a tumour biopsy and CSF pressure measurement and analysis. Ventriculography has to a large extent been superceded by C.T. Scanning.
   c. *Air encephalogram (AEG).* A lumbar puncture is necessary and with injection of air and carries risks. The information obtained relates to cisternal anatomy and anomalies of CSF flow, but is useful in patients without raised ICP.

STRATEGY FOR INTRACRANIAL LESIONS

All patients—plain X-ray and CT scan

Lateral supratentorial—isotope scan or EEG

Central supratentorial (sellar)—bilateral carotid angiogram to exclude aneurysm or AEG

Infratentorial—bilateral carotid angiogram and ventriculogram (raised ICP)

GENERAL PRINCIPLES OF SURGICAL MANAGEMENT

Anaesthesia

The aims of the anaesthetist are:

1. *To reduce ICP* by maintaining a patent airway, preventing coughing by spraying the vocal cords with local anaesthetic and avoiding volatile agents that increase cerebral blood flow (halothane). A combination of nitrous oxide and a neuroleptanalgesic (droperidine) is useful.
2. *To increase cerebral oxygenation.* This is aided by induced hypotension (reducing blood loss), hypothermia and barbiturate protection.
3. *To allow rapid recovery of consciousness.* The aim is for the patient to be lucid before leaving the operating theatre.

Pre-operative preparation

1. *Reduce ICP.* Three methods are available:

    a. *Osmotic diuretics.* Mannitol is the most useful. The full intravenous dose is 500 ml of 20% Mannitol over 20 minutes. The patient must have a urinary catheter.
    b. *Corticosteroids.* Useful both pre- and postoperatively, dexamethasone being the most efficacious.
    c. *Hyperventilators.* Induced hypocapnia reduces cerebral vasodilation and lowers ICP.

2. *Protecting the eyes.* Keratitis may develop in a cornea rendered anaesthetic and Vaseline is freely applied over the lids when the patient is asleep.
3. *Scalp preparation.* The head is completely shaved, defatted with ether, and antiseptic applied.

Operative procedures

1. *Exploratory burr hole* may be used to:

    a. Obtain biopsy
    b. Measure ICP
    c. Perform a ventriculogram
    d. Form part of a craniotomy incision

2. *Supratentorial exploration.* A frontal craniotomy, with a crescentic scalp incision within the hairline and reflection of a myoplastic (muscle-attached) bone flap, is preferred. This approach allows exposure of the frontal lobe, optic chiasm, pituitary and sellar regions and is ideal for aneurysm surgery particularly those procedures involving the circle of Willis (p. 91).

3. *Infratentorial (posterior fossa) exploration.* The scalp incision is vertical and midline; a bone flap is not reflected, but bone is nibbled away forming a craniectomy.
4. *Reduction of ICP*

    a. *Lateral decompression.* For supratentorial lesions, removal of the tumour mass reduces brain volume and may be supplemented by frontal, temporal or occipital lobectomy. For infratentorial decompression suboccipital decomposition is useful. This involves extending the craniectomy to include occipital bone, rim of foramen magnum and arch of atlas, thus reducing the effects of tonsillar coning. Raised ICP is a particular problem with posterior fossa lesions.
    b. *Short-circuiting.* Immediate but short-term reduction of ICP may be achieved by burr hole and ventricular drainage via a polythene drain tube.

    Ventriculo-atrial and ventriculo-peritoneal shunts may be used in the long term as a stop-gap measure to relieve raised ICP before and after definitive surgery.

Post-operative complications

1. *Intracranial clot* requires return to theatre and drainage
2. *Pyrexia* may be due to:

    a. Chest or urinary infection
    b. Wound infection
    c. CSF leak
    d. Cerebral abscess
    e. Osteomyelitis skull

3. *Epilepsy.* Fits in the first week usually resolve. Fits are more common following frontal approaches and if they have been present pre-operatively, and in these cases anticonvulsants are recommended.
4. *Eyes.* Peri-orbital swelling is common after frontal craniotomy and is best treated conservatively. Neuroparalytic keratitis and corneal ulcer due to trigeminal (fifth) nerve palsy is prevented by shielding the eye. When combined with a facial (seventh) nerve palsy, lateral tarsorrhaphy is indicated.

INTRACRANIAL TUMOURS

Surgical pathology

In all sense intracranial tumours could be considered malignant, because if left untreated they lead to death by causing raised ICP, brain shift and herniation. Brain tumours are the second most common cause of cancer-related death in children under 14 years. In adults 70% of tumours are supratentorial and 30% infratentorial, whereas in children the distribution is reversed. Brain tumours do not metastasize outside the central nervous system.

CLASSIFICATION

Intracranial tumours may be classified in terms of the cell or site of origin and for adults the commoner varieties are here noted in order of frequency:

1. *Metastatic*

2. *Neuroectodermal*
   a. Neuroglia—glioma
      astrocytoma
      ependymoma
      oligodendroglioma
   b. Neuronal—medulloblastoma

3. *Meningioma*

4. *Pituitary fossa tumours*

5. *Acoustic neuroma*

Metastatic tumours

These account for between 20–60% of brain tumours, depending on whether it is a surgical or pathological survey, as the majority of cases are not referred for neurosurgical treatment. Spread occurs via the arterial system and particularly the valveless cerebral veins. The commonest primary is bronchogenic carcinoma followed in order of frequency by breast cancer, renal cell carcinoma and malignant melanoma. The primary source is not discovered in 15% of cases and in most there are multiple metastases.

Treatment. When the primary site is known, surgical excision is indicated if symptoms are distressing. The results from palliative excision of a solitary metastasis are often very satisfactory. Dexamethasone may reduce symptoms of raised ICP but chemotherapy is of little value. Radiation therapy may improve the period of survival.

Glioma

SURGICAL PATHOLOGY

Neuroglia is the connective tissue of the brain and is composed of astrocytes, ependymal cells and oligodendrocytes. Gliomas are the malignant tumours of neuroglia and are graded I–IV on the basis of histological differentiation and the presence of haemorrhage and necrosis.

Astocytoma. These are the commonest and most aggressive of the gliomas, grow diffusely and are poorly encapsulated. The most anaplastic form, with areas of

haemorrhage and necrosis (Grade IV astrocytoma) is called glioblastoma multiforme and often involves the temporal lobe. Astrocytomas of the infratemporal region are usually less aggressive.

Ependymoma. The majority occur in children, often involving the floor of the fourth ventricle, but supratentorial tumours may involve the lateral ventricles. The tumour has a red, nodular, cauliflower appearance, is slow growing and is well encapsulated.

Oligodendroglioma. These often occur in the lateral supratentorial area and may invade the dura. Calcification is seen on plain X-ray in about 90% of cases, and the tumour has a tendency to form mucoid cysts and a liability to spontaneous haemorrhage.

TREATMENT

Despite being the commonest single type of brain tumour gliomas are the least satisfactory to treat and radical surgery is often misdirected.

Lobectomy. For well-circumscribed, low grade gliomas of frontal or occipital lobes.

Limited intracapsular removal. For palliation of symptoms or raised ICP because removing tumour mass will reduce brain volume.

Burr hole biopsy has the advantages of providing suitable material for histological grading and allowing drainage of cysts. Post-operative haemorrhage may be a problem and a rapid histological confirmation is useful in deciding whether to take further action.

PROGNOSIS

For Grade I astrocytomas the 3-year survival is about 60%, whereas it is only 4% for glioblastoma multiforme. Ependymomas and oligodendrogliomas behave like Grade I astrocytomas.

Medulloblastoma

Tumours of neuronal origin are much less common than of the neuroglia and occur only in children, being twice as common in boys. They arise in the posterior fossa, producing the typical clinical picture of a child with morning headache, vomiting and a staggering gait. Medulloblastomas are highly malignant, arising from the vermis of the cerebellum and the fourth ventricle, with subarachnoid seeding.

TREATMENT

Posterior fossa craniectomy. As much tumour as possible is excised without causing major cranial nerve deficits.

Radiotherapy. This is the most effective treatment, with irradiation of the whole neuroaxis in a spade-shaped field to cover the tendency for meningeal spread.

PROGNOSIS

Following surgery and radiotherapy 25–40% will survive 5 years but this may be improved in the future by the addition of chemotherapy.

Meningioma

SURGICAL PATHOLOGY

Meningiomas arise from meningothelial cells that occur in abundance at sites of arachnoid villi which accounts for their pattern of distribution which is (in descending order of frequency): parasagittal, convexity of cerebrum, sphenoidal wing, olfactory groove and suprasellar. Predisposing factors are trauma and female sex, and symptoms are exacerbated by pregnancy.

The tumour is well encapsulated, non-invasive and may grow to a large size without producing symptoms. The peripheral nature of meningiomas often causes bony changes with erosion, exostosis and increased vascularity.

TREATMENT

Total excision is often possible for parasagittal and convexity meningiomas. Haemorrhage from attached vessels, venous sinuses and hyperostotic bone is a common technical problem.

PROGNOSIS

80% of patients with a resected tumour will survive 5 years and recurrence is more a problem of incomplete excision than of spread of tumour.

Pituitary fossa tumours

SURGICAL PATHOLOGY

Chromophobe adenoma. 75% are non-functioning adenomas of polygonal cells, beginning in the pituitary gland and eroding the fossa. Some are cystic and may undergo necrosis and haemorrhage causing pituitary apoplexy.

Eosinophilic adenoma. These are comprised of granular cells, and most secrete growth hormone and increase in size and may grow large enough to cause chiasmal compression.

Craniopharyngioma (suprasellar cyst). Arise from Rathke's pouch, an embryological remnant of buccal ectoderm that forms the anterior lobe of the pituitary gland. The majority occur in children, are cystic and become calcified.

CLINICAL SYNDROMES

Hypopituitarism is more common than acromegaly, giantism (prepuberty) or Cushing's syndrome, because of the frequency of non-secreting chromophobe adenomas.

Bitemporal hemianopia follows bilateral medial compression of the optic chiasm.

Obstructive hydrocephalus and cavernous sinus syndrome may follow suprasellar extension of the tumour.

TREATMENT

Approaches may be:

1. *Frontal craniotomy* and retraction of frontal lobe with intracapsular aspiration or excision of tumour. This method is, however, associated with a high incidence of impaired visual acuity.
2. *Transethmoidal approach* using the operating microscope allows excision of any suprasellar extension with fewer visual and epileptic complications. CSF rhinorrhoea and meningitis are rare complications.
3. *Radiotherapy* is useful, as pituitary tumours are radiosensitive, and it is particularly valuable when surgical excision is not complete.

Acoustic neuroma

These arise in the neurilemmal sheath of the vestibular component of the eighth cranial nerve, within the internal auditory meatus growing slowly to fill the cerebellopontine angle, causing seventh, fifth and third pressure effects on the cranial nerves in that order. Patients present with tinnitus, deafness and vertigo, and often cerebellar ataxia and nystagmus can be demonstrated. An absent corneal reflex (V) is pathognomonic. Tomograms of the auditory meatus and CT scan are diagnostic.

TREATMENT

Posterior fossa craniectomy and total excision is the curative treatment, but makes seventh nerve palsy inevitable. There is a significant risk of brain stem damage, temporary bulbar palsy or ataxia. A total excision in two stages using the operating microscope gives better results in younger patients.

INTRACRANIAL ABSCESS

Surgical pathology.

Intracranial abscesses develop as the consequence of spread of infection from:

1. Chronic suppurative otitis media
2. Acute frontal sinusitis
3. Haematogenous spread from heart, especially congenital cyanotic heart disease

4. Trauma: surgical or open fracture

In a number of instances the abscess is cryptogenic—source unknown

Anatomically three intracranial planes may be involved:

1. *Extradural* due to osteomyelitis, otitis media or sinusitis
2. *Subdural* due to thrombophlebitis of superior sagittal sinuses with spread over the convexity of the brain
3. *Parenchymal* involving the brain substance and the result of trauma or haematogenous spread

The common causative organisms are streptococci (sinusitis), *B. proteus* and *Bacteroides* (otitis media) and *Staphylococcus* (trauma and haematogenous). Many abscesses are sterile following prolonged courses of antibiotics.

Clinical Features

Extradural (See Pott's puffy tumour p. 85).

Subdural. The patient is often quite toxic, dehydrated with signs of raised ICP and epilepsy.

Parenchymal. Generally a more subacute presentation, with general malaise, headache, irritability and pyrexia. Lateralizing signs give a clue to the diagnosis and the site of the abscess. The combination of cyanotic heart disease, pyrexia and neurological signs is pathognomonic.

Investigations

Lumbar puncture helps in excluding meningitis, and in abscess the protein is usually elevated.

EEG will demonstrate an abnormal focus.

CT scan. A contrast enhanced study shows a typical 'halo' of radiodensity around a radioluscent mass.

Treatment

All operative procedures are covered by parenteral antibiotics and these agents may also be used for wound irrigation post-operatively.

Extradural abscess. Excision of the osteomyelitic bone and drainage.

Subdural abscess. Multiple burr holes may be necessary for adequate drainage, combined with antibiotic lavage.

Parenchymal abscess. Burr hole aspiration which it is often necessary to repeat on two or three separate occasions. Excision and decompression of multiple small abscesses may be necessary.

Complications

Epilepsy is a common and troublesome sequel, particularly for frontal and temporal lobe abscesses.

VASCULAR DISORDERS

The consequences of an intracranial vascular disorder are inevitably some form of vascular accident or stroke which may be either haemorrhagic (subarachnoid or intracerebral) or ischaemic (vascular occlusion or perfusion failure). Lesions which may be surgically corrected include: aneurysms, arteriovenous malformations and occlusive vascular disease.

INTRACRANIAL ANEURYSMS

Surgical pathology

Saccular aneurysms account for the majority of cases, although atheromatous and mycotic aneurysms sometimes occur.

Factors relating to the propensity for aneurysm formation on the circle of Willis are:

1. Weakness of the vessel wall
2. Muscle deformity at junctions
3. Poorly-developed media
4. Single layer of internal elastic lamina

All these factors are aggravated by systemic hypertension and stresses of local haemodynamics.

Common sites of aneurysm formation are: anterior communicating arteries; junctions of middle cerebral and posterior communicating arteries; and basilar artery.

Supratentorially, the anterior communicating aneurysm is commonest and infratentorially, basilar artery aneurysms. 10–15% of patients have multiple aneurysms.

Clinical features

The presentation is a consequence of either rupture, or pressure effects from increase in size.

Rupture. Most rupture into the subarachnoid space presenting with sudden onset of severe headache and nuchal rigidity. Obstructive hydrocephalus may be a late sequel of subarachnoid haemorrhage.

Enlargement. Compression of neighbouring structures may cause signs e.g. aneurysms in the region of the cavernous sinus compress the fifth, third, fourth and sixth cranial nerves causing facial pain and extra-ocular myopathy.

Investigations

Lumbar puncture. Evenly bloodstained CSF is present with subarachnoid haemorrhage.

Bilateral carotid angiography. This is vital to confirm the presence of an aneurysm and determine operability for supratentorial lesions.

Vertebral angiography. Important to exclude the possibility of a basilar artery aneurysm which is less amenable to surgery.

Treatment

Conservative. Once the diagnosis of aneurysm has been established and the site is determined, the patient undergoes a period of conservative treatment, before surgery, which includes bed rest, control of hypertension and anti-fibrinolytic therapy (aminocaproic acid) in an attempt to consolidate any clot that has arrested the bleeding. Mortality from initial haemorrhage is 20% and a further 40% die in the subsequent 8 weeks from recurrent haemorrhage without adequate treatment.

Surgical. Operative treatment of the aneurysm, if accessible, is the ultimate treatment of choice. *Clipping the neck of the aneurysm* using a spring-loaded metal clip is the operation of choice. The operative mortality is 10% and the morbidity is low.

Wrapping the aneurysm with synthetic thrombogenic mesh or muscle or ligature of the proximal and distal feeding vessels are alternative procedures. For large aneurysms of the carotid siphon, ligation of the internal carotid artery in the neck may be necessary.

ARTERIOVENOUS MALFORMATIONS

Surgical pathology

These lesions are hamartomatous collections of capillaries with tiny arteriovenous communications, located almost exclusively in the cerebral hemispheres of the parietal and occipital lobes.

Clinical features

The majority of patients present with a haemorrhage, usually subarachnoid, but epilepsy or migrainous headaches may also occur. A cranial bruit is diagnostic and calcification is often present on a plain X-ray. Because the prognosis is much better it is important to differentiate malformations from aneurysms by bilateral carotid angiography.

Treatment

Surgical excision or ligation of the feeding vessels is performed depending on the site of the malformation.

VASCULAR OCCLUSIVE DISEASE

Transient ischaemic attacks (TIAs), which present as either temporary loss of sensation or power or amaurosis fugax, are most often caused by impaired cerebral perfusion or showers of thrombo-embolii. Lesions at the bifurcation of the internal carotid artery, either atheromatous stenosis or ulceration, may be demonstrated in these patients, and treated surgically by carotid endarterectomy (see also p. 279). However, as many as 20–30% of these patients may also have an incomplete occlusion of intracranial vessels especially the middle cerebral artery, demonstrable on carotid angiography. Such well-circumscribed stenoses of intracranial vessels may be treated surgically in an attempt to improve perfusion distal to the stenosis.

Extracranial–intracranial anastamosis between superficial temporal and middle cerebral arteries via a burr hole, and using a vein graft, is performed by a team of vascular surgeons and neurosurgeons. The early results are encouraging.

17

Face, lip, tongue, and mouth

Numerous conditions of the face, lip, tongue and mouth occur but only the more common disorders will be discussed in this chapter. In assessing lesions of this area, it is vital that a thorough examination of the mouth and both surfaces of the tongue is performed which, as with the anus, requires a good light and digital and bimanual examination.

CLASSIFICATION

Congenital disorders

Cleft lip and palate
Pre-auricular sinus
Tongue tie
Congenital fissured tongue

Inflammations

Facial infections
Glossitis
Stomatitis
Ulcers of the tongue

Cysts

Retention cyst of buccal mucous gland
Ranula
Sublingual dermoid

Carcinoma of the lip, tongue and floor of mouth

CONGENITAL DISORDERS

Cleft lip and palate

Cleft lip, cleft palate and combinations of the two are second only to club feet in frequency as congenital anomalies, the reported incidence being 1 in every 600–800 live births.

SURGICAL ANATOMY
The key to understanding the failure of embryological coalescence that results in cleft deformities is the *incisive foramen* which is in the hard palate just behind the incisor teeth. Anterior to the incisive foramen is the *primary palate* comprising the alveolus and lip. Posteriorly is the *secondary palate*, which is formed by medial growth of two shelves from the maxillary arches, comprising the hard and soft palate. The fusion of these shelves is usually complete by the 9th week in the foetus.

CLASSIFICATION
Clefts of the lip and palate may be:

a. *Partial or complete* depending whether primary or secondary palate is involved (partial) or both are involved (complete)
b. *Unilateral or bilateral*. Left clefts outnumber both right and bilateral clefts. The most common anomaly is a left complete cleft involving the lip, alveolus and hard and soft palate.

PREDISPOSING FACTORS
Factors known to be related to an increased incidence of clefts are:

a. Male sex
b. Previous family history
c. Exposure to X-rays, corticosteroids or viral infection (especially rubella) in the first trimester

PROBLEMS OF FUNCTION

1. **Feeding Difficulties.** Because with a cleft palate the baby cannot suck, breast feeding may be impossible and special teats, bottles and even an obturator may be required to aid feeding and sucking. Cleft lips do not usually present any major problem with feeding.

2. **Speech.** Consonants cannot be pronounced adequately with a cleft palate and speech therapy is required after closure.

3. **Dentition**. Abnormalities in the growth of teeth occur with alveolar deformity and corrective splints are required.

4. **Hearing**. Secondary oedema of the Eustachian tubes causes some hearing loss.

TREATMENT

Surgical reconstruction is the treatment of choice and satisfactory functional results are achieved in 70–90% of cases.

The aims of reconstruction are to:

a. Improve appearance, with restoration of the Cupid's bow of the lip
b. Correct any associated misshape of the nose
c. Achieve adequate speech and dentition

The timing of reconstruction depends on the anomaly.

1. **Cleft lip**. Use rule of tens; weight is greater than 5 kg, haemoglobin is at least 10 g/dl and baby is over 10 weeks old.

2. **Cleft palate**. The repair is performed when the baby is between 1 and 1½ years of age.

Principles of repair

1. **Cleft lip**. Millard's operation has stood the test of time and employs a medial Z-shaped incision in the cleft in order to rotate the Cupid's bow down to a normal position.

2. **Cleft palate**. Bilateral releasing incisions are made in the roof of the mouth, to allow extensive mobilization of the palatal muscles to achieve midline apposition. Revision procedures may be required in later years to improve appearance and function, especially for speech defects.

Pre-auricular sinus

This anomaly results from imperfect fusion of the tubercles of the first branchial cleft during formation of the pinna. The result is a discharging sinus or a cyst that forms at the root of the helix or on the tragus. Treatment involves complete excision of the sinus tract to prevent infective complications.

Tongue tie

A short fraenum linguae is a rare condition that produces more concern to the mother than the child. Despite its popular name—tongue tie—shortening of the fraenum effects neither speech nor feeding, and pleas of the mother to have it divided should be strongly resisted as sepsis, fibrosis and severe tethering of the tongue may occur post-operatively.

Congenital fissured tongue

Fissuring of the tongue is a feature of congenital syphilis, but a far more common cause is *congenital furrowing*. The syphilic fissures are longitudinal whereas congenital furrows are transverse and the latter may also be associated with *geographical tongue* due to hypertrophy of the filiform papillae around the periphery of the tongue.

INFLAMMATION

Facial infections

Though acne vulgaris is by far the most common type of infection of the face, the surgeon is rarely involved in its management. More important are boils and carbuncles that occur in the *danger or mask area* of the face. Deep venous communications of the anterior facial vein at the medial canthus, via the angular vein, with the ophthalmic veins and of the deep facial vein with the pterygoid plexus may result in spread of infection to the cavernous sinus. Thrombosis of the cavernous sinus causes localizing neurological signs (see p. 86) and in the pre-antibiotic era was fatal.

Treatment is prevention, achieved by the patient resisting the temptation to squeeze septic lesions, by improving skin hygiene and by administering broad spectrum antibiotics when infection of the mask area persists.

Glossitis

Acute superficial glossitis. This is caused by minor trauma and scalds or by a herpes simplex virus. Treatment is with mouth washes.

Acute parenchymal glossitis. Typically this follows an insect bite of the tongue with acute pain and swelling. Subcutaneous adrenalin relieves the allergic vasodilatation. Rarely pyogenic infections or Vincent's angina involve the tongue.

Furring of the tongue. May be present in dehydrated, malnourished patients with poor oral hygiene or those acutely ill with peritonitis. The furring is a consequence of accumulation of food debris and desquamated cells and an overgrowth of bacteria. The condition is more a sign of underlying disease than an entity in itself and treatment should be directed at the disease process.

Chronic superficial glossitis (leukoplakia). See below.

Stomatitis

VINCENT'S ANGINA

This condition is more accurately described as *ulcero-membranous stomatitis* and occurs exclusively in young adults, with their own teeth, as a consequence of poor oral hygiene and untreated dental caries. Bacteriologically there is an overgrowth of *Borrelia vincenti*, an anaerobic spirochaete and *Fusiformis fusiformis*, an anaerobic spindle-shaped Gram negative baccillus.

Clinical features

General malaise and pyrexia progress to toothache and bleeding gums. The patient has a foul-smelling breath and the gums are inflamed and covered with a yellow-white pseudomembrane, which when wiped off reveals superficial ulceration. There may be extension on to the cheek, fauces and palate, but rarely the tongue, and associated tender cervical lymphadenopathy. In neglected instances further spread takes place in the fascial planes of the neck and threatens the airway.

Treatment

Mouthwashes with dilute hydrogen peroxide and parenteral penicillin. When the acute phase has settled oral hygiene is improved and carious teeth are extracted. Incision is rarely needed.

APHTHOUS STOMATITIS

'Aphthous' is a term used to describe non-specific ulceration of the mouth, and translated literally from the Greek means 'mouth ulcers'. Three ages of man are inflicted by three different causes. Babies in the first few weeks of life may develop monilial stomitis, with white furry plaques on the mouth, tongue and lips. Treatment is with nystatin drops. In pre-school children aphthous ulcers caused by viral infections are not uncommon and are best treated symptomatically with a choline salicylate paste (Bonjela) to aid healing. Adults, particularly women, may develop recurrent ulceration of the cheek, tongue or lip which may also be associated with ulcers of the labia. The cause is unknown and the treatment symptomatic. Gonorrhoea and syphilis should be excluded in the promiscuous adult.

NUTRITIONAL STOMATITIS

Vitamin B complex and Vitamin C deficiencies, pellegra and scurvy respectively, will cause stomatitis and, though an uncommon presentation *de novo*, may be observed in malnourished patients on prolonged parenteral nutrition without adequate vitamin replacement.

CHEILOSIS

Another term of Greek derivation meaning 'lip ulcer' but commonly called *angular stomatitis*, cheilosis is common in the very young and the very old. In children streptococcal and monilial infections may be causative whereas in the elderly it is usually due to overclosure of the lips in the edentulous. Angular stomatitis may be a manifestation of syphilis.

Ulcers of the tongue

Carcinoma, syphilis and tuberculosis should always be considered possible diagnosis when managing a patient with an ulcer on the tongue. Therefore a biopsy, VDRL and Mantoux tests should be performed for deep ulcers, those with signs of proliferation and when neck glands are enlarged. Other common causes of tongue ulcers are:

a. *Dental ulcers*, caused by sharp teeth or illfitting dentures.
b. *Chronic non-specific ulcer*, usually on the tip of the tongue
c. *Apthous ulcers*

Local application of choline salicylate paste is the treatment of choice when a specific cause has been excluded.

CYSTS

Retention cyst of buccal mucous gland

Accumulation of fluid in an obstructed mucous gland causes a cystic swelling on the inner aspect of the lip. Treatment is excision.

Ranula

This is a transparent cyst which develops in the floor of the mouth, probably from embryological cellular rests or blocked minor salivary glands. A ranula may be *simple*, presenting in the floor of the mouth or *plunging* when it may present also as a neck swelling. Simple ranulae are best treated by marsupialisation via the mouth; plunging ranulae by excision via the neck (see p. 101).

Sublingual dermoid (see p. 100)

CARCINOMA OF THE LIP, TONGUE AND FLOOR OF MOUTH

These cancers are less frequent than formerly, which is due largely to better oral hygiene and a reduction in the incidence of syphilis. It is interesting to note however that whereas 50 years ago carcinoma in these regions was ten times more common in males the incidence is now equal in both sexes.

PREDISPOSING FACTORS

Leukoplakia

This simply means a 'white plaque' and is fundamentally an increased keratinizing process of the superficial cells of the epidermis which may be a local physiological response to a chronic irritant. The condition is premalignant and the frequency of neoplastic change is about 25%.

Macroscopically there are two outstanding features, a 'cracked white paint' appearance areas of grey white plaques of abnormal keratinizing epithelium; and the 'raw beef' appearance which represents areas of shed plaques.

Microscopically the epithelium shows hyperplasia and all degrees of cellular atypicality ranging from mild dysplasia to carcinoma-in-situ.

Chronic irritation

This may result from oral sepsis, stumps of teeth, smoking, spirits, syphilis, poorly fitting dentures, or check biting.

SURGICAL PATHOLOGY

Macroscopic features

1. Ulcer—with raised irregular rolled margin and red indurated base
2. Fissure—chronic in nature with no signs of healing
3. Protuberant lesion—varying from a small projection beyond the surface to a large verrucous or 'cauliflower-like' mass

Microscopic features

Virtually all are squamous call carcinomata with typical tongue-like projections of cells into the dermis or further. Transverse sections of these projections produce cell nests or epithelial pearls with their inner older cells showing keratinization and outer younger cells grouped in an 'onion-skin-like' manner.

Spread

1. Direct

a. Lip—through the substance of the lip and if untreated may involve the cheek, gum and alveolus
b. Tongue—through the substance of the tongue to involve the floor of the mouth, alveolus, tonsillar region and palate. Involvement of the lingual nerve may cause pain to be referred to the ear by way of the auriculo-temporal nerve.

2. Lymphatic

a. Lip—only 10% have evidence of spread to the submental or submandibular lymph nodes by one year. Drainage is sometimes contralateral.
b. Tongue—spread is earlier than with lip. The tip drains bilaterally to the submental lymph nodes and the posterior third of the tongue drains bilaterally to the upper deep cervical lymph nodes, while the anterior two-thirds drains unilaterally to the submandibular lymph nodes and thence to the deep cervical chain. Ultimately all lymph drainage from the tongue reaches the jugulo-omohyoid gland in the deep cervical chain (Fig. 17.1).

The submandibular lymph node is normally palpable if the bimanual method is used. However, it is soft and usually less than 1 cm in diameter.

Invasion of a lymph node by tumour cells causes it to be larger and firmer than normal. Later it becomes fixed to surrounding structures.

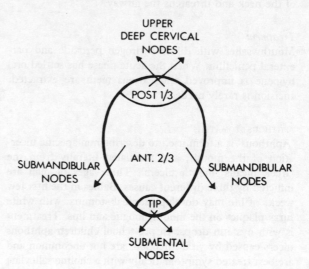

Fig. 17.1 Lymph drainage of the tongue

3. Blood

This is extremely rare, as local and lymphatic spread, and recurrence of disease, nearly always occur above the clavicles.

DIFFERENTIAL DIAGNOSIS

Lip

1. Benign chronic fissures and ulcers
2. Benign tumours; papilloma, haemangioma, lymphangioma, fibroma
3. Syphilitic chancre which is rare and usually on the upper lip

Tongue and floor of the mouth

1. Fissures—leukoplakia, congenital, tuberculosis, syphilitic
2. Dental ulcers—related to decayed or broken teeth or poorly fitting dentures
3. Dyspeptic (aphthous) ulcers—tiny punched-out white-based painful ulcers surrounded by erythema
4. Tumours—papilloma, haemangioma, fibroma, lipoma, rhabdomyoma, mixed salivary

TREATMENT

Prophylaxis

1. Remove the sources of chronic irritation
2. Biopsy suspicious lesions
3. Excise unresolving or suspicious areas of leukoplakia
4. Stop smoking

Curative treatment

1. *Early cases.* When the primary lesion is small, without infiltration of surrounding structures and when any involved lymph nodes are freely mobile then the following treatment is indicated:

   a. *Primary lesion.* Surgery or radiotherapy are probably equally effective. However, 'tridimensional excision' seems currently the treatment of choice.
   b. *Lymph nodes.* If cervical nodes remain enlarged and firm after the primary lesion has been healed for three weeks and if infection and post-irradiation effects on the nodes have been eliminated, then either a suprahyoid or complete neck dissection of the deep cervical lymph nodes is indicated.

   If cervical nodes are impalpable or clinically normal then 'prophylactic' excision is unnecessary but careful follow up is indicated.

2. *Late cases.* When there is massive growth and/or bony involvement, or recurrence after previous treatment then:

   a. *Primary lesion.* Surgery is indicated. This may entail resection and the use of full-thickness skin flaps for a lip lesion or an *en bloc* removal of half the tongue, mandible and floor of the mouth for a laterally-placed tongue lesion.
   b. *Lymph nodes.* If the deep cervical lymph nodes are fixed then surgery is contraindicated and radiotherapy is used. If the nodes are still mobile then they may be excised in continuity with the advanced primary lesion. A combined excision of primary tumour and block dissection of the deep cervical nodes, with the removal of part of the intervening body of the mandible, is called a *composite excision*. It is popularly refered to as a 'commando' operation and is best performed by a team of general, plastic and oral surgeons, the patient requiring a temporary tracheostomy and intensive post-operative physio- and speech therapy.

PROGNOSIS

Lip

There is an 80% 5-year cure with surgery or radiotherapy when cervical lymph nodes are not involved.

Tongue and floor of the mouth

This depends on the following factors:

1. *Site*
a. Anterior growth—50% 5-year cure
b. Posterior growth—10% 5-year cure
2. *Stage*
a. Early—60% 5-year cure
b. Late—15% 5-year cure
3. *Nodes*
a. Involved—15% 5-year cure
b. Not involved—60% 5-year cure

LYMPHATICS OF HEAD AND NECK

Lymphatic drainage from carcinoma of the head and neck ultimately reaches the deep cervical chain of lymph nodes which surround the length of the internal jugular veins from the base of the skull to the root of the neck. Jugular lymph trunks are then formed which empty into the thoracic duct on the left side and the internal jugular or innominate vein on the right side.

The arrangement of the head and neck lymphatics can be conveniently separated into two groups:

1. Vertical group

These are the deep cervical nodes. They are not arranged orderly about the internal jugular vein but three of them are named:

a. Jugulo-digastric node which lies below the posterior belly of the digastric muscle as it crosses the internal jugular vein. It is also called the tonsillar lymph node and receives lymph drainage from the tonsil.

b. Jugulo-omohyoid node which is behind the internal jugular vein where it is crossed by the inferior belly of the omohyoid muscle. All the lymph from the tongue ultimately reaches this node.

c. Supraclavicular nodes which extend from the nodes around the inferior part of the internal jugular vein, behind the sterno-mastoid muscle into the supraclavicular region.

2. Circular group

There are three 'circles' of lymphatics and with few exceptions they drain into the nearest nodes of the vertical group.

a. Innermost circle. This surrounds the pharynx and trachea and comprises the following nodes:

(i) Retropharyngeal
(ii) Paratracheal
(iii) Pretracheal

b. Inner circle. This is situated in the nasopharynx, is sometimes called *Waldeyer's ring* and comprises the following:

(i) Tubal tonsils
(ii) Nasopharyngeal tonsil (adenoids)
(iii) Pharyngeal tonsils
(iv) Lingual tonsil

Strictly speaking these are not lymph nodes but collections of lymphoid tissue.

c. Outer circle. This is made of superficially situated glands around the head and jaw and comprises the following:

(i) Occipital
(ii) Mastoid
(iii) Pre-auricular
(iv) Parotid
(v) Submandibular
(vi) Submental

BLOCK DISSECTION OF DEEP CERVICAL LYMPH NODES

In the slowly growing tumours of the lip and face and the more rapidly growing tumours of the tongue and floor of the mouth after radiotherapy, the lymph nodes of the neck should be removed if there is clinical evidence of nodal metastases, whilst the nodes remain mobile. Radiotherapy to nodes greater than 2 cm in diameter is unlikely to be successful. The presence of distant metastasis from the primary tumour obviates the operation.

The operation entails removal *en bloc* of the deep cervical lymphatic chain together with the internal jugular vein, sternomastoid, omohyoid and digastric muscles, the submandibular lymph and salivary glands, submental lymph glands, the lower pole of the parotid gland, the deep cervical fascia and cervical nerve plexus. The dissection extends from the midline of the neck up to the mandible, down to the clavicle and back to the anterior border of the trapezius muscle.

Special complications of block dissection

1. NERVES
Damage may occur to the following nerves:

a. Glossopharyngeal, vagus, hypoglossal or lingual nerves
b. Accessory as it penetrates the sternomastoid
c. Phrenic nerve
d. Mandibular branch of the facial nerve
e. Cervical sympathetics
f. Brachial plexus

2. THORACIC DUCT
A chylous (lymphatic) fistula may result

3. SKIN FLAP NECROSIS

4. SECONDARY HAEMORRHAGE
Infection and skin flap necrosis may result in the erosion of the underlying unprotected carotid artery.

5. VENOUS CONGESTION OF HEAD
Cyanosis and oedema of the face are likely to occur if a bilateral neck dissection is performed at one operation.

This fearsome list of complications notwithstanding, the surgery of malignancy of the head and neck has been made much more acceptable by primary repairs using skin flaps mobilized from the forehead and acromiothoracic region. The principle upon which these flaps are based is simple—they have a large artery and accompanying vein in their base so that they are both well vascularized and drained. Consequently, they can be made relatively long for their width. They are used both for *lining* inside the mouth and pharynx and for *cover* over large surface defects.

18

Neck swellings

Swellings in the neck are the result of a great variety of conditions, either specific to the region or part of systemic disease.

SURGICAL ANATOMY

The sternomastoid muscles on either side of the neck divide it into two anatomical triangles as they incline backwards from the clavicle and sternum inferiorly to the mastoid process of the temporal bone superiorly. (Fig. 18.1A)

These two triangles are further subdivided by two muscles which cross them—the anterior triangle is divided across by the anterior belly of the diagastric muscle, the space superiorly being called the submandibular triangle, the inferior space the carotid triangle. The posterior triangle is crossed by the amohyoid muscle which seperates the subclavian triangle from the occipital triangle (Fig. 18.1B).

The sternomastoid muscles are enveloped in the deep cervical fascia which splits to enclose them. By putting the muscles on the stretch it is possible to diagnose whether a swelling is superficial to or deep to the cervical fascia.

Swellings which are superficial to the deep fascia are not specific to the neck.

Swellings superficial to the deep fascia

1. Epidermoid (Sebaceous) cysts
2. Lipomata
3. Carbuncles
4. Neurofibromata

Masses deep to the deep fascia

1. Midline swellings
2. Lateral swellings

The former term may be slightly misleading as swellings nearly always deviate to one side or the other. It is

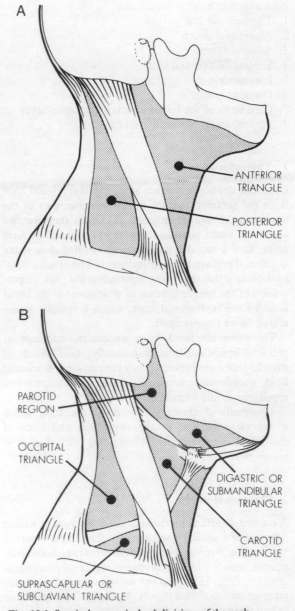

Fig. 18.1 Surgical anatomical subdivisions of the neck

A
ANTERIOR TRIANGLE
POSTERIOR TRIANGLE

B
PAROTID REGION
OCCIPITAL TRIANGLE
DIGASTRIC OR SUBMANDIBULAR TRIANGLE
CAROTID TRIANGLE
SUPRASCAPULAR OR SUBCLAVIAN TRIANGLE

better to think of masses arising from either *unpaired midline* structures or *paired lateral* structures.

PATHOLOGICAL FEATURES AND GENERAL MANAGEMENT

Table 18.1 summarizes the clinical features of the common neck swellings outlined below.

MIDLINE SWELLINGS

FROM UNPAIRED MIDLINE STRUCTURES

1. Thyroglossal cyst
2. Pharyngeal pouch
3. Subhyoid bursa
4. Sublingual dermoid cyst
5. Laryngocele
6. Plunging ranula
7. Carcinoma of the larynx, trachea and oesophagus
8. Perichondritis of the thyroid cartilage

1. Thyroglossal cyst

Cysts can develop anywhere along the thyroglossal tract from the foramen caecum in the posterior part of the tongue to the thyroid isthmus. However, they are rare above the hyoid bone and appear in childhood or early adult life as a rounded tense smooth swelling close to the midline. They are rarely translucent. The specific diagnostic test is that they move upwards in the neck on protrusion of the tongue because of attachment to the hyoid bone by the thyroglossal tract, which is usually degenerated into a fibrous band.

The cysts are lined by a squamous, columnar or cuboidal epithelium and occasionally small islands of thyroid tissue are present. They contain clear or mucoid fluid, occasionally clotted blood and are susceptable to sepsis and fistula formation.

Treatment of choice is Sistrunk's operation which incorporates excision of the cyst, tract and body of the hyoid in continuity, eliminating the chance of recurrence.

2. Pharyngeal pouch

A pulsion diverticulum through the dehiscence of Killian (triangle of Lannier) a weakness in the posterior part of the pharynx, between two components of the inferior constrictor muscle (thyro-pharyngeus and crico-pharyngeus muscles) (Fig. 18.2). Failure of relaxation of the lower component (crico-pharyngeus) during swallowing initiates pouch formation.

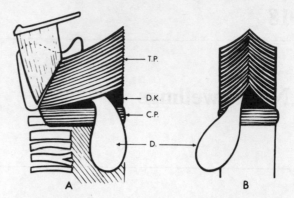

Fig. 18.2 Pharyngeal diverticulum *A*. Left lateral view: T.P. = thyropharyngeus part of the inferior constrictor; D.K. = dehiscence of Killian; C.P. = cricopharyngeus portion of the inferior constrictor; D. = pharyngeal diverticulum *B*. Posterior view

The pouch usually presents on the left side of the neck. It is a thin walled mucosal sac, only the neck of which has muscle. Depending on its size, it will be associated with regurgitation or obstruction. Rarely malignant change can occur.

Treatment is excision of the pouch and cricopharyngeal myotomy.

3. Subhyoid bursa

These are rarely enlarged. The bursa is found between the hyoid body and the thyro-hyoid membrane and may present as a soft fluctuant swelling just below the hyoid. When greatly enlarged it may become transversly sausage-shaped.

4. Sublingual dermoid cyst

Can be midline or lateral, above or below the mylohyoid muscle. When midline and sub-mylohyoid it may protrude beneath the symphysis menti. They are considered to be developmental abnormalities.

5. Laryngocele

This is not common but may occur in players of wind instruments. It arises as a herniation of the laryngeal mucosa through the thyrohyoid membrane and presents as a tense translucent swelling below the hyoid. It can be emptied by compression but re-inflates when the patient coughs. On occasion it can be so large as to extend over the front of the neck.

6. Plunging ranula

A term applied to a cystic swelling because of a salivary duct blockage in the floor of the mouth which is said to look like a frog's throat pouch. It is not necessarily a major salivary duct which is blocked but one of the accessory ducts. Therefore there may be no involvement of the salivary glands themselves. The ranula itself is a bluish-grey translucent fluctuant swelling covered by mucous membrane, which may burrow through between the muscle fibres of the mylohyoid and appear in the neck.

7. Carcinoma of the laryngx, trachea and oesophagus

This is a rare cause of midline or paramedian swellings and usually presents with primary features not related to the lump in the neck but of the more general features of a neoplasm affecting the laryngeal structures such as the vocal cords, with hoarseness, dyspnoea and occasionally dysphagia.

8. Perichondritis of the thyroid cartilage

A rare post traumatic affliction entirely benign and worthy of no further comment.

LATERAL SWELLINGS

FROM PAIRED LATERAL STRUCTURES
1. Lymph nodes
2. Thyroid swellings
3. Salivary gland swellings
4. Branchial cysts
5. Sternomastoid tumour
6. Cervical rib
7. Cystic hygroma
8. Aneurysm and a.v. fistula
9. Carotid body tumour
10. Actinomycosis
11. Muscle tumours
12. Clavicular tumours
13. Spinal abscesses

1. Lymph nodes

These form the commonest swellings in the neck. The involvement of nodes is usually secondary to either inflammatory or neoplastic process in the organs which they drain. Same conditions, though they are not necessarily confined to the neck e.g. lymphosarcoma, Hodgkin's disease.

INFLAMMATION

Acute lymphadenitis

Involvement of the deep cervical glands is common with infections of the face, gums, teeth and pharynx. The glands are painful and tender when acutely inflamed.

Chronic lymphadenitis

This is now uncommon in Western countries. Tuberculosis is the main cause. The node is part of a primary focus, with the tonsil the site of entry and the node usually being the jugulo-digastric. These nodes are painless, initially freely mobile but later becoming fixed and matted. If caseation occurs, the node may break down and form a *cold abscess*. If the abscess tracks to the skin of the neck it forms a subcutaneous collection which is called, because of the constriction at the point of penetration through the deep fascia, a 'collar stud' abscess.

NEOPLASM

Lymphatic metastases from scalp, face, lip, tongue, floor of mouth, tonsil, pharynx, larynx, thyroid, stomach, breast and lung result in hard fixed painless swellings. Of this group, two are worthy of particular note:

a. *'Lateral aberrant thyroid'*— so called because when excised the histology is difficult to distinguish from normal thyroid. However, the cause is a lymph node involved by papillary carcinoma of the thyroid gland.

b. *'Troisier's sign'*—an enlarged node in the left supraclavicular fossa in carcinoma of the stomach or other intra-abdominal organs. (Virchows node)

SYSTEMIC DISEASE

As part of a generalized lymphadenopathy the patient may have one of the following diseases.

a Lymphatic leukaemia
b Hodgkin's disease
c Lymphoma
d Lymphosarcoma
e Secondary syphilis
f Amyloid disease
g German measles
h Still's disease
i Glandular fever
j Plague
k Tubercle
l Sarcoidosis
m Toxoplasmosis
n Skin sepsis (e.g. scabies)
o Catscratch disease

2. Thyroid swellings

See Chapter 19.

Table 18.1 Diagnosis of neck swellings

		Lateral	Midline
A. History			
1. Age	Newborn	Sternomastoid tumour	
	Infancy	Cystic hygroma	
	Childhood	Lymphadenitis (including T.B.)	Thyroglossal cyst
			Sublingual dermoid
	Adults	Lymphadenitis	
		Salivary gland	Goitre
		Reticulosis	
		Carotid body tumour	
	Older adults	Secondary malignancy	Goitre
2. Duration	Days	Salivary calculus	Haemorrhage in
		Lymphadenitis	thyroid cyst
	Weeks	Chronic lymphadenitis	
	Months	Chronic lymphadenitis	
		Secondary malignancy	
		Reticulosis	
	Years	Branchial cyst	Goitre
		Pharyngeal pouch	Thyroglossal cyst
			Plunging ranula
			Dermoid cyst
3. Pain		Inflammation	
		Salivary calculus	Inflammation
4. Associated symptoms	Regurgitation	Pharyngeal pouch	
	Dysphagia	Secondary malignancy	
	Dysphonia		Goitre, particularly
	Dyspnoea		retrosternal
	Horner's syndrome		or
	Facial nerve lesion	Parotid carcinoma	malignant
	Brachial plexus lesion	Cervical rib	
		Subclavian aneurysm	
	Raynaud's phenomenon		
	Hemiparesis	Carotid body tumour	
	Exophthalmos		Toxic goitre
	Excessive sweating		
	Tremor		
	Nervousness		
	Weight loss		
B. Local examination			
1. Number	Multiple	Lymphadenitis	
		Reticulosis	
		Secondary malignancy	
2. Site	Behind ramus mandible	Parotid gland	
		Preauricular node	
	Level of greater cornu	Tonsillar node	Subhyoid bursa
		Branchial cyst	Laryngocele
	Beneath chin		Submental node
			Plunging ranula
			Sublingual dermoid
	Level of thyroid cartilage	Carotid body tumour	Goitre
			Thyroglossal cyst
	Supraclavicular	Supraclavicular nodes	
		Cervical rib	
		Subclavian aneurysm	

Table 18.1 (*continued*)

	Lateral		Midline
3. Size	Large	Hodgkin's disease	Goitre
4. Shape	May conform to an anatomical structure, e.g. thyroid gland, bifurcation of common carotid artery, parotid gland, submandibular gland		
5. Surface	Smooth with cysts, lipomata, lymph nodes Irregular and nodular with malignancy		
6. Swallowing	Midline swellings moving vertically with swallowing are usually thyroid or thyroglossal in origin		

7. Tenderness	Indicates inflammation
	    e.g. lymphadenitis
	        infected branchial or thyroglossal cyst
	        subacute thyroiditis		

8. Temperature	Indicates inflammation, but also may be present in highly vascular goitres.		
9. Transillumination	Of little value in neck. Cystic hygromas are brilliantly translucent, as are plunging ranulas in the mouth		
10. Tethering	To skin—consider sebaceous cyst, T.B., lymphadenitis To muscle—consider sternomastoid 'tumour' and malignancy To carotid artery—consider carotid body tumour		
11. Thrill	Vascular goitre. Aneurysm.		

12. Colour	Reddened skin over lump indicates inflammation
	    Consider—sebaceous cyst
	            lymphadenitis
	            branchial cyst
	            thyroglossal cyst.		

13. Consistency	Hard—calcified nodes, malignancy Tense—cyst Rubbery—branchial cyst, Hodgkin's disease Soft—lipoma		
14. Fluctuation	Some cysts		
15. Pulsation	Expansile pulsation may be elicited with vascular goitres, subclavian or innominate artery aneurysms Transmitted pulsation will occur with lumps situated over major vessels		
16. Percussion	Some laryngoceles may be tympanitic		
17. Protrusion of tongue	A thyroglossal cyst will usually move upwards when the tongue is protruded as it is attached by a fibrous cord to the hyoid bone		
18. Pressure over lump	If lump disappears with pressure, consider pharyngeal pouch, laryngocele or branchial cyst with a pharyngeal communication		
19. Auscultation	A bruit may be heard over a vascular goitre or over a stenotic carotid artery bifurcation		

20. Aspiration	This may be considered if a cystic swelling is present
	    Pus—suppurative adenitis or cyst
	    Pus-like—branchial cyst
	    Straw coloured or clear—cystic hygroma
	    'Toothpaste' like—sebaceous cyst.		

3. Salivary gland swellings

Swelling may be due to acute or chronic inflammation, neoplasm or retention of secretions. Mumps is the most common cause of salivary swelling.

NON-MALIGNANT LESIONS

Acute swelling. Acute parotitis due to the mumps virus is common, but post-operative parotitis is now seen very infrequently. It is thought that infection ascends the parotid duct from the mouth in association with poor oral hygiene and dryness of the mouth as the result of dehydration or drugs used for premedication.

Recurrent swelling, is usually due to salivary calculi (sialolithiasis) and the submandibular gland is affected most often, possibly because its secretions are more viscid. Infection and stenosis allow calcium phosphate and carbonate stones to form which cause periodic retention of salivary secretions. This results in pain and swelling of the gland.

Chronic swelling. This may be due to:

a. Chronic inflammation. Chronic non-suppurative infection usually affects the parotid. The condition is not apparently related to salivary calculi but is probably a combination of ascending infection from the mouth and dilatation of the ducts and acini in the gland (sialangiectasis).
b. Salivary tumours. These occur in the parotid gland in 90% of cases. They appear usually in adults over the age of 30 and most often are slow-growing and remain well localized for years.

NEOPLASMS

1. Benign
   a. Mixed salivary gland tumour.
   b. Benign muco-epidermoid tumour.
   c. Adenoma:

      (i) Papillary cyst adenoma lymphomatosum (Warthin's tumour)
      (ii) Serous cell adenoma
      (iii) Acidophilic cell adenoma

2. Malignant
   a. Epidermoid carcinoma (well or poorly differentiated)
   b. Muco-epidermoid carcinoma
   c. Adenocarcinoma:

      (i) Adenocystic carcinoma
      (ii) Acinic (serous) carcinoma
      (iii) Acidophilic cell carcinoma

   d. Unclassified carcinoma

Clinically, mixed salivary gland tumours are usually firm with an irregular surface and well defined border, situated just below the angle of the jaw. When a lump has been present for a short time and is associated with pain, rapid growth and a hard craggy surface, carcinoma must be suspected. Sometimes there is an associated facial nerve lesion and metastases in lymph nodes in the neck.

Microscopically, all show great variations and terms 'mixed parotid tumour' or 'pleomorphic adenoma' have been used to describe them. The epithelial elements in the tumours are spheroidal columnar, squamous, basal or glandular, while the stroma is fibrous or mucinous. The latter is probably a by-product rather than an independent tissue formation.

Primary carcinoma of the parotid gland may occasionally arise in a mixed parotid tumour. More often it occurs *de novo*. However, the epithelial and stromal elements show similar variations to a mixed tumour.

Warthin's tumour (adenolymphoma, papillary cystadenoma lymphomatosum) accounts for less than 5% of parotid tumours and may arise from the lymphoid tissue within the gland. It differs from a mixed parotid tumour in that it is softer, more mobile and situated superficially. It rarely gives rise to malignant changes or facial nerve palsy. It is easily removed and seldom recurs.

Microscopically, the outstanding features are cyst formation with a columnar epithelial lining supported by a lymphoid stroma. Sometimes the epithelial cells have intensely eosinophilic and granular cytoplasms with pyknotic nuclei (onkocytes).

Treatment of salivary gland tumours is by excision of the benign varieties and combinations of excision and X-ray therapy for malignant tumours. The latter carry a poor prognosis.

SPECIFIC SYNDROMES

In addition to the discrete swellings of the parotid gland mentioned above, there are two syndromes:

1. Sjögren's syndrome is an indeterminate entity which includes enlargement of the parotid and lachrymal glands together with polyarthritis and inflammatory lesions of the uveal tract, occurring nearly always in females close to the climateric. Microscopically, the parotid epithelium is atrophied and the stroma shows fibrosis and inflammatory changes.

2. Mikulicz disease is a term occasionally used to describe the enlargement of several pairs of salivary glands in young adults. Microscopically there is generalized lymphocytic infiltration with reduction in the amount of epithelial tissue. Sometimes the condition may be indistinguishable from a reticulosis or sarcoidosis.

4. Branchial cysts

These are of congenital origin arising from the remains of a branchial cleft.

A branchial cyst has the following characteristics:

a. Usually occurs in young people—rare over 40
b. Protrudes into anterior triangle from the angle of the jaw
c. Deep to and partially anterior to sternomastoid muscle, which makes palpation difficult if the muscle is tense
d. Rather soft and fluctuant
e. Usually too deep to transiluminate
f. If infected causes spasm and pain in the sternomastoid
g. Fluid contains cholesterol crystals

The treatment of a branchial cyst is excision, which may be a difficult procedure as the neck of the cyst often passes between the internal and external carotid arteries.

A branchial cleft which does not close over to form a cyst is not strictly a neck swelling but can be mentioned here. The unobliterated cleft communicates with the exterior, usually just medial to the sternal head of sternomastoid. Its internal opening is into the pharynx in the supratonsillar fossa. These branchial fistulae continuously discharge beneath the collar causing discomfort. Treatment is by complete excision.

5. Sternomastoid tumour

This is a fibrous mass in the sternomastoid muscle which is probably the result of either intrauterine or birth trauma. If left, the sternomastoid on that side becomes short and a wry neck develops. Secondary to this the child may develop facial asymmetry.

Treatment is always initially conservative. Only rarely is it necessary to detach the sternomastoid from its clavicular and sternal origin.

6. Cervical rib

A bony or fibrous extra rib may be associated with paraesthesia or paralysis of areas supplied by the first thoracic nerve. In addition, there may be autonomic and vascular phenomena.

Occasionally, a palpable pulsatile lump is present just above the clavicle. The pulsation is due to the elevated subclavian artery.

7. Cystic hygroma

Occurs in the neonate or may develop over the first few months of post-natal life. It is a failure of development of the lymphatic channels comparable to a vascular 'angioma' in which lymph spaces persist. Characteristically, the swelling is soft, diffuse, subcutaneous but infiltrating the deeper tissues so it is not easily moved.

The smaller examples are seen to be in the posterior triangle but the lesion may be so large that it involves the whole lateral aspect. Respiratory distress is common.

8. Aneurysms and arteriovenous fistulae

Lie along the line of the great vessels—common, internal and external carotid. Their general features are described in Chapter 36.

9. Carotid body tumour

An uncommon tumour of the chemo-receptors of the carotid body which presents in middle life as an oval painless lump in the line of the carotid sheath at the level of the upper border of the thyroid cartilage. It is rarely associated with pressure effects on the hypoglossal nerve, cervical sympathetics or internal carotid artery. There is a significant association with high altitudes.

The tumours are smooth or lobulated and display some lateral movement but restricted vertical mobility. They vary in size from that of a walnut to a hen's egg, but the majority grow slowly and remain confined to the neck. Malignant invasion of local structures and lymph nodes is rare. They are hard and white, or spongy and vascular, with dense fibrous septa.

10. Actinomycosis

Usually asymmetric though it can involve any of the fascial planes of the neck. In the early stage it is a diffuse woody swelling not conforming to any anatomical structure. Later pus and sinus formation ensues with the characteristic yellow 'sulphur granule' discharge.

11. Muscle tumours, clavicular tumours and spinal abscesses

These are all so rare that they do not merit separate description.

SEARCH FOR THE PRIMARY LESION

When a swelling in the neck appears to be a lymph node or group of lymph nodes, three questions must be asked:

1. Is it part of a local inflammatory process? Consider:
   a. Tonsillitis
   b. Pharyngitis
   c. Infected sebaceous cyst
2. Is it part of a generalized lymphatic process? Examine particularly the axilla and groin and palpate for an enlarged spleen. If there is evidence of lymphadenopathy or splenomegaly, such conditions as sarcoidosis,

glandular fever and the reticuloses have to be considered.

3. Is it part of a malignant process? Depending on the situation of the lymph nodes, cancer of the scalp, face, lips, tongue, floor of mouth, oropharynx, nasopharynx, larynx, thyroid, breast, mediastinum and stomach must be considered. All patients will require a general examination.

Special tests

To make the diagnosis some of the following special investigations may be necessary:

1. Laryngoscopy if laryngeal carcinoma is suspected
2. Bronchoscopy if lung carcinoma is suspected
3. Oesophagoscopy if oesophageal carcinoma is suspected
4. X-ray chest if lung, mediastinal disease, or some general process is being considered

5. Mammography if breast lesion is suspected
6. Full blood examination if a reticulosis is suspected
7. Excisional biopsy of the involved lymph node and histological section will usually be required when the diagnosis remains in doubt

TREATMENT

Excision will usually be indicated for branchial cyst, thyroglossal cyst, sebaceous cyst, lipoma, carotid body tumour, plunging ranula, sublingual dermoid, laryngocele, parotid tumour, pharyngeal pouch, cervical rib and submandibular gland calculus.

Excision en bloc with deep cervical lymphatics for certain cases of carcinoma of the tongue, lip, floor of mouth.

Radiotherapy and cytotoxic drugs may be used for the reticuloses and metastatic carcinoma.

19

Thyroid

SURGICAL ANATOMY

The adult thyroid gland has two symmetrical lobes. The upper parts embrace the thyroid cartilage on each side. The other parts of the two lobes lie to the sides of the larynx and trachea and are joined by an isthmus of gland tissue across the upper four tracheal rings.

The pyramidal lobe is a variable amount of glandular tissue extending upwards from the isthmus towards the hyoid bone. It represents the caudal or glandular part of the thyroglossal duct which is otherwise a fibrous or muscular structure (levator glandulae thyroidea).

The thyroid gland is invested in a delicate capsule and the pretracheal fascia. The latter is fixed to the trachea over the back of the isthmus.

Anteriorly the gland is covered by the strap muscles (sternothyroid, sternohyoid and omohyoid). These may be markedly attenuated and intimately attached to the gland when it is enlarged. The strap muscles are covered by the deep cervical fascia anteriorly and the sternomastoid muscles laterally. Superficial to these structures are the anterior jugular veins covered by platysma and skin (Fig. 19.1).

The parathyroid glands are four small pinkish structures which lie beneath the pretracheal fascia in close relationship to the thyroid gland. The superior parathyroid glands are usually situated on the middle third of the posterior border of the thyroid gland either in a groove in the thyroid or on a projecting nodule above the inferior thyroid artery, but occasionally behind it, or between it and the thyroid gland. The inferior parathyroid glands are usually situated at or just behind the lower pole of the thyroid gland, occasionally they are 1–2 cm below the lower pole and rarely as low as 10 cm below the lower pole in or near the thymus gland.

Blood supply

1. Superior thyroid artery, the first branch of the external carotid artery, reaches the superior pole in close relation to the external laryngeal branch of the superior laryngeal branch of the vagus nerve. The artery divides on the gland into the anterior and posterior branches (Fig. 19.2).

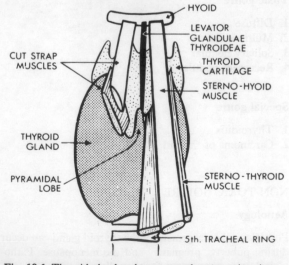

Fig. 19.1 Thyroid gland and strap muscles—anterior view

Labels: HYOID; LEVATOR GLANDULAE THYROIDEAE; THYROID CARTILAGE; STERNO-HYOID MUSCLE; CUT STRAP MUSCLES; THYROID GLAND; PYRAMIDAL LOBE; STERNO-THYROID MUSCLE; 5th. TRACHEAL RING

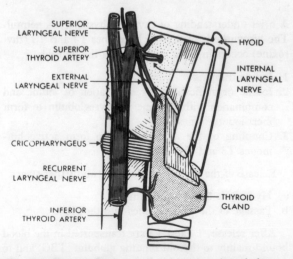

Fig. 19.2 Thyroid gland, nerves and arteries—lateral view

Labels: SUPERIOR LARYNGEAL NERVE; SUPERIOR THYROID ARTERY; EXTERNAL LARYNGEAL NERVE; CRICOPHARYNGEUS; RECURRENT LARYNGEAL NERVE; INFERIOR THYROID ARTERY; HYOID; INTERNAL LARYNGEAL NERVE; THYROID GLAND

2. Inferior thyroid artery, a branch of the thyro-cervical trunk which arises from the first part of the subclavian artery, ascends in the neck behind the common carotid artery to arch medially and divide into three or four branches before reaching the lower pole and freely anastomosing with the superior thyroid artery. The inferior thyroid artery has an intimate and important relationship to the recurrent laryngeal nerve. The artery may pass anterior, posterior or its branches may encircle the nerve before reaching the gland.

3. Thyroidea ima artery is an inconstant branch of the innominate artery or aortic arch which passes to the isthmus.

Venous drainage

1. Superior thyroid vein empties into the internal jugular vein
2. Middle thyroid vein empties into the internal jugular vein
3. Inferior thyroid vein or veins empty into the innominate veins

Lymphatic drainage

The lymphatics follow the arteries and ultimately reach the deep cervical lymph nodes about the internal jugular vein. Often the first node to be involved is that which lies in relation to the middle thyroid vein (Delphian node).

There is however a rich intraglandular network of lymphatics present which may explain why thyroid malignancies sometimes appear to be multi-focal.

PHYSIOLOGY

A brief understanding of thyroid physiology is helpful. The biosynthesis of thyroid hormones T4 and T3 (thyroxine) occurs in three stages within the thyroid:

1. Iodine trapping
2. Iodine organification, by oxidization of iodine and combination with tyrosine in thyroglobulin to form inert iodotyrosines
3. Coupling of the iodotyrosines to form active hormones T3 and T4

Release of the hormones involves two further stages:

a. Hydrolysis of thyroglobulin
b. Passage of the iodotyrosines into the blood

After release, T4 and T3 are transported in the blood bound mainly to thyroid binding globulin (TBG) and to a lesser extent thyroid binding pre-albumin. Only a very small amount, 2%, of T3 and T4 is free in the blood. T3 is the biologically active hormone, T4 is largely inactive and serves as a prohormone, being converted to T3 peripherally.

Thyroid function is controlled within precise limits by two feedback loops, a central positive and a peripheral negative loop.

1. Central control is maintained by the hypothalamus, mediated by thyroid releasing hormone (TRH) which maintains a positive feed back on to the pituitary, causing release of thyroid stimulating hormone (TSH); this in turn acts on the thyroid to synthesize and release more of the thyroid hormones.
2. The peripheral levels of T3 and T4 in the circulating blood act via another feedback loop on the pituitary, stimulating TSH secretion when T3 and T4 concentrations are low and inhibiting TSH secretion if T4 and T3 concentrations are high.

GOITRE

The term 'goitre' is used here to describe enlargement of the thyroid gland due to any cause.

CLASSIFICATION

Non-toxic goitre

1. Diffuse
2. Multinodular
3. Solitary nodular
4. Recurrent nodular (following surgery)

Toxic goitre

1. Diffuse
2. Multinodular
3. Solitary nodular
4. Recurrent nodular

Special goitre

1. Thyroiditis
2. Carcinoma of thyroid

NON-TOXIC GOITRE

Aetiology

Physiological enlargement of the thyroid gland can occur during puberty, pregnancy and the menopause. Pathological goitre may occur for the following reasons.

1. IODINE DEFICIENCY

The result of a low dietary intake of iodine (less than 100 μg per day) and is a major factor in the production of endemic goitres. It can be overcome by iodinization of salt or bread. Relative iodine deficiency occurs during pregnancy and a 'physiological goitre' may occur as one of the early signs of pregnancy.

2. GOITROGENIC SUBSTANCES

Dietary. There is some evidence that goitrogenic substances may be present in turnips, swedes, Tasmanian weeds used for cow feed, soya beans and the drinking water in Himalayan India.

Fluoride excess has been incriminated for the production of goitre in the Punjab and calcium excess in Columbia, Cape Province, Burma, and West China.

All these substances may prevent the proper uptake of iodine into the thyroid gland or the synthesis of thyroxine.

Drugs. Over treatment of hyperthyroidism with thyroid blocking drugs may result in goitre formation. Similarly thiocyanates which have been given for hypertension, iodides for asthma, para-aminosalicyclic acid for tuberculosis and resorcinol when administered over a time may cause goitre formation.

Goitre and hypothyroidism may occur in infants if the mother has taken antithyroid drugs during pregnancy or lactation.

3. GENETIC DEFECTS

In a small percentage of cases the susceptibility to goitre is probably due to an autosomal, non-sex-linked, not fully recessive gene defect. This supposedly leads to a defect in an enzyme system which is necessary for thyroxine synthesis.

Five distinct biochemical defects resulting from the inheritance of an abnormality of a single gene have been described:

a. Inability to concentrate iodide in the thyroid
b. Inability organically to bind iodine which, in its most complete form, results, in congenital hypothyroidism with goitre. In some cases congenital deafness may be associated (Prendred's syndrome).
c. Inability to couple iodotyrosines to form iodothyronines
d. Inability to retain iodine in iodotyrosines due to lack of the deiodinase enzyme. This results in loss of iodine in its organic form in the urine.
e. Capability of producing an abnormal iodinated protein which resists the normal process of hormone synthesis

Whatever the aetiological factor may be, if insufficient iodine is available for thyroid hormone production, or if there is an increased demand for thyroid hormone, the thyroid gland undergoes initial hyperplasia with multiplication of the acini as the result of increased TSH stimulation. This produces what is described as a 'parenchymatous' goitre.

When the process is controlled or the demand for the thyroid hormone ceases, then colloid may collect in the previously hyperplastic acini with the production of a colloid goitre.

Multinodular or clinically solitary nodular goitres may develop if iodine lack is not corrected. Then the initial diffuse hyperplastic process becomes localized to a few or even a single area of activity which later undergo haemorrhage and subsequent resolution resulting in the formation of new follicles, collections of colloid, or cysts. Then activity moves to some other area and the process is repeated and multinodularity is gradually developed.

Treatment

1. DIFFUSE GOITRE

This may be parenchymatous or colloid. Physiological diffuse goitres do not require any treatment but pathological goitres will require the administration of iodized salt if iodine lack is apparent. For large diffuse goitres, thyroxine 0.1–0.3 mg daily is given and continued for 1 year if signs of reduction are apparent and then gradually withdrawn. Thyroidectomy is indicated only if pressure effects develop or if the gland is of such dimensions to be unacceptable for cosmetic reasons.

2. MULTINODULAR GOITRE

Until recently there has been conflicting evidence concerning the incidence of thyroid cancer in nodular and parenchymatous goitres. However, modern views are that thyroid cancer is more common in areas where goitres are endemic.

Thyroidectomy is therefore possibly indicated for multinodular goitres because of their malignant potential, as well as for pressure and cosmetic reasons.

3. SOLITARY NODULAR GOITRE

After radioactive thyroid scan to confirm the solitary nature and degree of uptake

1. If nodule is 'hot'—may attempt to suppress by giving thyroxine. If no effect after one month's treatment proceed to operation—usually removal of nodule.
2. If nodule is 'cold'—investigate by needle aspiration under local anaesthetic:

   a. If solid—cytology of cells and proceed to operation
      (i) If benign adenoma, then simple excision
      (ii) If malignant—thyroidectomy

b. If cystic—cytology of fluid and review nodule
   (i) If cells benign and nodule disappears, keep under review for 1 year
   (ii) If cells malignant or nodule does not disappear, operation indicated with frozen section analysis on table

Ultrasound scan may be used as an adjunct to needle aspiration in differentiating solid and cystic nodules (Fig. 19.3).

4. RECURRENT NODULAR GOITRE

After previous thyroidectomy for nodular goitre a recurrent thyroid nodule should be scanned for its ability to take up radio-active iodine as it may be the only remaining functioning thyroid tissue in the neck.

Further surgery may be difficult or hazardous, particularly if recurrent laryngeal nerve damage is evident and the intact nerve is situated on the same side as the recurrent nodule. Surgery would certainly be contra-indicated if there is no other functioning thyroid tissue present. In this situation continued observation together with the administration of thyroxine would be indicated.

TOXIC GOITRE

Aetiology

The cause of hyperthyroidism remains unknown. It is not simply the end result of overproduction of the thyroid-stimulating hormone by the anterior pituitary. Genetic predisposition, provocative and unidentified circulating substances, or auto-immune reactions may prove to be initiating factors in some cases.

The long-acting thyroid stimulator (LATS) is a gamma globulin which can be isolated from the serum of patients with hyperthyroidism in many cases. It is now known that LATS causes hyperthyroidism by its action on the thyroid gland.

Surgical pathology

1. DIFFUSE TOXIC GOITRE (Graves' disease, primary toxic goitre)
The thyroid gland is enlarged and smooth and its cut surface is reddish and firm.

Microscopically the outstanding features are:

a. Epithelial proliferation with papillary projections.
b. Increased stromal vascularity.
c. Lymphocytic infiltration of the stroma. This may be part of a focal thyroiditis associated with the production of auto-antibodies. Occasionally the thyroiditis takes on a slowly progressive course with increasing fibrosis and the eventual development of Hashimoto's disease.

2. MULTINODULAR TOXIC GOITRE (secondary toxic goitre)
A goitre has usually been present for many years before hyperthyroidism develops. The gland is irregularly enlarged and its cut surface shows many nodules which may be solid, cystic or colloid-filled.

Microscopically areas of epithelial hyperplasia can usually be found.

3. SOLITARY NODULAR TOXIC GOITRE (toxic adenoma 'hot' nodule)
The distinction between multinodular and solitary nodular toxic goitre may not be a real one. However, on rare occasions a single nodule appears to be the cause of hyperthyroidism.

Microscopically the area of epithelial hyperplasia is confined to the nodule while the remainder of the gland consists of acini in the resting phase.

4. RECURRENT NODULAR TOXIC GOITRE
After thyroidectomy for hyperthyroidism, further toxic nodule formation may occur.

Clinical features

1. DIFFUSE TOXIC GOITRE
Outside features include: weight loss despite a good appetite, preference for cold weather, sweating, tremor of hands, nervousness, emotional instability, palpitations, diarrhoea, menorrhagia, loss of hair, muscle weakness and exophthalmos.

The thyroid gland itself is usually symmetrically enlarged, and, because of its increased vascularity, a palpable thrill and audible bruit are present in about half of the cases.

Eye signs which may be present include:

a. Lid retraction
b. Lid lag
c. Proptosis
d. Oedema of eyelids
e. Congestion of the conjunctiva
f. Ophthalmoplegia (paralysis of extrinsic eye muscles)

2. MULTINODULAR TOXIC GOITRE
Hyperthyroidism due to multinodular toxic goitre differs from that due to diffuse toxic goitre in the following ways:

a. Onset later in life
b. Eye signs are slight
c. Cardiac arrhythmias and cardiac failure are frequent
d. The goitre may displace the trachea

LABORATORY ASSESSMENT OF THYROID DISORDERS

THYROID FUNCTION TESTS

These can be divided into two main groups:

1. In vitro
2. In vivo

In vitro tests involve:

a. Measurement of hormone concentrations by radio-immunoassay (RIA)
b. Indirect measurement of thyroid hormone binding, T3 resin uptake
c. Direct measurement of thyroid binding globulin (TBG) by RIA
d. Calculation of free thyroxine index (FTI)

In vivo tests involve:

a. Isotope uptake
b. Thyroid antibody estimation
c. TRH stimulation
d. TSH stimulation
e. T3 suppression test

In vitro

The concentration of the thyroid hormones T3 and T4 and also TSH can be measured in peripheral venous blood samples employing RIA techniques. Most of these measure both bound and free hormone which is usually adequate in the clinical context. Full details of RIA techniques will not be given—they can be found in many text books.

The binding of active hormones in peripheral plasma can be measured by a resin uptake test. This is often called T3 uptake, but a more exact name is resin uptake. The basis of the test is the addition in vitro of isotopically labelled T3 to patient's serum which is then incubated with an insoluble particulate matter, for example resin, capable of competing with the hormone binding proteins, binding unoccupied labelled T3. After a standard interval the proportion of labelled hormone bound by the particulate material is determined, thus giving an indirect measure of thyroid hormone binding. More recently it has become possible to measure TBG directly using an RIA.

The product of the in vitro uptake value and the serum total T4 concentration provides the so called 'free thyroxine index' or FTI, which is analogous to and varies with the absolute concentration of free T4.

In vivo

a. Isotope uptake studies
Two isotopes are used, either I^{131} which is trapped by the gland or ^{99m}Tc which is also trapped only by the thyroid. An external scintillation counter is passed over the neck to provide an image of the thyroid gland. This provides a record of thyroid anatomy, useful for delineating thyroid nodules, and can also provide a measure of the rate of uptake of the labelled substances.

b. Thyroid auto-antibodies
Two thyroid antibodies can be routinely measured in blood. These are antithyroglobulin, measured by tanned red cell agglutination or RIA, and antimicrosomal antibodies by complement fixation test (CFT) or RIA.

c. Thyroid releasing hormone stimulation
After the administration of synthetic releasing hormone, samples of blood are collected at regular intervals for thyroid stimulating hormone estimation. This gives an assessment of the integrity of the hypothalamic pituitary thyroid axis and also assesses the pituitary reserve of TSH. It can be used to exclude thyrotoxicosis when the diagnosis is doubtful after T3 RIA and when diagnosis of hypothyroidism is in doubt.

d. TSH stimulation
TSH is injected intramuscularly for 3 days and a further Scintiscan of the thyroid after the dosage has been given. This test enables agenesis of the thyroid gland to be distinguished from hypofunction.

e. T3 suppression test
T3 is given in quite large doses for 10 days and the Scintiscan is repeated. This differentiates an autonomous 'hot' nodule on the scan and can be used to predict the likelihood of relapse of thyrotoxicosis after discontinuation of anti-thyroid drugs.

SUGGESTED SCHEME FOR INVESTIGATIONS OF THYROID DISORDERS

1. Thyrotoxicosis

The diagnosis can usually be achieved by resin uptake test, T4 RIA and if the diagnosis is still in doubt T3 RIA.

2. Hypothyroidism

A general screen is provided by resin uptake test and T4 RIA. Once myxoedema is proven using these methods a TSH estimation can differentiate between primary or secondary hypothyroidism.

3. Hashimoto's thyroiditis

The levels of hormone are unpredictable varying from case to case between extreme hyperthyroidism through euthyroidism to hypothyroidism. There are, however, extremely elevated titres of thyroid antibodies, particularly the anti-thyroglobulin antibodies.

4. Thyroid nodules (see Fig. 19.3)

All nodules in the thyroid should be Scintiscanned. They can then be divided into:

a. cold

b. warm

c. hot

Cold nodules. Ultrasound is of value in defining whether the lesion is solid or cystic. It is permissable to put a needle into a cystic nodule, empty it and send the aspirate for cytological examination. Very rarely this will show malignant cells which will then mean treatment as for thyroid cancer (p. 118). More commonly the cytology will be negative then; as Figure 19.3 shows, further management depends upon whether the cyst refills. Approximately two thirds do so and will then require excision. Solid cold nodules should be operated upon forthwith to exclude neoplasm.

Warm spots should be treated as if they were cold and the distinction is only made because reporting techniques in nuclear medicine departments frequently identify this group separately.

Hot spots. If the patient is clinically or biochemically toxic, the nodule should be removed. If euthyroid, then a T3 suppression test may be carried out, but it is then difficult to decide unequivocally whether the patient is best served by operative or nonoperative treatment.

Current clinical practice—the foregoing not withstanding—is to remove a single thyroid nodule if there is the slightest doubt about it being benign. In effect, such doubt virtually always exists and, other things being equal, nearly all patients should be recommended to have a lump which has been established as single by scanning removed. The nodule should be excised intact and this usually means a formal lobectomy. Immediate examination by frozen section is then done if the facilities exist. However, frozen sections may be difficult to interpret and if there is doubt it is better to terminate the operation and wait for a definite answer from the paraffin section before deciding on further surgical management.

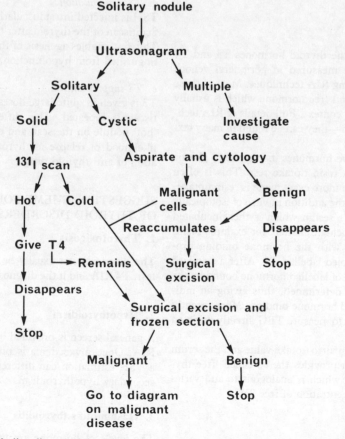

Fig. 19.3 Approach to a clinically solitary nodule

TREATMENT OF THYROTOXICOSIS

The treatment of thyrotoxicosis does not remove the cause of the disease and so long as we attack the thyroid alone by the crude methods of cutting (thyroidectomy), poisoning (anti-thyroid drugs) or *in situ* cell destruction (radioactive iodine) we should talk of the management of the thyrotoxic patient rather than the treatment of thyrotoxicosis.

There are few disorders in which the choice of treatment is so delicately balanced as in thyrotoxicosis and often this choice is determined by the available facilities, the experience of the physician or surgeon and the wishes of the patient.

Antithyroid drugs

Carbimazole. 10 to 20 mg eight-hourly depending on severity with 0.1 mg thyroxine eight-hourly. Once euthyroid (1 to 2 months), the dosage is halved and a maintenance dose of 10 mg per day for about 18 months to 2 years is aimed for and then the drug is gradually withdrawn.

Advantages
1. Avoid the hazards of surgery.
2. Avoid the hazards of radio-active iodine

Disadvantages
1. Relapse rate is high even in the best hands (about 70%)
2. Reactions to drug in about 10%. The most serious of these is agranulocytosis and aplastic anaemia which occur in about 1% of patients.
3. Resistance to the drug may occur
4. Repeated follow up over 1–2 years is essential and this may be unreliable, uneconomic, or unacceptable to the patient

Indications
1. Children
2. Mild thyrotoxicosis in adolescents
3. Recurrence after surgery, as an alternative to radio-iodine
4. Decompensated thyrocardiacs in combination with radio-iodine
5. Pregnancy, as an alternative to surgery
6. Hyperthyroidism in association with high titre of thyroid antibodies indicating thyroiditis

Radio-active iodine

Advantages
1. Simply given as a drink
2. Avoids the hazards of surgery
3. Avoids the hazards of antithyroid drugs

Disadvantages
1. Slow in producing an effect
2. Hypothyroidism rate is increasing with time (35% after 10 years)
3. Genetic effects in reproductive age
4. Danger of carcinogenesis—so far unestablished

Indications
1. Adults over 40 years and not pregnant
2. Recurrent thyrotoxicosis after surgery particularly if associated recurrent nerve damage
3. Severely ill thyrocardiacs

The beta-adrenergic receptor antagonist propranolol (40 mg, four times daily) may be given in conjunction with radio-active iodine to alleviate some of the sympathetically mediated manifestations of thyrotoxicosis until the radio-active iodine has suppressed thyroid function.

Surgery

Advantages
1. Rapidly effective
2. Low incidence of recurrence

Disadvantages
1. In unskilled hands it is a dangerous procedure
2. In skilled hands the most serious complications which occur infrequently are hypoparathyroidism, recurrent nerve lesions and late hypothyroidism (up to 25% at 10 years)

Indications
1. Nodular toxic goitre (with or without cardiac failure)
2. Large toxic goitres with pressure symptoms
3. Social and economic factors, when the patient is unable or unwilling to undergo long-term supervision with medical treatment
4. Failure of antithyroid drugs due to resistance, relapses or reactions
5. Intrathoracic toxic goitre (rare)

SPECIAL CONSIDERATIONS

1. Thyrocardiac. If the thyrotoxic and cardiac components (cardiac failure, arrhythmias) are readily controlled with drugs then surgery is advised.

If cardiac failure cannot be adequately controlled then continuation of medical treatment is preferred and radio-active iodine is usually given after initial control of the thyrotoxic component with antithyroid drugs.

2. *Pregnancy.* This is not really a special consideration and thyroidectomy is usually preferred as there is little risk to the pregnancy if the operation is done in the second trimester. The mother can later breast-feed her child which would be inadvisable if she were receiving antithyroid drugs as these are secreted in the milk.

If for any reason antithyroid drugs are preferred then the lowest dose possible should be used so that the fetal thyroid is not threatened.

3. *Exophthalmos.* This may get better or worse whether the hyperthyroidism is controlled by surgery, drugs, or radio-iodine. Whatever form of treatment is used, thyroxine should be given to counteract any possible hypothyroidism and to damp down TSH production.

SURGICAL MANAGEMENT

Pre-operative preparation

This can be performed without admitting the patient to hospital and must include the following:

1. X-ray chest for tracheal deviation, intrathoracic extension (20% of goitres)
2. Indirect laryngoscopy for assessment of vocal cord movement
3. Full blood examination, particularly if patient receiving antithyroid drugs
4. Sedation
5. Drugs to render patient euthyroid. These are two groups of patients:

    a. *Mildly toxic* (sleeping pulse between 90 and 110 BMR not more than +50%).

    There is no need for antithyroid drugs and Lugol's iodine (5% iodide in 10% potassium iodide solution) 10 drops three times per day in milk is given.

    Operation is performed when the pulse rate has been lowered, the gland is smaller and the general state of the patient improved. This usually takes about 10–14 days. Lugol's solution is continued postoperatively as long as the patient is in hospital (5–6 days).

    b. *Severely toxic* (sleeping pulse 11C or over or BMR more than +50%).

    Antithyroid drugs must be used and the course should be as short as possible to avoid inducing a hypothyroid state with its associated dangers of glottic oedema and a large and vascular over-treated 'drug goitre'.

    Carbimazole is usually preferred and it must be taken exactly 8-hourly as it is rapidly excreted; 10 mg three times a day is usually adequate.

In addition thyroxine 0.1 mg or diotroxine 0.1 mg (a mixture of 90% thyroxine and 10% tri-iodothyronine) may be given with each dose of carbimazole to prevent a drop in plasma thyroxine which may stimulate TSH production and cause an increase in the size and vascularity of the gland.

It takes 4–8 weeks to achieve the euthyroid state.

At this stage the surgeon may:

1. Operate without pre-operative Lugol's iodine. Some consider that the increased rigidity of the gland caused by iodine may make thyroidectomy more difficult.
2. Add Lugol's iodine, 10 drops three times a day, to the carbimazole and thyroxine or diotroxine for 10 to 14 days in the hope that vascularity of the gland will be reduced before operation.
3. Cease anti-thyroid drugs and give Lugol's iodine for 10 to 14 days.

An alternative form of preparation is propanolol—the beta adrenergic antagonist. The advantage is the very short time required—no more than a week—the avascular gland and the absence of side-effects. The method is rightly gaining popularity but requires skill and judgement in its use.

Operation

A sub-total thyroidectomy is performed. How much thyroid tissue is left behind will depend on the severity of the toxicity, the degree of nodularity of the gland, the age of the patient, and presence or absence of lymphoid tissue in the cut surface of the gland. The latter may suggest the presence of an associated thyroiditis and the possibility of post-operative hypothyroidism if too much gland is removed. In general however the older the patient and the more nodular the gland the more thyroid tissue is removed.

Postoperative care

1. Analgesics for pain
2. Continue Lugol's iodine, 10 drops 3 times a day for 4 to 5 days
3. Continue propanolol if this has been used pre-operatively

POSTOPERATIVE COMPLICATIONS

Thyroidectomy is associated with excellent results in the majority of cases. There are however certain potentially dangerous local and special complications which demand elaboration.

LOCAL COMPLICATIONS

1. Haemorrhage

This is usually reactionary and a major concern within the first 24 hours after operation. It may be profuse if the ligatures slip off the divided superior thyroid vessels. Haemorrhage may also occur from the cut surface of the thyroid gland or from the middle thyroid or inferior thyroid veins. Superficially, haemorrhage can occur from the anterior jugular veins and skin.

When haemorrhage is allowed to continue in the neck after thyroidectomy then blood may collect deep to the deep cervical fascia and cause respiratory obstruction and death.

The drain tubes used after thyroidectomy are placed deep to the deep cervical fascia and are intended to collect and drain blood from this area. They are, however, notoriously unreliable and, if too small, may become clotted and obstructed.

Haemorrhage may be:

a. Into the dressings. Skin bleeders may be controlled by placing an extra clip or stitch in position. If this fails then two clips or stitches are removed and the skin gently everted and the offending vessel ligated. If these methods fail then the patient is returned to theatre and the wound explored and haemostasis secured.

b. Into the subcutaneous tissues. This is usually harmless, but hideous bruising may develop after a few days and extend from the neck to the chest wall. Close observation is usually all that is necessary.

c. Beneath the deep cervical fascia. The condition is recognized by the patient's pallor and signs of respiratory obstruction. There may be obvious swelling in the neck.

Treatment is urgent; in the ward the skin clips or sutures are removed and the deep fascia is opened and the clot is evacuated to relieve compression. The patient is returned to the theatre and under general anaesthesia the bleeding vessel is found and ligated. Blood replacement may be necessary.

Tracheostomy will be required if respiratory embarrassment continues.

2. Liquefying haematoma

Seven to ten days after operation a lump may develop in the neck. This is initially firm but later it softens as liquefication occurs.

Prophylaxis
As for haemorrhage.

Treatment
1. Reassurance
b. Observation
c. Aspiration occasionally

3. Wound infection

This is uncommon after thyroidectomy.

4. Tracheitis

This may result from operative manipulation or from the endotracheal tube.

Treatment
Soothing linctus.

5. Pneumothorax and mediastinal emphysema

Air may enter the extrapleural space or tissues about the neck and mediastinum from a damaged trachea or pleura, or through the drain tube openings. Severe mediastinal emphysema may cause respiratory obstruction.

Prophylaxis
a. Careful intubation
b. Careful surgery

Treatment
a. Expectant usually
b. Tracheostomy if respiratory obstruction
c. Intercostal catheter if large pneumothorax

6. Air embolism

Air may enter major veins during operation. Positive pressure anaesthesia minimizes this risk.

7. Unsightly scar

Most neck wounds heal well and present good cosmetic results.

Prophylaxis
Good surgical technique and proper siting of the incision.

Treatment
Excision of the scar and careful resuture may be indicated.

SPECIAL COMPLICATIONS

1. Glottic oedema

Over-treatment in the pre-operative period with antithyroid drugs causes hypothyroidism and oedema and thickening of the vocal cords which may result in post-operative respiratory obstruction.

2. Tracheal collapse

The trachea may be softened and distorted by a long-standing and large goitre which when removed allows the trachea to collapse and cause respiratory obstruction. Collapse may be accelerated post-operatively by blood clot beneath the deep cervical fascia. Tracheostomy will be required.

3. Nerve injuries

These may be unilateral, bilateral, transient or permanent.

THE RECURRENT LARYNGEAL NERVES

These may be injured from bruising, stretching, ligature or division. Damage is most likely to occur during operations for multinodular or recurrent goitres when the nerves may be displaced by nodules or scar tissue.

The recurrent nerves supply all the muscles of the larynx except the cricothyroid muscles which are supplied by the external laryngeal nerves. The recurrent laryngeal nerves also supply sensation to the laryngeal mucosa below the level of the vocal cords.

If one recurrent nerve is paralysed the vocal cord on that side becomes motionless and the voice is weak and hoarse.

If both recurrent laryngeal nerves are paralysed then laryngeal stridor may occur due to a sudden and unopposed adductor action of the cricothyroid muscles which tense and lengthen the cords and close the glottis. Tracheostomy will then be necessary. However, the effects may be more gradual in onset when the cords become immobile and positioned midway between the normal and the cadaveric position. Phonation is lost and though respiration is possible dyspnoea occurs with exertion.

Transient recurrent laryngeal paralysis may occur days after operation. Phonation is lost and the cords are adducted and recovery is complete days, weeks or months later; presumably the effects are due to bruising or oedema to the nerves.

Treatment of recurrent nerve lesions includes:

Prophylaxis
a. A knowledge of the variable relationship of the nerves to the inferior thyroid arteries
b. Visualization of the nerves. Some advise that they should always be identified but a search and dissection must be weighed against the possibility of

inadvertently stroking or stretching the nerves or producing a haematoma in the region.
c. Meticulous and gentle technique
d. Immediate control of haemorrhage which otherwise may obscure or spoil tissue planes
e. Care to avoid excessive traction on lobes
f. Ligation of the inferior thyroid artery must be performed as far away from the gland as possible

Treatment
a. If injury detected at operation—nerve suture
b. Tracheostomy if severely dyspnoeic
c. If injury detected after operation—probably best to wait 6–9 months before labelling as a permanent paralysis, especially if only one nerve is involved. Operations which may then be employed include:
    (i) Exploration and resuture of nerve
    (ii) Arytenoidectomy with lateral fixation of cord
(iii) Anastomosis of hypoglossal and recurrent nerves

THE SUPERIOR LARYNGEAL NERVES

These are rarely damaged at thyroidectomy but, as they and their external laryngeal branches are closely related to the superior thyroid arteries, injury may result when the superior pole is mobilized and divided. The internal laryngeal nerve is unlikely to be damaged as it leaves the vicinity of the superior thyroid artery early to pierce the thyro-hyoid membrane.

Superior or external laryngeal nerve damage may cause voice weakness and huskiness.

Prophylaxis
Ligature of superior thyroid artery and vein as close to the superior pole of the gland as possible.

Treatment
Expectant

THE CERVICAL SYMPATHETICS

These may be stretched by deep and forceful retraction of the common carotid artery to cause a Horner's syndrome. Spontaneous recovery will occur.

4. Endocrine abnormalities

HYPOPARATHYROIDISM

This probably occurs as a transient or permanent complication in 2 to 3% of thyroidectomies and is caused by removal of, or damage to, the parathyroid glands resulting in a lowering of the serum calcium and if this is marked then muscle spasm will occur. This is most apparent in the hands, particularly when the circulation to the arm is occluded (Trousseau's sign), or the facial muscles, when tapping over the facial nerve will cause them to contract (Chvostek-Weiss sign).

Prophylaxis

a. Avoid removal of parathyroids at operation. All four lie on or in the thyroid gland inside the pretracheal fascia.
b. Some surgeons consider that ligation of the inferior thyroid artery, which is standard practice with thyroidectomy, may devascularize the parathyroids and cause hypoparathyroidism.

Treatment

a. For minor degrees of hypocalcaemia, which are often transient, calcium tablets 4–16 g daily is usually sufficient. If the serum calcium does not return to normal levels, Vitamin D (Calciferol) is added.
b. For more severe hypoparathyroidism, 10 ml of 10% calcium gluconate or 5 ml parathormone by injection may be needed.

HYPOTHYROIDISM

Tiredness, lethargy, coldness, puffy eyelids and weight increase may occur within a few months after thyroidectomy in about 5% of patients. Too much thyroid gland has been removed. Hypothyroidism is also likely to occur when operation has been performed for autoimmune thyroiditis. There is an increasing incidence (to 25%) over the next 10–15 years.

Prophylaxis

Removal of seven-eighths of the thyroid gland for thyrotoxicosis is usually adequate. Occasionally mild and transient hyperthyroidism is due to thyroiditis and, if high thyroid antibody titres are present, then antithyroid drugs are preferred to surgery.

After partial or total thyroidectomy for thyroid carcinoma, replacement therapy with thyroxine is usually indicated.

Treatment

Replacement therapy with thyroxine.

RECURRENT THYROTOXICOSIS

This is unusual after thyroidectomy but may occur if insufficient gland has been removed or if hyperplasia has occurred in its remnants.

Prophylaxis

a. Removal of pyramidal lobe and any retrosternal extension in thyrotoxic patients
b. Removal of seven-eighths of the main lobes

Treatment

Further surgery can be dangerous or difficult, especially if no thyroid tissue is palpable, or if a recurrent laryngeal nerve lesion is already present.

Antithyroid drugs or radioactive iodine are preferred, particularly in those over 40 years.

PROGRESSIVE EXOPHTHALMOS

Active exophthalmos may get better or worse after thyroidectomy for thyrotoxicosis. Therefore, it is wise to prefer the antithyroid drugs for treatment initially and if thyroidectomy is indicated later the post-operative administration of thyroxine will ensure that there is no sudden drop in plasma thyroxine which may worsen the exophthalmos. In severe and progressive cases, tarsorrhaphy or orbital decompression may be required.

THYROID CRISIS

This is very rare but was common when thyrotoxic patients were not adequately controlled before surgery. Tachycardia, fever, restlessness and delirium may occur and treatment includes heavy sedation, Lugol's iodine, steroids, fluid replacement, and particularly the administration of a beta adrenergic blocker such as propanolol.

SPECIAL CONDITIONS

THYROIDITIS

This term embraces a group of conditions which may or may not be stages in a chain of events that result from auto-immunizing processes. Excluded is acute bacterial thyroiditis which is a rare condition of the thyroid gland caused by streptococcal, staphylococcal and other organisms.

Classification

1. Hashimoto's disease
2. de Quervain's disease
3. Riedel's thyroiditis

Surgical pathology

1. HASHIMOTO'S DISEASE (Lymphadenoid goitre, autoimmunizing thyroiditis).

The condition is thought to result from autoimmunization to the patient's own thyroglobulin with the production of a self perpetuating destructive process. However, as auto-antibodies can now be demonstrated throughout the whole spectrum of thyroid disease, the situation is not absolutely clear.

The thyroid gland becomes diffusely enlarged over a 1 to 2 year period and as the disease progresses it may become stony hard, white and fibrotic.

Microscopically there are two basic changes:

a. Epithelium—the cells become swollen, plump and 'liver like'
b. Stroma—is infiltrated with lymphoid and fibrous tissue, and round cells

2. DE QUERVAIN'S DISEASE (Subacute thyroiditis, giant cell thyroiditis, pseudo-tuberculous thyroiditis, granulomatous thyroiditis.)

A much less common clinical entity and thought by some to be due to the mumps virus.

The thyroid gland is slightly enlarged and tender.

Microscopically there are two basic changes:

a. Epithelium—the cells are acutely disrupted and their nuclei are extruded into the vesicles giving a pseudo-giant cell appearance.
b. Stroma—shows inflammatory cellular infiltration with polymorphs and round cells. Micro-abscesses may form and later fibrosis and scarring occurs.

3. RIEDEL'S THYROIDITIS (Woody thyroid, ligneus thyroiditis)

Very rare and most consider that a critical analysis should be made before accepting this condition as a separate entity because both Hashimoto's and de Quervain's disease can end up with a very hard and densely fibrotic gland fixed to the trachea and cervical muscles in the manner described by Riedel.

Clinical features

1. HASHIMOTO'S DISEASE

The typical features are:

a. Middle age
b. Predominantly women
c. Goitre present for 1–2 years which is firm, symmetrical and affecting every part of the gland
d. Little or no involvement of extrathyroid tissues
e. Discomfort in the neck
f. Possibly moderate dyspnoea
g. Never serious pressure effects
h. Hyperthyroidism occasionally
i. Hypothyroidism commonly
j. High titre of thyroglobulin and complement fixing antibodies. In over 90% of cases the tanned red cell agglutination test is positive (thyroglobulin-coated red cells which have been treated with dilute tannic acid will agglutinate when placed in contact with antibodies in patient's serum). This test is about 1000 times more sensitive than the complement fixation test.

2. DE QUERVAIN'S DISEASE

The typical features are:

a. Usually young women
b. Abrupt febrile episode with sore throat, malaise and fever
c. Painful, tender and swollen thyroid
d. Tests show an elevated erythrocyte sedimentation rate and a lowered uptake of radio-active iodine

3. RIEDEL'S THYROIDITIS

In this situation a dense, hard, and fixed thyroid gland will cause pressure symptoms or concern as to the possibility of malignancy.

Treatment

1. HASHIMOTO'S DISEASE

Treatment consists of thyroid replacement for life (laevothyroxine 0.3–0.4 mg/day). Biopsy may be necessary if the diagnosis is in doubt.

2. DE QUERVAIN'S DISEASE

There is no place for surgery but dramatic results are obtained with corticosteroids or the antithyroid drugs.

3. RIEDEL'S THYROIDITIS

Biopsy for diagnosis is usually necessary, and division of the isthmus to prevent suffocation is occasionally indicated.

CARCINOMA OF THE THYROID

This is a rare but interesting disease which can sometimes be modified by the administration of hormones.

Classification

1. Papillary
2. Follicular
3. Anaplastic
4. Medullary

Predisposing factors

1. Goitre. There is a positive correlation between sporadic or endemic goitres of the multinodular type and follicular and anaplastic carcinomata and an increased secretion of TSH (thyroid stimulating hormone) may play a part in the occurrence of these tumours.

2. Radiation. Exposure of the fetal or growing thyroid to radiation can lead to thyroid cancer.

3. Genetic. There may be a hereditary factor in some thyroid cancers and there is undoubtedly so in medullary cancer.

Surgical pathology

1. PAPILLARY CARCINOMA

This is the commonest and usually occurs in young adults.

a. Macroscopically there is a complex mass of papilliferous material lying in cystic spaces.

b. Microscopically there are 'glomerulus-like' papillary processes often arranged like a Christmas tree. Many show some areas of follicular patterns. There are no signs of encapsulation.

The tumour is slow growing but has a special tendency to spread via the lymphatics through the thyroid gland and outside it to nodes about the superior and inferior thyroid arteries, the pretracheal nodes and, in particular, those about the middle thyroid veins (Delphian nodes) and the deep cervical chain.

The primary tumour in the thyroid may be minute and easily overlooked even when lymph nodes are involved.

2. FOLLICULAR CARCINOMA

Less common and usually occurs in middle-aged females.

a. Macroscopic. Initially well encapsulated but local invasion and breach of the capsule is always likely. The cut surface of the tumour shows fleshy, haemorrhagic and cystic areas.

b. Microscopic. There may be colloid follicles filled with masses of epithelial cells or solid masses or trabeculae of cells, some of which assume a liver cell like appearance. Many show papillary patterns as well.

There is a special tendency for follicular carcinoma to spread by the blood stream and about 50% of all patients present with metastases, particularly in bones and the lungs.

3. ANAPLASTIC CARCINOMA

Is uncommon and occurs particularly in females over the sixth decade. Sometimes there has been a goitre present for many years. The tumour grows rapidly and survival for longer than six months is unusual.

a. Macroscopically the thyroid is hard and irregular.

b. Microscopically there is considerable cell variation of giant cells, small round cells, or spindle cells.

Rapid spread is predominantly by direct infiltration to local structures with the production of respiratory obstruction, dysphagia and recurrent and sympathetic nerve lesions. Some anaplastic 'cancers' seem to be indistinguishable from lymphomas.

4. MEDULLARY CARCINOMA

This is a rare tumour of intermediate malignancy (about 10% of all thyroid cancers) but one which has caused a great deal of interest because it is quite distinct from the other varieties. It occurs at any age and is very slow growing.

a. Macroscopically it is solid and circumscribed and its cut surface is grey or yellow.

b. Microscopically there is always a variable amount of amyloid surrounding undifferentiated cells which may be plump and polygonal with clear or eosinophilic cytoplasm, or spindle shaped and closely packed.

Spread is characteristically by the lymphatics to the neck and mediastinal nodes.

The tumour is of interest in that it is thought probably to arise from parafollicular or C-cells of the thyroid gland which are responsible in part for the production of calcitonin. Patients with widespread medullary carcinomas have been shown to have enormously high levels of serum calcitonin.

In some cases the tumour is familial and associated with parathyroid adenomas, phaeochromocytomas and multiple neuromas of mucous membranes.

Clinical features

Thyroid carcinoma usually presents in one of the following ways:

1. As an involved lymph node in the lateral side of the neck
2. As a solitary thyroid nodule
3. As a clinically malignant thyroid, when the gland is hard and irregular and there is evidence of direct spread and fixation or distortion of the strap muscles, oesophagus or trachea
4. Occasionally, distant metastases, particularly in bones, are the first signs. Then a search for a primary lesion must be made and the breast, thyroid, lungs, kidneys, adrenals, and the prostate must receive special attention.

Malignant potential of solitary thyroid nodules

About 50% of clinically solitary nodules prove to be part of a multinodular process. The incidence of malignancy in truly solitary nodules varies considerably in different reports from 1–15%, probably according to the population sampled.

Management and outcome of thyroid cancer

Papillary. Because of the multifocal nature of the disease, total thyroidectomy is usually advised. If there are obviously enlarged nodes in one or other side of the neck these are dissected to reduce tumour bulk. The patient is then placed on thyroxine which is thought to have a suppressive effect.

Recurrences are treated by radioactive iodine for which the tumour cells usually have a greater avidity once the gland has been removed. Local deposits may also be managed by radiotherapy. The outlook in papillary carcinoma is quite favourable and even if recurrence takes place it can often be controlled for many years.

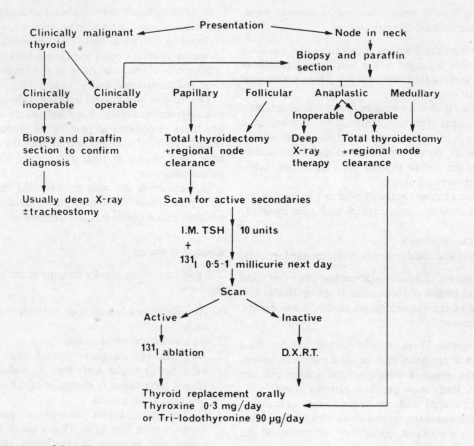

Fig. 19.4 Management of thyroid cancer

Follicular. Total thyroidectomy is the treatment of choice, accompanied by block dissection on the affected side. The five year survival is less, but as with papillary growths radioiodine and radiotherapy may be useful.

Medullary. The tumour and its lobe are excised with the regional lymph node field. There is insufficient experience of this growth to give a percentage prognosis. However, the outlook is generally regarded as poor. Radiotherapy and radioiodine are not helpful.

Anaplastic. This is an almost uniformly fatal lesion. Total thyroidectomy, which is theoretically the treatment of choice, is seldom possible because the growth has infiltrated the neck by the time the patient presents. These tumours are often highly radiosensitive and the distressing demise that accompanies tracheal strangulation can be avoided. However, the relief is usually short lived.

The management of thyroid cancer—a confusing subject at best—is summarized in the flow sheet (Fig. 19.4).

20

The breast

Carcinoma is the only capital disease of the breast and is the commonest malignancy in women. It accounts for about 20% of all female deaths due to cancer.

Improvement in the prognosis of patients with breast cancer can be expected with earlier diagnosis and as the majority of breast lumps are discovered by the patients themselves it is desirable that self examination of the breast be encouraged in women over 35 years.

It is also advisable that women with a past or family history of breast cancer or those with fibroadenosis should be selected for careful and regular follow up as they have a greater than average risk of developing breast cancer.

SURGICAL ANATOMY

Though the shape of the female breast varies considerably, its base is constantly situated over the second to the sixth ribs in the midclavicular line, the pectoralis major and the serratus anterior muscle laterally, while the variably sized tail extends over the serratus anterior towards the axilla.

The parenchyma of the breast contains 15–20 main or lactiferous ducts which open independently and radially onto the nipple. Each duct is formed from lobular ducts which drain the alveolar system of a sector of the breast.

The lymphatic drainage

Cancer of the breast spreads readily to the regional lymphatics and present treatment of this condition is influenced by the anatomy of the lymphatics.

Surgical dissection and clinical experience have shown conclusively that there are three primary pathways for lymph drainage from the breast:

1. 75% to the axillary nodes
2. 20% to the internal mammary chain of nodes
3. 5% to the lymphatics near the neck of the ribs (posterior intercostal nodes)

It has also been shown that:

1. The main lymphatics tend to accompany the major blood vessels of the breast
2. There is no significant drainage of the lymph from the breast to contralateral nodes in normal circumstances
3. The subareolar plexus plays no important role
4. The submammary plexus on the pectoral fascia plays no part in the main pathway of lymphatic drainage in the normal or early malignant breast

Axillary lymph nodes

These are:

1. Medial group (lateral thoracic or pectoral) which is situated on the medial wall of the axilla in close relationship to the lateral thoracic vessels at the lower border of pectoralis minor
2. Lateral group (humeral) which is situated on the medial side of the axillary vein close to the upper end of the humerus
3. Posterior group (scapular or subscapular group) which is situated around the sub-scapular vessels on the posterior wall of the axilla
4. Central group which is situated on the floor of the axilla in relation to the intercosto-brachial nerve
5. Apical group which is situated at the apex of the axilla on the medial side of the axillary vein close to the first rib. It receives lymph from all other groups and then drains into the supraclavicular nodes at the root of the neck.

When lymph nodes become invaded with cancer they become hard, irregular and eventually fixed to surrounding structures. These features may, but cannot always, be detected on clinical examination. It is important to realize that one's clinical impression of the nature of axillary lymph nodes is likely to be accurate in no more than 50% of cases.

BREAST DISORDERS

COMMON BREAST DISORDERS

1. Fibroadenosis
2. Retention cysts
3. Fibroadenomata
4. Abscess and mammillary fistula
5. Carcinoma

LESS COMMON BREAST DISORDERS

1. Duct papilloma and papillomatosis
2. Mammary duct ectasia
3. Fat necrosis
4. Galactocele
5. Paget's disease of the nipple
6. Sarcoma

Fibroadenosis

This is a diffuse and painful condition of the breast in young and youngish women (25–45 years) characterized by remissions and exacerbations which may later become painless and nodular with or without cyst formation.

The condition is not due to bacterial infection, neoplasm, or fat necrosis and though there is no evidence of any hormonal imbalance it probably represents an abnormal expression of the physiological proliferative and involutionary changes which normally occur in the breast.

There are four main pathological processes in fibroadenosis:

1. *Adenosis.* An increase in the number of normally patterned ductules.
2. *Epitheliosis.* An increase in the number of cells lining a ductule which causes the epithelium to become heaped up into papillary processes. This hyperplastic process may be premalignant.
3. *Fibrosis.* An increase in fibrous tissue in the stroma of the breast.
4. *Cysts.* These are most probably retention cysts; a duct may be obstructed by fibrosis or intraduct papillary changes, causing it to distend and become cystic. The cysts contain clear, yellow, or blue-green fluid.

The four processes may be present in the one breast in various combinations.

The clinical diagnosis of fibroadenosis is not usually difficult but to achieve the diagnostic certainty necessary to exclude cancer may require excision biopsy of a doubtful area. The patient presents with *pain*, a lump, or both. The pain is usually cyclical and may begin about halfway between periods, rising to a crescendo just before menstruation begins. The pain is usually mild but some few unfortunate women have severe pain and such tenderness that they are acutely uncomfortable when their breasts are touched or accidentally bumped. Lumps may be single or multiple and may come and go with the menstrual cycle. A rapidly appearing, tender lump frequently turns out to be a cyst.

Clinical examination shows a breast which is irregular and 'lumpy'. A discrete lump is uncommon and sometimes irregularity is segmental in distribution. A cyst has all the characteristics of such a lesion but when embedded in abnormal breast tissue may be difficult to distinguish. Mammography may be helpful in fibroadenosis but careful interpretation and a cautious attitude are vital.

Fibroadenosis is treated conservatively once the diagnosis is made. However, the condition may so closely mimic cancer that an excision biopsy is required.

Retention cysts

These are managed by needle aspiration. The wall collapses and it is unusual for the cavity to refill. However, further cysts may occur until the menopause, either in the same or the contralateral breast. A haemorrhagic aspirate should be examined for malignant cells and, if after aspiration of a cyst, the lesion does not completely disappear, excision biopsy is undertaken.

Fibroadenomata

Though pericanalicular and intracanalicular solid lesions which have the microscopic appearances of fibrosis intermingled with scanty adenomatous tissue may occur in fibroadenosis, a discrete benign tumour is also found at any age from menarche to menopause in otherwise normal breasts. It may well represent a highly localized dysplasia rather than a true tumour. The clinical features of a fibroadenoma are characteristic. The lump is discrete, firm to hard, highly mobile (a 'breast mouse') and often almond-shaped. The rest of the breast is normal. Some neglected fibroadenomas grow to a great size and may then resemble sarcoma (see p. 130). Small fibroadenoma can be watched and some will disappear. Larger ones are excised through a cosmetic incision (periareolar or submammary).

Mammillary fistula

Atkins used the term to describe an uncommon uni- or bilaterally occurring condition in the breasts of women in their mid thirties in which a track lined by granulation tissue communicates between the skin close to the areola and an abnormal major duct which may become lined by squamous epithelium and patchy inflammatory changes.

The usual natural history is long and most often para-areolar abscesses have been incised or have pointed and discharged spontaneously with the development of recurrent sinuses. Most often the nipple is inverted and it is usually possible to pass a probe along the track through the communicating major duct and out through the nipple.

The aetiology is disputed but the two popular theories are as follows:

a. *Congenital.* A congenital abnormality of the ampulla of a major duct in which its unnatural lining of squamous epithelium leads to blockage by a plug of cornified cells causing stagnation, abscess and then fistula formation. They also considered that the surrounding major ducts were normal.

b. *Acquired.* The view that mammillary fistula is nothing more than a variant of duct ectasia. In support of this there is convincing evidence of dilatation and stagnation of other major ducts in the area together with periductal mastitis and para-areolar abscess formation.

Treatment is by excision of the fistula and related duct segment.

Abscess

The common cause is a cracked nipple and ascending infection with *Staphylococcus aureus* in the puerperium. The infection is initially cellulitis in a subsegmental compartment of the breast with acute pain, tenderness and considerable systemic disturbance. Because the breast is broken up into relatively rigid compartments by a fibrous tissue stroma, tension rapidly rises in the inflamed area. Necrosis takes place and pus forms. The abscess then ruptures into an adjacent compartment and the process repeats itself.

The patient should stop feeding from the affected breast. Antibiotics are prescribed in the early stages but drainage is needed *early*. All loculi are opened up and slough removed.

Duct papilloma

The true papilloma is usually single and occurs in a major duct in the subareolar area in women aged 35–55 years. It is initially pedunculated and branching but as growth continues it loses its villous appearance and becomes more solid.

The tumour consists of a single layer of hyperplastic columnar epithelium and the stroma has a rich and delicate branching blood supply which causes a characteristic blood-stained and recurrent nipple discharge.

Occasionally many ducts show more extensive hyperplastic changes forming multiple papillomata (duct papillomatosis).

There is little convincing evidence that duct papillomata are premalignant. Management is by identifying the duct and excising the breast segment.

Mammary duct ectasia (secretory disease)

This condition is rare and usually occurs in women at or near the menopause. It begins as a dilatation of the major subareolar ducts, usually bilaterally but asymmetrically. Secretions stagnate and the ducts become filled with a thick greasy material containing neutral fat, crystalline bodies, and lipid-containing macrophages (colostrum corpuscles). The cause of this stagnation within the duct system is not known. In any event the condition tends to spread peripherally so that distended and discoloured ducts ramify throughout the breast. It may declare itself by a yellow, green, brown or thick and sticky 'toothpaste-like' nipple discharge. Sometimes the dilated ducts can be palpated as worm-like thickenings beneath the areola. Later the walls of the stagnant ducts thicken and probably shorten so as to lead to nipple retraction which may be the outstanding physical sign (to be compared with carcinoma). Concurrent with duct wall thickening the lining epithelium becomes attenuated and atrophic and it is probable that the stagnant contents pass into the stroma of the breast inciting an inflammatory reaction (periductal mastitis) which contains various combinations of plasma cell (plasma cell mastitis) and lipid-containing macrophages. This stromal reaction may represent some auto-immune process which proceeds acutely, subacutely or chronically. When it is acute it may present as an abscess but incision and drainage will produce little if any pus and cultures are usually sterile. Secondary infection, however, may occur in the dilated duct system and lead to a true pyogenic reaction. When the response is more chronic, fibrosis predominates causing nipple retraction, skin tethering and deep fixation, all of which are also features of breast malignancy. Serous nipple discharge is, however, the commonest symptom.

Treatment is essentially conservative provided the diagnosis can be made with confidence.

Fat necrosis

Fat necrosis occurs after trauma (often quite trivial). The process is a slow one, a dense area of sterile inflammation developing over 6 months or so. The problem is distinction from carcinoma and a biopsy is usually required. The condition eventually resolves.

Galactocele

Galactocele usually follows pregnancy and is essentially a cyst with a milky content. It is aspirated.

Paget's disease of the nipple

This is a rare condition of middle-aged and elderly women which begins as a dry, red and granular eczema of the nipple and slowly progresses to erode the nipple and areola. The condition must be suspected in all cases of persistent nipple scabbing, when biopsy is essential to exclude this insidious form of cancer.

Microscopically the epidermis is ulcerated superficially and proliferates deeply with an increase in size of the inter-papillary processes in which large hydropic round cells (Paget cells) appear.

Paget's disease is always associated with breast cancer and there are two theories concerning the development of the nipple eczema:

1. Intradermal lymphatic obstruction due to deep seated breast cancer.
2. Duct epithelium hyperplasia (epitheliosis) allowing Paget cells to invade the epidermis and be the cause of ulceration and to invade the breast stroma to give rise to a cancer.

CARCINOMA

There is no known certain causative factor for the development of breast cancer. However, it is clear that there is an increased incidence of the condition in the following situations:

1. A previous cancer in the opposite breast. It has been calculated that there is a six times greater risk of cancer developing in the 'normal' breast of women who have been apparently cured of cancer in the opposite breast when compared with women without a previous breast cancer.
2. A family history of breast cancer. There is a three to four times greater chance of a woman developing breast cancer if there is a family history of the condition.
3. Previous benign breast lesions. There is a four times greater chance of breast cancer developing in a patient with previous benign breast disease than in an individual without benign breast disease.

Breast cancer occurs almost always in women (males 1%).

It is commonest between 40 and 60 years of age and 60% are situated in the upper and outer quadrant.

Practically all arise from the epithelium of the duct system of the breast. Initially hyperplastic epithelium may proliferate to form a duct papilloma and possible intraduct carcinoma though this is debatable. In most instances the basement membrane of the duct is disrupted and malignant epithelial cells enter the stroma to become spheroidal in shape.

Various pathological types of adenocarcinoma of the breast are described according to the microscopic appearance of the cells and the stroma which vary according to the functional activity of the breast. Thus there may be:

1. Scirrhous carcinoma occurring in an atrophic breast with a dense fibrous stroma
2. Encephaloid carcinoma occurring in a softer, younger, and more vascular stroma. It grows rapidly and disseminates early. Acute cancer of pregnancy and lactation is an extreme variety of the encephaloid type in which the stroma is very vascular and hot. It is highly malignant and dissemination often leads to early death.
3. Mucoid carcinoma indicates that mucoid degeneration with signet ring cell formation has occurred in sufficient amount to produce a soft and bulky tumour
4. Medullary cancer in which the tumour is surrounded by a marked inflammatory infiltrate, and the cells are arrayed in clusters

Squamous carcinoma of the breast is rare but it may arise from the nipple, areola, or the termination of the major ducts.

Breast cancer spreads: directly to the skin and neighbouring muscles; by the lymphatics to axilla and less commonly to the internal mammary nodes; and by the blood stream particularly to bone but also almost anywhere in the body. The old idea was that spread was sequential—initially locally, then to the lymph nodes and then via the blood stream. Now it is believed that there is early dissemination of small clumps of cells which may or may not express themselves as metastatic deposits: micrometastases. Upwards of 30% of women at initial presentation must have such deposits because at least that number of stage 1 (see p. 128) patients will die within 10 years of effective *local* treatment.

Clinical features of carcinoma of the breast

Nearly all cancers present as a lump. Nipple bleeding, retraction or ulceration are less common. Occasionally an occult cancer is found after a metastasis has provided the presenting feature (e.g. pathological fracture).

Examination of the breast has one major objective in view and that is to confirm or exclude the presence of carcinoma. The clinical features of breast cancer are recognized earliest chiefly by the accompanying and visible effects of fibrosis; the density of the lump—hard rather than firm; its irregularity; dimpling of the skin because of infiltration of the fibrous stroma of the breast; superficial and deep tethering of the lump; and nipple retraction.

When the spread of carcinoma causes intradermal lymphatic obstruction a tough and incompressible oedema of the skin results (orange skin—*peau d'orange*) and if this is allowed to progress the entire skin of the breast and sometimes the chest wall and neck becomes rigid (*cancer en cuirasse*). These signs together with ulceration, skin nodules and fixed axillary and supraclavicular nodes, which are pathognomonic of breast cancer, are really 'too late' signs.

Method of examination

INSPECTION

Four positions should be used:

1. Standing or sitting 'square', unclothed to the waist. Look for:

   a. Breast colour
   b. Breast contour—lumps and dimples
   c. Nipple levels
   d. Nipple retraction
   e. Nipple eczema and ulceration
   f. Areolar pigmentation
   g. *Peau d'orange*
   h. *Cancer en cuirasse*

2. Raising the arms above the head—when breasts normally carried cranially—may accentuate or make obvious lumps or dimples. Deep attachment may make one breast less mobile.
3. Pressing on the hips and contracting pectoralis major may accentuate attachment of the lump
4. Bending forward—when deep attachment may cause failure of breasts to 'fall away' equally from anterior chest wall

PALPATION

The patient is supine and the body is rotated so that the nipple is at the highest point on the chest wall. To accomplish this the arm and shoulder of the potentially affected side are placed on a pillow.

The examination is performed in some orderly sequence such as:

1. Affected breast
2. Potentially affected axilla
3. Potentially affected side of neck and deep cervical lymph chain
4. Opposite breast
5. Opposite axilla
6. Opposite side of the neck

Breast palpation is performed quadrant for quadrant initially with the flat of the hand and any lump felt in this way must be considered highly suspicious of malignancy until proven otherwise.

Next, palpation with finger and thumb is performed and any lump, not only in the breast, is accurately described, viz. number, site, size, shape, colour (skin),

contour, consistency, tenderness, temperature, tethering (attachments), and transillumination.

Local examination of the breast must always be accompanied by the usual general examination but particular emphasis is placed on the skeleton, lungs and liver.

Mammography

Carefully performed plain X-rays of the breasts using special techniques may tip the diagnosis balance in a doubtful lump and also detect unsuspected lesions in apparently normal breasts or in large obese breasts. When performed properly, mammography has an accuracy rate close to 90%.

The mammographic findings of benign lesions are as follows:

1. Homogeneously dense, rounded or smoothly lobulated lesion
2. Surrounding halo of a thin radiolucent layer of fat
3. Coarse calcification in 30% of cases

The mammographic findings of malignant lesions are as follows:

1. Lesion is dense in centre and has an irregular spiculated border
2. Calcification in the lesion is stippled or punctate, resembling grains of salt. It occurs in about 30% of cases and is practically pathognomonic of carcinoma.
3. Secondary breast changes of localized or diffuse skin thickening, nipple retraction and increased vascularity

Screening for breast cancer

The relatively poor results of treatment of established clinical breast cancer have focussed attention on the possibility that the disease might be detected at an earlier stage by screening women at risk—ie, those over the age of 35. There is one encouraging result from New York that suggests that 10-year survival was slightly but definitely improved by detection of cancer (using mammography) at the asymptomatic stage, and other studies are in progress. There are three main methods of screening:

1. Self examination regularly, usually best done just after menstruation
2. Periodic physical examination by skilled or semi-skilled people
3. Imaging—mammography as already described, thermography (increased heat production by cancer) or ultrasonography. Only the first has so far shown sufficient precision to be of value. Another possibility is to concentrate screening on *high* risk patients and to endeavour to develop markers for such patients.

Much work has been done on hormonal profiles but so far has failed to identify anything sufficiently specific for clinical use.

Management

It is a good axiom to start with the view that any patient with a persistent lump in the breast, particularly one that is easily felt with the flat of the hand, should have that lump removed and subjected to histological scrutiny. However, there are ways in which it is possible to get closer to a diagnosis in pathological terms before biopsy is done. These can never absolutely replace a histopathological statement, which is the final arbiter, but they can help guide other investigation and also allow the surgeon to prepare and counsel his patient in what is often a situation fraught with anxiety. In addition, a firm diagnosis of cancer allows a discussion of surgical treatment rather than the unpleasant statement: 'We'll put you to sleep, cut the lump out and if necessary go on to remove your breast'.

Cytology. A fine needle aspiration will produce cellular fragments which can be examined by the cytologist. Note that the diagnosis then rests on the characteristics of the cells and not on the architecture of the tissue which may also be important in saying whether any lesion is benign or malignant. Though cytology cannot be used as a final means of making a diagnostic decision, it is in experienced hands remarkably accurate (90–95%).

Needle biopsy. In this procedure a little local anaesthetic is infiltrated into the skin, a 2 mm incision made and a special needle inserted. The needle cuts a core of tissue from the lump which can then be submitted to histopathological examination. Though it is said that cancer can be disseminated by this process, this is almost certainly not so. In patients who ultimately turn out to have cancer a biopsy of this kind is positive in 60–70%. Clearly it is of no value if it is negative and the patient must proceed to open excisional biopsy. However, a positive diagnosis:

1. Permits discussion of the problem with the patient
2. May obviate an operation to obtain a 'tissue diagnosis' in a patient with an advanced or disseminated growth
3. Saves operation time by making a 'frozen section' (see below) unnecessary

Dissemination and its detection. Obviously if dissemination has occurred local treatment can only help in controlling the local disease and thus it may not be appropriate in an individual case to carry out the standard local treatment aimed at cure. Also the identification of disseminated disease may indicate the necessity for systemic treatment (considered below). For both these reasons it is highly desirable to detect dissemination which can be done in the following ways radiologically:

1. *Chest X-ray*—pulmonary and pleural metastases.
2. *Skeletal scintigraphy*—the uptake of radionucleotide by bone. This is dependent on change in vascularity in the bones associated with osteolysis. Therefore 'hot spots' are non-specific but if they occur in bones that are radiologically normal nearly always mean tumour deposits.
3. *Skeletal survey*—skull, spine, ribs, proximal parts of arms and legs, pelvis. Osteolytic metastases—rarely osteoblastic. Somewhat insensitive as quite marked bone disease can be present without radiological appearances. Useful to confirm scintigraphy.
4. *Liver scintigraphy* occasionally (no more than 5%) shows deposits and is probably no more sensitive than
5. *Liver function tests*: characteristic finding in metastases—raised alkaline phosphatase.
6. Bone deposits cause breakdown of collagen in bone matrix. *Urinary hydroxyproline* is therefore raised in bony disease. Not often used.

General assessment prior to treatment

This entails a consideration of the patient and the primary lesion.

THE PATIENT

1. Age and general health. Age itself is no contraindication to surgery but in the very old and feeble with a short life expectancy when a slowly growing scirrhous lesion is present then a simple mastectomy or no treatment only may be seriously considered.

2. Pregnancy and lactation. A rapidly growing, vascular ('inflammatory') cancer appearing during pregnancy or lactation is associated with a high mortality. Radical surgery for the primary lesion is then contraindicated; the pregnancy should be terminated and systemic therapy used.

3. Metastases. The presence of skeletal, visceral or other metastases will preclude curative surgery for the primary. However, local control may still be necessary.

4. Oestrogen receptor values in the cytoplasm. The ability of the cell to take up oestrogens is related to:

a. The differentiation of the tumour (more differentiated, the more likely to be oestrogen positive)
b. Prognosis—see below
c. Response to endocrine therapy—see p. 128.

Thus it is valuable to have this information where facilities are available. It can be obtained *before* definitive treatment only if an excision biopsy is done for diagnostic purposes.

The primary lesion

1. Site and size. Inner hemisphere and central growths are associated with a 40% chance of internal mammary lymph node involvement. Therefore, a mastectomy with removal of the axillary lymph nodes is certain to be effective in many cases. Usually simple mastectomy and radiotherapy is the treatment of choice.

Bulky four-quadrant growths over 5 cm in diameter are considered to have involved the internal mammary chain and beyond. Surgery for cure is contra-indicated.

2. Stage. Clinical staging is of limited value for no reliance can be placed on the stage of either the axillary or the internal mammary lymph nodes. Staging is also a 'clinical impression' and therefore subject to varying human interpretations. This is particularly so with an obese patient in whom fat conceals the axillary nodes from accurate palpation and assessment. In such a situation one has only about a 50% chance of being correct in estimating whether malignancy is present or not.

Similarly in large fat pendulous breasts it may be extremely difficult to assess accurately whether the primary lesion is attached deeply or even superficially.

The value of clinical staging is to eliminate some patients from ineffective surgery and to provide common documentation. The TMN classification is now universally accepted.

TNM classification

T = Size of primary tumour
T1—Up to 2 cm in its greater dimension
T2—Between 2 and 5 cm
T3—Between 5 and 10 cm
T4—Over 10 cm

N = Regional lymph nodes
N0—No palpable homolateral axillary nodes
N1—Mobile homolateral axillary nodes
N2—Fixed homolateral axillary nodes
N3—Palpable homolateral supraclavicular nodes

M = Distant metastases
M0—No evidence of distant metastases
M1—Distant metastases, including the skin of chest wall and contralateral axilla

Treatment

Textbooks and research papers are full of confusing and contradictory information on the treatment of breast cancer. Part of this stems from an ignorance of the biology and natural history of the disease and part from the fact, already mentioned, that upwards of 30% of patients have disseminated disease at the time of presentation. The principles of management are:

1. To control local disease in a way that
   a. avoids local complications and
   b. ensures cure if the disorder is truly localized.
2. If there is dissemination, to achieve local control and achieve as great a quantity as possible of good quality survival.
3. In the presence of incurable disease to ensure maximum comfort for the patient and, as with all malignant disease, 'death with dignity'.

Effective local treatment. Though the spread of breast cancer is centrifugal (i.e. both to axillary and to internal mammary nodes), removal of the growth, the affected breast and either removal of axillary nodes or their treatment by irradiation constitute effective local treatment for outer quadrant tumours.

Irradiation therapy can also deal with the internal mammary nodes. Thus, treatment is either

1. Radical mastectomy—tumour, breast, and axillary nodes. The usual technique preserves the pectoral muscles.
2. Simple (total) mastectomy and radiotherapy to axilla and internal mammary nodes. Various subdivisions of this have been proposed—e.g. simple mastectomy without radiotherapy for those who have no evidence on node sampling of spread to the axilla and delayed treatment of axillary nodes should they enlarge. None of these is established as satisfactory.
3. Wide local excision with or without nodes plus radiotherapy.

The advantage of taking nodes from the axilla is less for cure than for staging the disease—see prognosis below. Also when nodes are involved there is an increased likelihood of local recurrence and thus there is a case (not completely established) for giving radiotherapy.

Adjuvant therapy in 'curable' breast cancer. The knowledge that up to a third of patients with what seems to be curable disease will succumb within 5 years because of established dissemination has led to the suggestion that systemic therapy should be used in an attempt to destroy small collections of tumour beyond the reach of surgery. This policy is attractive in patients with node involvement who have a particularly poor prognosis. Four regimens have shown promise in increasing the disease free interval:

1. Oophorectomy in premenopausal women
2. Phenyl alanine mustard systemically for 1 year
3. Combination chemotherapy with 5-flourouracil, vinca-alkaloid and cyclophosphamide
4. Antioestrogen therapy with the agent tamoxifen

Evidence of real improvement in survival is yet to be produced but there is prolongation of the disease-free interval in some circumstances—e.g. in premenopausal women with (1), (2) and (3), and postmenopausal women with (4). Needless to say, (2) and (3) have some element of complication from side effects of the drugs.

Prognosis

Breast cancer is unique amongst the common cancers in that it continues to claim victims for 20 years or more after effective local treatment. This is because of the micrometastates already referred to (p. 124). At the end of a quarter century only 20–25% of an unselected series of patients will be alive. Some of the factors which determine outcome have been mentioned but they are summarised here:

1. *Stage.* A $T_1N_0M_0$ growth will have an 80–90% chance of a prolonged disease-free interval. By contrast, lymph node involvement (particularly greater than 3) decreases 5-year survival to less than 50%. Few patients with established distant metastases (M_1) survive 5 years.
2. *Histopathological state.* The more differentiated the tumour the better the chance of a long disease-free survival.
3. *Oestrogen receptor status.* The same arguments as for differentiation apply—perhaps for the same reason.
4. *Age.* Postmenopausal patients are said to do better than premenopausal but there is some doubt about this.

Advanced carcinoma of breast

Blood-borne and lymphatic metastases from breast carcinoma may result in distressing symptoms such as pain or hypercalcaemia from destruction of bone, dyspnoea from mediastinal, pulmonary or pleural involvement, coma from cerebral secondaries and discomfort and misery from extensive local disease. In these situations palliative treatment is obligatory.

SURGICAL PHYSIOLOGY

Normal breast epithelium is dependent on hormones for development. Normal mammogenesis passes through three phases. Firstly, proliferation of ducts is under the influence of growth hormone from the anterior pituitary and oestrogens from the ovary and adrenal cortex. The latter are stimulated by FSH and ACTH respectively from the anterior pituitary. During the reproductive years the major source of oestrogens is the ovary but after the menopause the adrenal cortex source assumes a major role. Secondly, the formation of glands is supported by growth hormone and prolactin from the anterior pituitary, together with oestrogens and progesterone. Thirdly, the establishment and maintenance of lactation is especially influenced by prolactin.

About 50% of breast cancers are potentially hormone-dependent because they are capable of retaining characteristics of normal breast epithelium. With a change in the hormonal environment it may be possible therefore to exploit an inherited characteristic of the malignant cell and so arrest its growth. However, ultimately control is lost, the tumour becomes independent and a state of uncontrolled carcinomatosis is reached.

Though growth of breast cancer may be dependent on hormones in 50% of cases, fewer than 30% of patients show clear objective evidence of a response to hormonal manipulations. When a response is produced its average duration is about 18 months. If a tumour is oestrogen receptor negative response is most unlikely.

PREDICTION OF A RESPONSE TO HORMONE MANIPULATIONS

There are three possible groups of predictors which may give some indication as to the likelihood of a response of a breast cancer to hormone manipulation.

1. Clinical predictors

a. The 'free interval'. The time from the primary treatment to the appearance of metastases is termed the 'free interval'. The chance of success with palliative therapy increases as the free interval lengthens. When this time is less than 2 years then the chances of producing a remission are slight.

b. The site of the first metastases. Visceral deposits, particularly brain, lung and liver are less likely to regress than skeletal, skin or lymph node deposits.

c. The menopausal status of the host. Premenopausal women fare better than others. Those within 5 years after the menopause fare worst of all and in this group any form of endocrine therapy is likely to produce a response no greater than 20%. However, from about 5 years after the menopause and onwards the response, especially to tamoxifen, becomes worthwhile and it approaches something like 30%.

d. Pregnancy. Tumours appearing during pregnancy and lactation may be unfavourably affected. Paradoxically, however, pregnancy is said to afford some degree of protection to a woman who has already had primary treatment for a tumour.

e. Extent of the disease. Terminal disease, as evidenced by jaundice, ascites, hepatomegaly and cachexia, indicates a hopeless situation but when the disease is progressive and symptomatic and not affecting general health then palliative treatment is warranted.

f. The response to previous endocrine therapy. Premenopausal women who have responded previously to oophorectomy are more likely to gain a further remission with other endocrine therapy.

2. Histological predictor
Poorly-differentiated tumours and those without any lymphocyte infiltration respond poorly.

3. Endocrine predictors
There is said to be some correlation between the presence of oestrogen and responsivity.

THERAPEUTIC MEASURES AVAILABLE
Until more carefully controlled prospective and comparative clinical trials are available, together with more detailed critical analyses of the many factors which influence a response, treatment will remain largely 'hit or miss'.

It is also important to remember when considering treatment for advanced breast cancer that survival of the patient has two components—quantity and quality. Ablative procedures like adrenalectomy and hypophysectomy may produce a short-lived regression but the patient may still be unable to enjoy any home life because she is bedridden from pathological fractures, cerebral secondaries or liver failure. In some circumstances, therefore, it may be appropriate to institute no special therapy whatsoever but merely aim, with the aid of sympathetic nursing, to keep the patient comfortable and free of pain during the terminal phases of the disease.

Specific treatment for advanced breast cancer may be considered as follows.

Local therapy
This is often of value in relieving distressing symptoms and it includes:

1. *Surgery.* This may be indicated for:

   a. Solitary skin secondaries
   b. Local recurrence on the chest wall
   c. Untreated fungating primary disease
   d. Inadequately performed initial surgery to the primary lesion, when completion of the mastectomy may be considered
   e. The effects of distant metastases such as paraplegia from vertebral involvement when laminectomy may be indicated, or for pathological fractures when internal fixation of a long bone or even joint replacement may be advisable

2. *Radiotherapy.* This is the treatment of choice for untreated and inoperable primary lesions and for pain due to isolated bone secondaries. It may also be considered for mediastinal and cerebral secondaries causing compression. Radiotherapy takes 2–3 weeks to show an effect.

3. *Cytotoxic drugs.* Pleural involvement is best treated by aspirations and the instillation of a sclerosant. The antimalarial mepacrine is very effective.

Systemic therapy
Metastases are rarely, if ever, single and systemic treatment must also be given unless the patient is in the terminal stage of the disease.

Treatment is based largely on the menopausal status of the patient and it is usual to establish a sequential plan of treatment. Haphazard polytherapy is to be condemned.

An accepted plan of attack would be as follows:

Pre-menopausal and early post-menopausal women. The rationale of oestrogen therapy or withdrawal is that in some way the steroid molecule affects genetic programming in the nucleus of the cancer cell. Thus, in a pre-menopausal woman the tumour is 'accustomed' to oestrogens and removal of these by castration or other endocrine ablation embarrasses the gene. In a postmenopausal woman the cancer is growing in an oestrogen-poor environment and addition of these substances or their analogues has the same disruptive effect.

The situation is made more complex by so-called oestrogen antagonists (e.g. tamoxifen) which by presenting the gene with an oestrogen-like molecule may cause arrest of tumour growth in either pre-menopausal or post-menopausal patients. Such oestrogen antagonists have largely replaced the use of both oestrogens and androgens which have undesirable side-effects.

Response to therapy of the above kind is absolutely dependent on the presence of oestrogen receptors in the cytoplasm of the malignant cell which can then translocate the steroid molecule to the nucleus. Presence of such receptors is *not* a guarantee of response, but absence means response is highly unlikely and that cytotoxic therapy should be used.

Castration. Oophorectomy is the simplest and most reliable first step for women showing ovarian activity. Relief of pain and recalcification of lytic bone secondaries may then follow; sometimes the effect lasts for years.

Surgical castration rather than radiotherapy, is recommended. The presence or absence of abdominal metastases can be established. Radiation castration is equally effective, but it takes 2–3 months to produce an effect. The response rate for castration is about 30% and its average duration is 18 months.

'Anti-oestrogen' therapy. Tamoxifen is virtually free from side-effects and is thus the best first-line treatment. Failure to respond is now taken as an indication for chemotherapy.

Adrenalectomy or hypophysectomy. These operations are now only rarely performed. Following a relapse or if there has been no previous response to other measures, then either may be considered. The choice of operation is debatable and depends largely on the experience of the specialists available. There is little to choose between adrenalectomy or hypophysectomy performed by means of the transnasal route or by yttrium implantation into the pituitary fossa.

It is known, however, that these operations are probably not worthwhile if there has been no previous response to castration. Hypophysectomy may be superior to adrenalectomy on logistic grounds.

The mortality from either operation is about 10%, and there is a 30% chance of producing a remission for 20 months in carefully selected patients.

Cytotoxic drugs and prednisolone.
Cytotoxic drugs are withheld if endocrine therapy controls the disease. Systemic chemotherapy with a wide variety of agents may then be used but all are likely to produce gastro-intestinal symptoms and bone marrow depression.

Though single agent chemotherapy may control the disease in some instances, better response rates, though not necessarily prolongation of life, are obtained with combination chemotherapy, using up to four different agents. A bewildering variety of such regimens is available with none showing significant superiority over another.

The cytotoxic drugs may act synergistically with prednisolone, particularly in the presence of brain, lung and peritoneal secondaries. Prednisolone is the drug of choice when hypercalcaemia occurs as the result of androgen or oestrogen therapy.

Prednisolone is given orally, and the usual dose is 1 mg three times a day. However 20–30 mg thrice daily may be indicated in an emergency to control hypercalcaemia or pressure effects arising from cerebral or mediastinal secondaries.

There is no correlation between the likelihood of a response to corticosteroids and that achieved from a previous hormone response.

Post-menopausal women. After 5 years of the menopause or when there is no evidence of urinary oestrogen excretion by the ovaries, then the following sequential therapy is suggested:

Tamoxifen is the first choice, particularly in the elderly patient. *Cytotoxic drugs and prednisolone* would be indicated when tamoxifen had failed to control the disease. From the above it can be seen that endocrine and cytotoxic therapies are essentially palliative procedures which produce a favourable effect in the minority of patients, the chances of achieving such an effect being about 30% and the duration of the increased survival time about 18 months. However, such therapy may not be considered justifiable if it is at the expense of severe physical or mental disability or at the risk of a high operative mortality.

Male breast cancer

This is uncommon—1.5–3% of all breast cancer. It is usually not diagnosed until advanced. Treatment is on the same lines as breast cancer in the female.

Sarcoma of the breast

This is rare. One variety, cystosarcoma phylloides, may grow to a great size while still remaining quite local. The problem is usually to distinguish one malignant lump from another and the diagnosis is usually made only at biopsy. Treatment is by surgical excision.

21

Intrathoracic conditions

In the past 25 years the incidence of many intrathoracic lesions has changed. Infective lesions—pulmonary tuberculosis, lung abscess and bronchiectasis—previously common surgical conditions are now rarely seen. Instead, thoracic surgery is increasingly concerned with surgery of the heart and great vessels and carcinoma of the lung.

The commoner surgical intrathoracic conditions will be dealt with in this chapter under the following sections:

1. Chest wall
2. Pleural cavity
3. Lung
4. Mediastinum

Chest injuries, pulmonary embolism, oesophageal surgery and diaphragm are dealt with in separate chapters.

I. CHEST WALL

CLASSIFICATION

1. Congenital pectus excavatum and carinatum
2. Chest injuries (p. 44)
3. Soft tissue tumours:

   a. Lipomas, neurofibromas
   b. Fibrosarcomas, liposarcomas

4. Skeletal tumours:

   a. chondromas, fibrous dysplasia (bone cyst);
   b. osteosarcoma, myeloma.

5. Metastatic chest wall tumours.
6. Sternal and rib osteomyelitis.
7. Tietze's syndrome.
8. Thoracic outlet syndrome.

For details of soft tissue and skeletal tumours, a specialized text is recommended.

SURGICAL PATHOLOGY

Pectus excavatum ('tunnel chest'). There is varying degree of depression of the sternum and caving inward of adjacent costal cartilages. Deformity is noted at birth and progresses at a varying rate.

Pectus carinatum ('pigeon breast'). A rare deformity with a keel-like protrusion of the sternum. In some cases may be associated with Marfan's syndrome (a widespread disorder of elastic tissue).

Metastatic chest wall tumours. The involvement of ribs and sternum by a wide variety of metastatic growths is far more common than primary neoplasms of the bony thoracic cage. Direct extension occurs with breast and lung carcinomas. Lesions are often multiple and other primary sites include kidney, thyroid, prostate, stomach, uterus or colon.

Osteomyelitis of the sternum and ribs used to be complications of tuberculosis and typhoid fever. The majority of sternal and rib infections now occur as complications of sternotomy and thoracotomy incisions. Rib infections may occur adjacent to a draining empyema.

Tietze's syndrome is a painful non-suppurative swelling of unknown cause of one or more costochondral cartilages. The natural history of the condition is self-limiting, though recurrence is possible.

Thoracic outlet syndrome refers to a group of disorders associated with abnormal compression of the neurovascular structures at the base of the neck. The brachial plexus alone, the subclavian vessels alone, or both, may be affected.

The abnormal compressing structure may include:

1. Cervical rib
2. Scalenus anterior (scalenus anticus syndrome)
3. Anomalous ligament (costoclavicular syndrome)
4. Positional changes which alter the normal relation of the first rib to the structures that pass over it (hyperabduction syndrome)

The pathogenesis of arterial symptoms is due to post-stenotic dilatation, aneurysm formation, microembolism and eventually arterial occlusion.

CLINICAL FEATURES

Thoracic outlet syndrome

HISTORY

The primary cause of symptoms in most patients is inter-mittent compression of the lower trunk (C8–T1) of the brachial plexus resulting in pain, paraesthesias and a feeling of numbness over the ulnar nerve distribution. When arterial involvement occurs, there may be symptoms of episodic digital ischaemia (secondary Raynaud's phe-nomenon) or upper limb claudication with exercise. In chronic cases, moderate to severe permanent ischaemia may lead to loss of digits from gangrene.

EXAMINATION

Peripheral sensory or motor deficits are rare and usually indicate severe compression of long duration. A bruit may be audible over the subclavian artery above the centre of the clavicle with the arm abducted. The Adson manoeuvre—diminished radial pulse by abduction of the arm, with the head rotated to the opposite side—is often positive in completely normal persons. Distention of superficial veins and oedema from axillary vein throm-bosis is a rare finding.

DIFFERENTIAL DIAGNOSIS

a. Cervical disc and arthritis of the cervical spine
b. Carpal tunnel syndrome
c. Raynaud's disease
d. Buerger's disease

SPECIAL TESTS

1. *Chest X-ray*: may demonstrate a cervical rib or an anomalous first rib. The incidence of cervical rib is 0.5 per cent of the normal population, and in at least 70 per cent of patients cervical ribs are symptomless.
2. *Nerve conduction test*: to differentiate from carpal tun-nel syndrome.
3. *Arteriography*: when vascular complications supervene and arterial surgery contemplated.

MANAGEMENT

Mild neurological symptoms will usually respond to non-operative management by postural correction and physiotherapy directed at strengthening the shoulder girdle musculature.

If vascular complications are present, treatment of cervical rib and the scalenus anticus syndrome is sur-gical. Controversies exist in the method of approach (supraclavicular, transaxillary) and the surgical pro-cedures done for thoracic outlet syndrome (resection of cervical rib, resection of the first rib and mid-portion of clavicle, scalenotomy, division of fibrous band). Arterial reconstruction of the subclavian artery may be necessary. Results also vary widely in different series.

2. PLEURAL CAVITY

The pleural cavity is a potential space in which normally no appreciable amount of fluid is found. This state of affairs represents an equilibrium between absorption and transudation.

CLASSIFICATION

1. Malignant pleural effusion
2. Benign pleural effusion

   a. Hydrothorax
   b. Pyothorax (epyema) (p. 77)
   c. Haemothorax (p. 46)
   d. Chylothorax (p. 47)
   e. Secondary pleural effusion
        Pancreatic
        Meigs' syndrome—ovarian tumour plus pleural effusion

3. Primary pleural tumours—mesothelioma
4. Secondary pleural tumours
5. Pneumothorax (p. 46)

   a. Iatrogenic
   b. Traumatic
   c. Spontaneous

SURGICAL PATHOLOGY

Malignant pleural effusion

About 50% of all patients with carcinoma of the breast or lung develop pleural effusion during the course of their disease. Other primary sites include ovarian carci-noma and gastrointestinal tract tumours. Though in many instances there are associated pulmonary met-astases, in some cases the intrathoracic metastatic lesions may be limited to the pleural cavity. Malignant pleural effusions are often bloodstained (serosanguineous) and cytology is positive in at least 70% and pleural biopsy in 80% of malignant effusions.

Chylothorax

Congenital chylothorax due to abnormal development of the lymphatic system is relatively rare. Leakage of lymph from the thoracic duct may result from penetrating or blunt injuries, or follow complications of cardiovascular or oesophageal surgery.

Pancreatitic pleural effusion

In acute pancreatitis, a left-sided effusion may be present. The amylase content in the pleural fluid is usually above that in the serum.

Meigs' syndrome

The triad of ovarian fibroma, ascites and hydrothorax constitute the Meigs' syndrome. Other benign ovarian tumours have also been associated, such as thecomas, granulosa cell tumours. The pleural fluid resolves when the ovarian tumour is removed.

Mesothelioma

The localized form is usually benign, composed mainly of spindle cells and well encapsulated. Diffuse malignant mesothelioma proliferates rapidly and is often associated with bloodstained effusion. There is a recognized association with exposure to asbestos.

CLINICAL FEATURES

Symptoms of pleural disease

1. *Pleuritic pain*—pain associated with respiratory excursion, usually felt in the shoulder over the distribution of C3–5 segments. Pleuritic pain may diminish when an effusion forms.
2. *Dyspnoea*—the extent of shortness of breath is dependent upon the size of the effusion and the degree of pulmonary reserve
3. *Haemoptysis*—may be present with malignant infiltration
4. *Cough*—may be productive, particularly with complicated empyema

Signs of pleural disease

1. On inspection—respiratory movements may lag on the affected side
2. On palpation—tenderness, local swelling, redness and heat with empyema

   —tactile fremitus is diminished with effusion
   —with longstanding pleural disease, there may be immobility of the hemithorax

3. On percussion—dullness to percussion with effusion
4. On auscultation—breath sounds may be exaggerated and bronchial
5. Fever—particularly with empyema, and also malignancy

Special tests

1. *Chest X-ray*: will demonstrate the extent of an effu-

sion, and there may be evidence of underlying lung disease
2. *Bronchoscopy*: may be useful in determining the primary disorder
3. *Thoracentesis*: identification of the specific type of effusion—depends on examination of the fluid, which should be sent for bacteriology and cytology
4. *Pleural biopsy*: especially if thoracentesis unsuccessful, biopsy may be obtained either by needle or by an open method

MANAGEMENT

Malignant pleural effusion. Though the prime objective is to obtain lung expansion and obliteration of the pleural space, this is limited by the very poor overall prognosis. The average duration of life in patients with malignant effusions is approximately 6 months. Closed intercostal tube drainage, maintained for several days, may permit re-expansion of the lung and result in obliteration of the pleural space. Instillation of various sclerosing agents may help. Repeated needle aspirations are unpleasant and recurrence of effusions is inevitable.

Chylothorax. In most instances repeated thoracenteses result in obliteration of the pleural space, as spontaneous closure of the leak occurs. Rarely, surgical division and ligation of the thoracic duct is required.

Pancreatitic pleural effusion. If of sufficient size to compromise pulmonary function, then needle aspiration may be needed.

Mesothelioma. The localized form may be resected, and the prognosis is good. The prognosis of malignant mesothelioma is poor with either surgical or radiation therapy.

3. LUNG DISORDERS

CLASSIFICATION

1. Congenital bronchogenic cysts
2. Lung infections:
   a. Lung abscess
   b. Tuberculosis
   c. Bronchiectasis
   d. Mycotic (fungal)
   e. Parasitic (hydatid)
3. Pulmonary embolism (p. 270)
4. Lung trauma (p. 46)
5. Hamartoma
6. Pulmonary metastases
7. Carcinoma of the lung

For details of lung cysts and infections, the student is referred to a specialized text.

CARCINOMA OF THE LUNG

This is the most common malignancy to cause death in men. The incidence in females is rising so that it is the second commonest cancer next to that of the breast.

Aetiological factors

1. Cigarette smokers are statistically more likely to develop a bronchial carcinoma
2. Several environmental factors are known to be causally related: asbestos, arsenic, nickel, chromium, uranium, cobalt
3. The epidemiology of the disease indicates that genetic factors may be important (the highest incidence of bronchial carcinoma in the world is in Scotland)

Surgical pathology

1. Squamous cell carcinoma. Approximately 60% of all lung tumours are derived from the squamous cell. They may be centrally located near the hilum, or peripheral. The degree of differentiation depends upon the presence of keratinization, formation of epithelial pearls, cell size and number of mitoses.

2. Adenocarcinoma. This group represents about 15% of lung carcinomas. Histologically, glandular elements are seen and may be acinar or papillary in type. Loss of differentiation produces pleomorphic or multinucleated cells. They often spread along vascular channels. Adenocarcinoma is more often seen in women, and is more often peripheral in location.

3. Undifferentiated large cell carcinoma comprises another 15% of malignant lung tumours, dependent on the series of origin. Histologically, there is abundant cell cytoplasm and the cell pattern is highly variable, with anaplastic or squamous-cell features. This group of tumours also tends to be peripheral.

4. Oat cell carcinomas are more often central in location and the frequency is about 10%. These are the most malignant of lung tumours, and on histology show small round or oval cells. They are the best-known group of tumours to produce ectopic endocrine disturbances (secretion of ACTH or ADH). Oat cell carcinoma most frequently invades the lymphatics and has the highest incidence of pleural effusion.

Clinical features

HISTORY
1. Age—over 50 years old in both men and women, the incidence of bronchial carcinoma is still rising
2. Personal history—heavy cigarette smoking

3. Occupation—exposure to known hazards, e.g. asbestos, cobalt

SYMPTOMS
1. No symptoms—about 10–20% discovered as a chance finding on routine chest X-rays
2. Thoracic
   a. Cough, haemoptysis, dyspnoea
   b. Pain   —chest pain
            —pleuritic pain with pleural extension
            —retrosternal pain with mediastinal involvement
   c. Hoarseness of voice from recurrent laryngeal nerve involvement
   d. Pain and loss of strength in the arm—Pancoast's syndrome when an apical lung carcinoma involves the brachial plexus with or without involvement of the sympathetic ganglia at the base of the neck (Horner's syndrome: ptosis, miosis, anhidrosis, enophthalmos)
3. Extrathoracic
   a. Metastatic—bone pains, symptoms of brain metastases, liver and adrenal metastases
   b. Non-metastatic—Progressive weight loss
                    —Anaemia with lethargy
                    —Hyperadrenocorticism (ectopic ACTH)
                    —Inappropriate antidiuresis (ectopic ADH)

SIGNS
1. Pleural effusion
2. Supraclavicular and cervical lymphadenopathy
3. Pancoast's syndrome, Horner's syndrome
4. Swelling of the upper body and distended superficial veins from superior vena caval obstruction
5. Hypertrophic pulmonary osteoarthropathy
6. Bony, liver and other organ metastases

Special tests

1. *Chest X-ray.* This remains the most important method of diagnosis for lung carcinoma. Posterio-anterior and lateral views are essential to delineate which lobe the tumour occupies. Almost a third of thoracotomies performed are based on radiological findings, and errors are infrequent.
2. *Bronchoscopy and biopsy.* Rigid bronchoscopy is favoured for biopsies and to assess operability.
3. *Mediastinoscopy* through a small suprasternal incision allows direct biopsy of paratracheal and carinal lymph nodes. This technique is often used together with bronchoscopy to assess operability.
4. *Scalene node biopsy.* This has been largely replaced by mediastinoscopy.
5. *Lung biopsy* using a needle is occasionally indicated

where there is a doubt whether a peripheral shadow in the lung is due to tuberculosis or to some other non-malignant condition. Carcinoma has been established by this method in expert hands.

6. *Computerized tomography*. Though increasingly used to evaluate thoracic lesions, the value of CT scanning in primary lung carcinoma is not yet objectively established but may aid guided biopsy.

7. *Cytology*. The reliability of sputum cytology or brushings taken via the bronchoscope depends very largely upon the enthusiasm of those concerned for cytological diagnosis.

Differential diagnosis

'Coin lesion'—the solitary pulmonary nodule.

These are peripheral circumscribed pulmonary lesions that may be:

1. Non-specific granuloma
2. Hamartoma (mixed tumour)
3. Primary carcinoma
4. Metastatic carcinoma
5. Tuberculous granuloma

It is generally advised that after all diagnostic procedures are done, it is still unwise to adopt a watch-and-wait policy in a peripheral coin lesion. This is based on the calculation that the risk of thoracotomy in the average patient is less than one per cent, and the risk of malignancy 5%. The probability of cure will outweigh the risk of thoracotomy.

Principles of treatment

1. Though the overall results are depressing, the only treatment presently available for patients with lung carcinoma which offers hope of survival is *surgical resection*.

2. *Radiotherapy* is of great value in the treatment of distressing symptoms—pain from bony secondaries, superior vena caval obstruction, haemoptysis.

3. Approximately *two-thirds of patients are incurable* when first seen, because of:

   a. Malignant pleural effusion
   b. Enlarged supraclavicular nodes
   c. Superior vena caval obstruction
   d. Recurrent laryngeal nerve paralysis
   e. Distant metastases

4. In otherwise resectable tumours, the commonest contra-indication to operation is poor respiratory reserve.

5. If there is no evidence of incurability, the surgical treatment of lung carcinoma consists of thoracotomy and resection of the involved lung with regional nodes or contiguous structures.

6. Where possible, lobectomy is the procedure of choice.

Pneumonectomy is used when the tumour is sited at a fissure or in such a way as to require wide excision.

7. 30% of patients who have undergone resection are likely to live 5 years, and 15% are likely to live 10 years.

8. The best results are achieved with squamous cell carcinoma; next come those with undifferentiated large cell carcinomas, then adenocarcinomas, and there are very few survivors after two years with oat cell carcinoma.

9. The presence of metastases in hilar glands considerably worsens the prognosis.

PULMONARY METASTASES

Secondary carcinoma of the lung is found in about 30 per cent of all patients with malignancy.

Surgical pathology

Pulmonary metastasis may be solitary (see 'coin lesions') or multiple (particularly from genito-urinary tract primaries giving rise to 'cannonball' lesions). Common primary sites include colon, kidneys, uterus and ovaries, testes, malignant melanoma, pharynx and bone.

Management

As long as the initial primary is controlled and there is no evidence of further metastases, it is reasonable to recommend surgical resection for solitary pulmonary metastasis. About 80% of solitary pulmonary metastases are found to be resectable, producing 5-year survival figures of up to 35%.

4. MEDIASTINUM

This is the midline space between the pleural cavities and may be divided anatomically into four sections: superior, anterior, middle and posterior.

Surgery of the mediastinum is concerned mainly with the heart and great vessels, mediastinal mass lesions and occasionally, trauma.

CLASSIFICATION

1. Mediastinal mass lesions

   a. Neurogenic tumours
   b. Teratodermoids
   c. Lymphoma
   d. Thymoma

e. Intrathoracic goitre (p. 108)
f. Mediastinal cysts
g. Ganglioneuroma

2. Congenital heart disease

a. Coarctation of the aorta
b. Patent ductus arteriosus
c. Fallot's tetralogy
d. Septal defects

3. Acquired heart disease

a. Valvular heart disease
b. Ischaemic heart disease

4. Aneurysm

a. Thoracic aortic aneurysm
b. Dissecting aneurysm

5. Pericarditis

a. Effusion
b. Cardiac tamponade (p. 47)

6. Atrial myxoma

SURGICAL PATHOLOGY

Mediastinal mass lesions

1. Neurogenic tumours. These are the most common tumours of the mediastinum and found almost exclusively in the posterior mediastinum. Ten per cent of neurogenic tumours are malignant, malignancy being more frequent in children. The most common variety is the nerve sheath tumour, neurilemmoma (schwannoma) and neurofibroma, usually attached to intercostal nerves or the sympathetic nerves. Neuroblastoma and ganglioneuroblastoma are malignant varieties. Neurogenic tumours may be multiple and may erode into the vertebral foramina with intraspinal extension.

2. Teratodermoids. These are the most common mass lesion of the anterior mediastinum and tend to be more frequent in the young. They range from solid tumours with a single epithelial lining (dermoids) to both solid and cystic tumours with elements of all three germ layers present (teratomas). Calcifications are often present and may contain hair or teeth. Occasionally they rupture into the lung, pleura or pericardium.

3. Lymphoma. Mediastinal lymphoma is usually associated with concurrent disease outside the mediastinum. At times, Hodgkin's disease, lymphosarcoma or reticulum cell sarcoma arises as a primary mediastinal growth.

4. Thymoma is more common in adults and rare in children. About 30% of patients with thymoma have myasthenia gravis, and about 15% of patients with myasthenia develop a thymoma. The relationship is incompletely understood. Thymomas may be difficult to differentiate from lymphoma on histology and furthermore it is extremely difficult to distinguish benign from malignant thymoma. Gross tumour invasion of adjacent structures defines malignancy in thymoma. About one-third of thymomas are malignant. Metastatic deposits may settle on the pleura.

Congenital heart disease

1. Coarctation of the aorta. In the majority the coarctation is located adjacent to the ligamentum arteriosum or ductus arteriosus. It occurs twice as frequently in males as in females. The obstruction to flow is by-passed by collaterals opening up from the subclavian arteries to those from the intercostals.

2. Patent ductus arteriosus. Failure of normal obliteration, which normally occurs at birth, results in a patent ductus arteriosus. With a patent ductus after birth, blood is shunted from the aorta to the pulmonary artery with consequent increase in pulmonary resistance, and pulmonary hypertension.

3. Fallot's tetralogy is the most common lesion in the group of disorders where there is a right-to-left shunt with a combination of an obstructive lesion of the right heart and a septal defect. The four characteristic features are:

a. Right ventricular outflow obstruction
b. Ventricular septal defect
c. Right ventricular hypertrophy
d. An aorta which overlies both ventricles

Acquired heart disease

1. Valvular heart disease. Usually attributed to past rheumatic fever, but may be simply degenerative or late manifestation of congenital defects. The aortic and mitral valves are most commonly affected, with either stenosis or insufficiency. In many instances, the anatomical abnormality consists of a fixed orifice that may both restrict forward flow and fail to prevent backward flow.

2. Ischaemic heart disease. Atherosclerosis of the coronary vessels impairs myocardial perfusion with consequent myocardial ischaemia. The effects of myocardial ischaemia include:

a. Depressed ventricular contractility
b. Exertional chest pain—angina pectoris
c. Rest pain
d. Unstable angina—prolonged chest pain at rest with-

out electrocardiographic or serum enzyme changes of infarction

e. Myocardial infarction

f. Deaths from arrhythmias or low cardiac output

Dissecting aneurysm

A split in the wall of the aorta usually arises from an intimal tear either just distal to the aortic valve or adjacent to the origin of the left subclavian artery. Blood dissects along a plane of cleavage in the media. Ruptures may be:

1. Internal: into the true aortic lumen, thus decompressing itself
2. External: either into the pericardium with cardiac tamponade, or into the mediastinum or into the abdominal cavity

The pathogenesis is cystic medial necrosis. Predisposing factors are Marfan's syndrome, atherosclerosis and hypertension.

Atrial myxoma

This accounts for almost 80% of primary benign cardiac tumours. Macroscopically it may be a smooth, firm, encapsulated mass, or a cystic gelatinous mass. The majority are found attached to the left atrial septum.

DIAGNOSIS AND MANAGEMENT

Mediastinal mass lesions

Repiratory symptoms may be the presenting feature, particularly in children, but in adults mediastinal tumours are frequently discovered on incidental chest X-rays. Symptomatic tumours in adults are more likely to be malignant with symptoms related to compression of surrounding structures. Though computerized tomography may prove to be useful in evaluating mediastinal lesions, an extensive diagnostic work-up for mediastinal lesions is usually not productive and surgery is then required to establish the diagnosis. Most mediastinal tumours can and should be removed surgically. Adjuvant radiotherapy or chemotherapy may be indicated for malignant lesions.

Coarctation of the aorta

Infants with coarctation may have life-threatening heart failure. There may be other associated cardiac lesions. Hypertension in a child or young adult should raise the suspicion of coarctation. There may be diminished or delayed femoral pulsations in relation to upper limb pulses. A systolic murmur may be audible in the chest. Chest X-ray shows left ventricular enlargement, and rib-notching may be seen due to large intercostal collaterals. *Operative repair* consists of excision and anastomosis or prosthetic replacement of the diseased aortic segment. The results of coarctation repair are good.

Patent ductus arteriosus

A machinery-like murmur is best heard over the second left interspace. Pre-term infants may present with heart failure. Left untreated, some 5% of full-term infants die from heart failure and pulmonary complications in the first year of life. The remainder are usually asymptomatic. Apart from *chest X-ray*, which may reveal left ventricular enlargement and increased pulmonary arterial markings, *cardiac catheter studies* are usually not required unless other congenital lesions are suspected. Treatment is surgical obliteration of the ductus by ligation or division. More recently indomethacin, a prostaglandin E_1 inhibitor, has been shown to produce ductus closure in infants.

Fallot's tetralogy

The cyanotic or hypoxic appearance is diagnostic of a right-to-left shunt in congenital cardiac disorders. *Chest X-ray* shows a small heart size with diminished pulmonary markings. *Cardiac catheter* studies are essential to asses the feasibility of a one-stage total correction under total cardiopulmonary by-pass or a two-stage procedure with initial palliative shunting. The overall success rate for surgical correction is reported to be about 90%.

Valvular heart disease

Cardiac catheter studies and *cineangiocardiography* are almost invariably performed to assess significant valvular heart disease. They provide precise delineation of the degree of stenosis and regurgitation. Non-invasive *echocardiography* is useful in the initial assessment. Since the disease is one of mechanical failure of the valve, definitive therapy is necessarily surgical. Apart from some fairly limited indications for mitral valvotomy (i.e. splitting the valve), replacement of the diseased valves is recommended for valvular heart disease. Valve replacement may be of two types:

1. *Mechanical prosthetic valves*

—advantage: excellent durability
—disadvantage: require lifetime anticoagulation

2. *Tissue valves*

—advantage: less thrombogenic

—disadvantage: may require replacement 5–10 years later

Ischaemic heart disease—angina pectoris

HISTORY

Substernal chest pains radiating to the arm, neck or jaw, occurring with exertion or exposure to cold; symptoms promptly disappear with rest and relief with nitroglycerin.

EXAMINATION

Usually unremarkable; may be known hypertensive.

SPECIAL TESTS

ECG—graded exercise ECG may show ischaemic changes (ST segment depression) during or immediately following exercise; ST segment depression on resting ECG during episodes of chest pain indicates more severe coronary insufficiency.

MANAGEMENT

1. Medical

—nitroglycerine or β-adrenergic blockers for pain relief
—control of hypertension or hyperlipidaemia if present
—stop smoking
—attain ideal weight

2. Surgical

Indications

—disabling angina pectoris refractory to medical management
—unstable angina
—post-myocardial infarction angina
—block of the main stem of the left coronary artery

Pre-operative: coronary angiography and left ventriculography. Ideal conditions for recommending surgery are: greater than 70% stenosis of one or more major coronary arteries, satisfactory distal vessels and acceptable left ventricular function.

Operation. Cardio-pulmonary by-pass, using hypothermia and cardioplegia, is employed. Autogenous saphenous vein grafts are anastomosed from ascending aorta to the coronary arteries. Coronary endarterectomy may be necessary.

Prognosis. The saphenous graft patency rate is about 80% at one year, and prospective randomized studies show improved survival with surgery in patients with lesions of the left main stem coronary artery.

Dissecting aneurysm

HISTORY

Acute onset of chest pain ('tearing') with extension into the back and abdomen.

SIGNS

Absent or diminished peripheral or distal pulses. Shock from rupture, e.g. cardiac tamponade.

SPECIAL TESTS

Chest X-ray may show mediastinal widening

Aortography to confirm the diagnosis and to locate site of intestinal tear

CT-scan is increasingly useful as a non-invasive means to monitor patients with dissection

DIFFERENTIAL DIAGNOSIS

Myocardial infarction; a normal ECG and abnormal pulses suggest dissection.

PRINCIPLES OF MANAGEMENT

1. Control of hypertension in the acute stage
2. If the ascending aorta is involved, emergency operation may be needed as there is a high risk of rupture and cardiac tamponade. A tube graft replacement of the ascending aorta is required and aortic valve surgery may also be needed.

Atrial myxoma

This acts as a ball-valve effect and mimics mitral stenosis or regurgitation. Peripheral embolisation may be the presenting feature, which is verified on histology following embolectomy. Echocardiograms and angiography may be needed to clinch the diagnosis. Treatment is surgical removal.

22

Oesophagus and diaphragm

OESOPHAGUS

The main purpose of the oesophagus is to transport food from the mouth to the stomach and disorders which interfere with this function most commonly present with *dysphagia*. Though there are many non-malignant conditions of the oesophagus which cause difficulty with swallowing and which are amenable to treatment, a common cause is carcinoma which still carries a grave prognosis.

SURGICAL ANATOMY AND PHYSIOLOGY

The oesophagus is a muscular conduit from the pharynx to the stomach. In the adult the length of the oesophagus, as measured from the upper incisor teeth to the cardio-oesophageal junction, is about 40 cm. It extends through the superior and posterior mediastinum and lies in close proximity to the thyroid gland, trachea and carotid arteries in its cervical portion. In the thorax, the oesophagus passes behind the aortic arch and the left main stem bronchus, enters the abdomen through the diaphragm between the crura of the oesophageal hiatus, and joins the stomach at an angle in its cardiac portion. About 4 cm of oesophagus normally lie below the diaphragm.

The musculature of the pharynx and upper third of the oesophagus are composed of striated muscle, while the distal two-thirds of the oesophagus are smooth muscle. Whereas the upper oesophageal sphincter (cricopharyngeus) is a distinct anatomical entity, the lower sphincter is anatomically indistinct, but with a highly sensitive physiological response.

Three anatomical areas of narrowing occur in the oesophagus:

1. At the level of the cricoid cartilage.
2. In the mid-thorax, from compression by the aortic arch and left main stem bronchus
3. At the level of the oesophageal hiatus of the diaphragm

Blood supply

Cervical segment: branches from the inferior thyroid arteries

Thoracic segment: from bronchial arteries; oesophageal branches directly from the aorta

Abdominal segment: inferior phrenic arteries; oesophageal branches of the left gastric artery

Venous drainage

Upper two-thirds: to the azygos vein

Lower one-third: to the oesophageal tributaries of the coronary vein, a tributary of the portal vein which forms the connection between the systemic and the portal venous systems. When there is a rise in portal venous pressure, as in cirrhosis of the liver, blood is shunted upward through the coronary vein and the oesophageal venous plexus, with the subsequent development of oesophageal varices (p. 222).

Structure

The mucosal lining of the oesophagus consists of stratified squamous epithelium. While the oesophagus is remarkably distensible it is also notably friable and its wall is thin and lacks the protective covering of the peritoneum. For these reasons surgery of the oesophagus demands meticulous technique.

Motility

The peristaltic contractions of the oesophagus serve two main purposes:

1. To propel food from the pharynx to the stomach
2. To prevent reflux of gastric contents into the oesophagus

As a bolus of food enters the oesophagus, a peristaltic wave sweeps distally at a speed of 4–6 cm per second.

Primary peristalsis: the wave of contraction initiated by swallowing which begins in the upper oesophagus and travels the entire length of the organ.

Secondary peristalsis: local stimulation by food residues, distension or gastro-oesophageal reflux.

Tertiary waves: stationary non-propulsive contractions considered abnormal but may be present in elderly subjects who have no symptoms of oesophageal disease.

CLASSIFICATION OF DYSPHAGIA

Conditions causing difficulty with deglutition, such as local disease of the mouth, tongue and pharynx, are excluded and only lesions involving the oesophagus will be considered.

Lesions in the lumen of the oesophagus

Foreign bodies, including food.

Lesions in the wall of the oesophagus

1. Stricture

   a. Trauma
   b. Corrosives
   c. Reflux oesophagitis

2. Carcinoma (including carcinoma of cardia)
3. Benign tumours
4. Paterson-Kelly syndrome (sideropenic dysphagia)
5. Schatzki's ring with hiatus hernia
6. Scleroderma
7. Dermatomyositis
8. Crohn's disease
9. Motility disorders

   a. Achalasia of the cardia
   b. Cricopharyngeal spasm
   c. Diffuse oesophageal spasm

10. Tetanus
11. Bulbar paralysis (including post-diphtheritic)
12. Myaesthenia gravis
13. Post-vagotomy
14. Globus hystericus
15. Congenital atresia (tracheo-oesophageal fistulae)

Lesions outside the wall of the oesophagus

1. Pharyngeal pouch
2. Para-oesophageal hiatus hernia
3. Retrosternal thyroid
4. Mediastinal lymph nodes and tumours
5. Aortic aneurysm
6. Dysphagia lusoria
7. Peri-oesophagitis after vagotomy
8. Tight oesophageal hiatus repair

The *commoner* conditions are:

1. Carcinoma of the oesophagus
2. Carcinoma of the cardia
3. Reflux oesophagitis with stricutre formation
4. Achalasia of the cardia

SURGICAL PATHOLOGY

Carcinoma of the oesophagus

This occurs particularly in males over 65 years but there is a higher incidence in females with long-standing sideropenic dysphagia or in people suffering from long-standing chronic irritation of the oesophagus in association with reflux oesophagitis, leukoplakia and achalasia. The disease is interesting in having strong geographic links: Southern Africa, the Caspian and parts of mainland China. In Africa at least, iron brewing pots and nitrosamines are held to blame.

Macroscopically, the malignancy presents as an ulcer, a protuberant lesion or a stricture and the lower third, the middle third and the upper third of the oesophagus are involved in about 50%, 35% and 15% of cases respectively.

Microscopically, most are squamous-cell carcinomata but with little keratinization or cell nest formation. Adenocarcinomas involving the lower oesophagus are largely of gastric origin. Adenocarcinoma may develop in the lower part of the oesophagus if it contains gastric mucosa (Barrett's oesophagus).

Spread of the carcinoma longitudinally in the submucous plane usually occurs while direct spread through the wall of the organ can lead to involvement of vital structures such as the lung, bronchi and aorta.

Lymphatic spread to regional lymph nodes is present in about 60% of all operative cases but blood-borne metastases are uncommon. Metastases from upper oesophageal lesions may skip to the supraclavicular lymph nodes whereas lower oesophageal lesions may involve sub-diaphragmatic and coeliac nodes.

Complications arising as the result of oesophageal carcinoma include obstruction, ulceration, and perforation, while spread to vital structures may lead to recurrent laryngeal and phrenic nerve paralyses, tracheo-oesophageal fistula, empyema, lung abscess, pneumonia, pericarditis and superior vena cava obstruction.

Reflux oesophagitis with stricture formation

Reflux of gastric content into the oesophagus usually occurs in association with a sliding hiatus hernia but may be independent of it. Severe oesophagitis may then result because the oesophageal mucosa has no protective mechanism against the digestive action of gastric juice and in longstanding cases fibrous stricture formation can occur.

Achalasia

Failure of relaxation of the lower oesophagus (achalasia, cardio-spasm, mega-oesophagus) is considered to result from a neuromuscular disorder which may be associated with degeneration of the intramural plexus of Auerbach. The gullet becomes dilated, elongated and often hypertrophied above the obstructing segment while the muscle layers at the site of the obstruction may be atrophic normal or hypertrophied.

The condition usually occurs in middle age in patients of either sex but they may not present with symptoms until later in life, when regurgitation, aspiration and painless dysphagia become prominent symptoms.

Diffuse muscle spasm is a variant of this disorder in which varying lengths of the oesophagus are involved.

Paterson-Kelly syndrome (Plummer-Vinson syndrome, sideropenic dysphagia)

Some women with long-standing iron deficiency anaemia develop epithelial changes causing glossitis, angular stomatitis, koilonychia, pruritus ani and vulvae, gastritis and atrophy of the pharyngeal and cricopharyngeal mucosa. At the latter site, folds or webs of mucosa may develop as the result of chronic inflammation and hyperkeratinization and together with spasm of the cricopharyngeus muscle cause dysphagia (post-cricoid dysphagia).

Oesophageal webs can also develop in the absence of any typical anaemia and may be congenital or traumatic in origin.

The Schatzki ring

This is a rare abnormality in which a circumferential web-like obstruction occurs at the cardia in association with a hiatus hernia. It is presumably the result of inflammation of the oesophageal wall.

Post-vagotomy dysphagia

Following abdominal vagotomy, dysphagia may result from medistinitis and perioesophagitis, transient achalasia or subsequent hiatus hernia formation with reflux oesophagitis. The latter is alkaline. All these are rare.

Dysphagia lusoria

Anomalous right subclavian artery or aortic arch formation may compress the oesophagus and cause dysphagia.

Globus hystericus

The rather poor name given to dysphagia occurring in moments of tension. It expresses the patient's personality and there is no physical lesion.

Oesophageal laceration and perforation

Mallory-Weiss syndrome (see p. 223).
Perforations of the oesophagus may be:

1. *From within*

   a. Foreign bodies including food
   b. Instrumental perforations are most likely to occur in the cervical oesophagus, particularly when the posterior wall is pressed against osteoarthritic spurs of the cervical vertebrae. In the intrathoracic oesophagus, peforations are most common at the natural sites of anatomic narrowing.

2. *From without*: penetrating and missile injuries (rare)
3. *Postemetic*: so-called 'spontaneous' perforation most frequently occurs in the left posterolateral aspect of the lower oesophagus. Following on an alcoholic debauch with excessive food intake, there is violent vomiting or retching: a paroxysmal rise in intragastric tension occurs so that a pressure cone is driven up into the lower oesophagus resulting in full thickness rupture into the pleural cavity. Borehave's

DIAGNOSIS AND MANAGEMENT

The establishment of a diagnosis for dysphagia is usually possible after a consideration of the history, radiological and endoscopic findings. However, occasionally special tests such as exfoliative cytology, manometry and cineradiography may be helpful.

The diagnosis is made from a consideration of the usual triad: history, examination and special tests.

History

AGE:
30–40 years—suggests achalasia
Menopause—suggests Paterson-Kelly syndrome
50–70 years—suggests carcinoma of the oesophagus

SEX

Paterson-Kelly syndrome occurs almost exclusively in females.

SYMPTOMS

Dysphagia

1. A sudden onset may suggest foreign body obstruction or acute oesophagitis. Occasionally foreign body obstruction may be the first evidence of carcinoma of the oesophagus.
2. A slow onset is more likely with carcinoma of the oesophagus, achalasia and stricture formation.
3. Progressively worsening dysphagia, going on to total dysphagia, is typical of carcinoma and stricture. With spastic lesions there may be periods of remission.
4. Difficulty in swallowing solids initially is typical of malignancy, while fluids may cause symptoms initially with achalasia.

Pain

Pain from oesophageal disease may be located from the high cervical area to the epigastrium. Location of pain can be misleading.

Dysphagia together with a burning retrosternal pain suggests reflux or peptic oesophagitis. There is frequently a past history of dyspepsia. Pain is also characteristic of diffuse muscle spasm when it is severe and may be confused with myocardial disease.

Retrosternal or back pain following recent instrumentation or violent vomiting may indicate oesophageal perforation.

Regurgitation

This is characteristic of long-standing achalasia but it is also present, with stooping or straining, when a sliding hiatus hernia is present. Pharyngeal pouch formation, when large enough, causes regurgitation and spasms of coughing. It may be associated with a visible lump in the neck which may be emptied with pressure.

PREVIOUS DISODERS

1. Anaemia, glossitis, and stomatitis in a female suggest oesophageal web formation.
2. Instrumentation or swallowed corrosives suggest benign stricture formation.
3. Vagotomy for duodenal ulcer may indicate that perioesophagitis is the cause for the dysphagia.
4. Hiatus hernia repair and post-operative dysphagia may suggest that the oesophageal hiatus has been repaired too tightly.
5. Poliomyelitis or diphtheria may have resulted in oesophageal paralysis.

SPECIAL QUESTIONING

When no apparent clue has been forthcoming from the interrogation then other possibilities would be considered, e.g.:

1. Psychiatric disorders may suggest globus hystericus.
2. Peripheral arterial disease may lead to an aortic aneurysm being suspected.
3. Some bowel disorder may suggest the rarity—Crohn's disease of the oesophagus.

Signs

Most often, examination reveals remarkably little. However, malignancy may be evidenced by weight loss, palpable cervical lymph nodes, hepatomegaly or ascites. Crepitus in the cervical region and surgical emphysema in the acute case indicate oesophageal perforation.

Special tests

Barium swallow, barium meal and oesophagoscopy are most frequently helpful.

BARIUM SWALLOW

This will be of particular value in the following conditions:

1. Pharyngeal pouch will be visualized as a rounded pouch or as a 'teapot-spout' or 'cup and spill effect' when the barium overflows into the gullet.
2. Achalasia of the cardia produces dilatation of the oesophagus which may be fusiform, sausage-shaped or tortuous. In some cases contractility can be seen, but always the lower end tapers to a smooth point. As the oesophagus never empties adequately, the normal gas bubble in the stomach fundus is absent. Evidence of lung infection, as the result of repeated aspiration, may also be present.
3. Paterson-Kelly syndrome may show spasmodic stricturing in the upper end of the oesophagus, with or without webs.
4. Carcinoma of the oesophagus will appear as an irregular filling defect. There may be barium in the air passages if an oesophago-bronchial fistula is associated.
5. Reflux oesophagitis, stricture and hiatus hernia may be associated with free reflux, ulceration, stricture formation or a sliding hiatus hernia.
6. Perforation of the oesophagus may be demonstrated by swallowing a small quantity of water-soluble contrast, especially in regard to its site.

BARIUM MEAL

This is particularly helpful in determining the presence or absence of associated gastric disorders such as carcinoma of the cardia extending into the stomach, hiatus hernia or peptic ulceration.

OESOPHAGOSCOPY

An examination with a rigid instrument must be considered a potentially dangerous procedure which should be performed only by those experienced in its use. In the aged, with degenerative cervical spinal disease, rupture of the oesophagus is a particular hazard. The modern flexible fibreoptic panendoscope has however abolished many of the problems associated with the rigid instrument.

Typical oesophagoscopic features include the following:

1. *Carcinoma of oesophagus*. Ulceration, stricture formation of a protuberant lesion may be demonstrated. Haemorrhage may occur at these sites as the instrument is passed.
2. *Reflux oesophagitis*. The lowest part of the gullet wells up with gastric juice and the mucosa may be hyperaemic, ulcerated, haemorrhagic, strictured or covered with areas of leukoplakia.
3. *Achalasia*. The oesophagus is seen to be dilated and filled with stagnant food which when washed out reveals a remarkably normal-looking mucosa.
4. *Paterson-Kelly syndrome*. Cricopharyngeus muscle spasm may cause the passage of the oseophagoscope to be difficult. Webs and atrophic muscosa may be seen.

In all cases, biopsy of any doubtful lesion must be performed.

CYTOLOGY

Either at the time of oesophagoscopy or independently, cytology may detect some early oesophageal cancers.

MANOMETRY

Most beneficial in the detection of early achalasia.

TREATMENT

Prophylaxis

1. Careful instrumentation of oesophagus to avoid trauma
2. Correction of anaemias which may be associated with epithelial changes such as stomatitis, glossitis, pruritis
3. Control of reflux oesophagitis by medical or surgical means, e.g. repair of a hiatus hernia, reduction in acid output by vagal section or H_2 receptor blockade (p. 150)

Curative treatment

1. Pharyngeal pouch. Excision.

2. Corrosive stricture. Early oesophagoscopy (the flexible scope is preferred) is useful to determine extent of injury and to guide further management. Initially nothing by mouth and broad-spectrum antibiotics and corticosteroids are often prescribed. There is no objective evidence that steroids are necessary. In very severe corrosive burns with transmural involvement and mediastinitis, total parenteral nutrition may be life-saving. Subsequently narrowing and stenoses of the oesophagus require repeated dilatation but ultimately by-pass, usually with a segment of colon, will often be necessary.

3. Achalasia. Antispasmodics are of little value. The condition may sometimes be cured or relieved for a long time by a forcible if gradual dilation using a hydrostatic bag. However, the best treatment is division of all the muscle layers at the oesophago-gastric junction (Heller's cardiomyotomy). A similar technique may be applied to diffuse muscle spasm.

4. Paterson-Kelly syndrome. Correction of anaemia, repeated dilatation and regular follow-up for possible developing oesophageal carcinoma is required.

5. Carcinoma of the oesophagus. In all cases the prime aim is to restore the power of swallowing. About 70% of patients are fit enough for operation but in only 40% of these is there no evidence of spread beyond the oesophagus. In addition the mortality from oesophagectomy is still of the order of 15% and the average survival time after operation is about 15 months. Few cases can be cured.

When malignancy is confined to the oesophagus and not associated with evidence of local or distant spread, an oesophago-gastrectomy may be performed for carcinoma of the lower third of the oesophagus and a partial oesophagectomy for carcinoma of the middle third. For carcinoma of the upper third of the oesophagus resection would entail a near total oesophagectomy, the alternative being radiotherapy which in expert hands can give comparable results to surgery.

Post-cricoid carcinoma in relation to Paterson-Kelly syndrome is more susceptible to cure but this usually means pharyngo-oesophagectomy and the anastomosis of the mobilised stomach to the mid or upper pharynx. Permanent tracheostomy is necessary.

When the malignancy cannot be resected, restoration of swallowing may be obtained with a by-pass operation utilising an isolated limb of small bowel; alternatively, and usually preferably, the tumour may be intubated with a plastic tube. Either a laparotomy is done and the tube threaded down the oesophagus or, particularly where the disease reaches epidemic proportions and many cases have to be dealt with, the stricture is dilated and the tube pushed down on the end of the endoscope.

6. Stricture formation with reflux oesophagitis. The treatment depends on the cause. Many patients' symptoms can be controlled by medical means because the lesion is not a true stricture, more in the nature of inflammatory oedema. When antacids or H_2 blockers fail, reduction of a hiatus hernia usually combined with vagal section is most commonly done. If there is an established fibrous stricture a variety of complex operations may be needed.

7. Oesophageal perforation. Following supportive therapy of intravenous fluids and antibiotics to combat mediastinitis, the mainstay of treatment is thoracotomy, mediastinal drainage and suturing of the tear if feasible.

DIAPHRAGM

Diaphragmatic herniae constitute the main surgical condition of this structure.

CLASSIFICATION OF DIAPHRAGMATIC HERNIA

1. Congenital
   a. hernia through the foramen of Morgagni
   b. hernia through the foramen of Bochdalek
   c. eventration of the diaphragm
2. Traumatic
3. Hiatus hernia
   a. sliding
   b. para-oesophageal (rolling)
   c. combined sliding and para-oesophageal

SURGICAL PATHOLOGY

1. Congenital diaphragmatic herniae

Embryologically the diaphragm is developed by fusion of:

   a. the septum transversum
   b. the dorsal mesentery
   c. the pleuro-peritoneal membranes
   d. a peripheral rim from the body wall (somatomes)

Foramen of Morgagni hernia—failure of fusion of the sternal and costal portions of the diaphragm anteriorly in the mid-line creates the defect. It is more common on the right side.

Foramen of Bochdalek hernia—failure of fusion of the pleuro-peritoneal canal so that a free communication exists between the abdominal and pleural cavities.

Abdominal viscera sometimes nearly fills up the hemithorax.

Eventration of the diaphragm may occur as the result of anomalous development of the diaphragm or its innervation. The affected hemidiaphragm is raised and immobile.

2. Traumatic diaphragmatic hernia

Rupture of the diaphragm is usually the result of severe blunt external trauma or crushing injuries and sometimes from penetrating wounds. Apart from penetrating injuries, the left hemidiaphragm is more commonly ruptured. Herniation of abdominal viscera into the chest either occurs immediately or there may be a lapse of some time—even months or years.

3. Hiatus hernia

This is a prolapse of any part of the stomach through the oesophageal diaphragmatic hiatus into the thorax. Hiatus herniae are common, but probably only 30% are associated with more than slight symptoms.

PREDISPOSING FACTORS

It is commonly held that these herniae arise as a result of progressive weakening of the oesophageal hiatus due to the following factors:

   a. *Degeneration or disruption of the oesophageal hiatus musculature*
      (i) Fatty infiltration with obesity
      (ii) Normal ageing processes
      (iii) Wasting diseases
      (iv) Multiple pregnancies
   b. *Raised intra-abdominal pressure*
      (i) Chronic cough
      (ii) Constipation
      (iii) Bladder neck obstruction
      (iv) Pregnancy
   c. *Raised intra-gastric pressure*
      (i) Pyloric narrowing, particularly due to duodenal ulcer
      (ii) Pyloro-spasm in association with duodenal ulcer or cholelithiasis

Sliding hiatus hernia

This is really a *hernia-en-glissade* (comparable in anatomical principle to a sliding inguinal hernia, see p. 233) and it represents about 80% of all types.

As the name implies the upper part of the stomach and the cardia slide up and down in the posterior mediastinum in association with an empty left-sided peritoneal

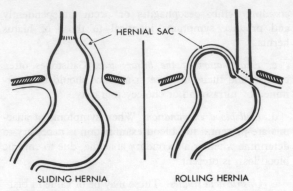

HERNIAL SAC

SLIDING HERNIA   ROLLING HERNIA

Fig. 22.1 Types of hiatus hernia

sac the apex of which corresponds to the level of the cardia (Fig. 22.1).

Under normal conditions there is a difference of pressures between the oesophagus and stomach and reflux of gastric content into the lowest oesophagus is prevented by a mechanism which is complex and ill-understood.

The following are thought to be relevant factors:

a. The valve-like effect of the angulation of the oesophago-gastric junction
b. The sphincteric action of the circular muscle of the lowest oesophagus (inferior oesophageal sphincter)
c. The 'cork in a bottle' action of the mucosal folds and thickened muscularis mucosae at the cardia
d. The 'pinch cock' action of the right crus of the diaphragm

Once the cardia and portion of the stomach are allowed to remain in the chest, then protective mechanisms are lost and reflux of gastric juices occurs; the severity of the effects is dependent on the degree of acidity of the juice and the susceptibility of the oesophageal squamous epithelium, not on the size of the hernia.

Reflux leads to oesophagitis of the lowest oesophagus and superficial and multiple ulcers occur; if the process is allowed to continue, haemorrhage, fibrosis, stricture formation and peri-oesophagitis will result.

Para-oesophageal hiatus hernia

In contrast to the sliding type, the para-oesophageal or rolling hiatus hernia is really a hernia of the greater curvature of the stomach, carrying with it a peritoneal sac to the right or left side of the oesophagus (Fig. 22.1). It is therefore a true hernia and accounts for about 10% of hiatus hernias (the remaining 10% being combinations of the sliding and rolling types).

Unlike sliding herniae, para-oesophageal herniae are liable to obstruct or strangulate. Because the cardia remains an intra-abdominal structure at all times, reflux oesophagitis does not occur.

CLINICAL FEATURES

1. Congenital diaphragmatic herniae

Foramen of Morgagni hernia may not develop any symptoms until later in life as the defect is usually small. The vast majority of Morgagni herniae are detected incidentally on routine chest X-ray as asymptomatic anterior cardiophrenic masses.

Foramen of Bochdalek hernia often presents as an acute respiratory emergency at or shortly after birth, depending upon the amount of herniated abdominal viscera present in the hemithorax. Rarely Bochdalek herniae remain undetected till later childhood. The affected hemithorax is usually dull to percussion with evidence of shift of mediastinal structures to the opposite side. The diagnosis is almost always apparent on chest X-rays which often demonstrate gas-filled intestines. Colon, small bowel, stomach, omentum and portions of liver have been encountered. Symptoms are uncommon with eventration of the diaphragm which is usually discovered on incidental chest X-ray.

2. Traumatic diaphragmatic hernia

The amount of herniated abdominal viscera present in the thorax following injury determines the degree and onset of symptoms. With massive herniation, cardiorespiratory function is impaired and life may be threatened. Haemorrhage and intestinal obstruction leading to strangulation may occur.

Gas-filled or homogenous shadows, along with mediastinal shift on chest X-rays following injury, are strongly suggestive of ruptured diaphragm. Occasionally contrast studies of the gastrointestinal tract are required to establish a diagnosis.

3. Hiatus hernia

Hiatus herniae tend to occur in the middle-aged and elderly and particularly in obese females.

It is important to remember that a hiatus hernia can exist without the production of symptoms; even large herniae which are associated with little or no incompetence are often associated with trivial or no symptoms.

When symptoms do occur, they often closely resemble those produced by biliary, gastric, duodenal or pancreatic disease and when X-rays demonstrate a hiatus hernia it should not necessarily be accepted as the cause for the symptoms until other causes have been eliminated.

Symptoms can be described under the following headings:

a. Those due to reflux and oesophagitis. As a result of incompetence of the cardia in association with a sliding hernia the following occur:

(i) *Reflux.* Fluid often reaches the mouth where the acid taste of gastric juice is recognised.

(ii) *Heartburn.* This may be present as a sensation of retrosternal heat or rawness, or a burning pain which is aggravated by lying down or stooping. The pain may radiate through to the back or be referred to the jaw or arms, simulating cardiac ischaemia.

(iii) *Belching.* The upward passage of 'wind' is common and occurs most often at night.

b. Those due to the complications of reflux oesophagitis.

(i) *Dysphagia.* The result of oedema initially but later due to fibrosis of the lower oesophagus.

(ii) *Haematemesis.* Peptic ulceration of the oesophagus.

(iii) *Anaemia.* Chronic blood loss from the ulcerated oesophagus: rare and other causes should be sought.

c. Those due to the presence of the hernia in the chest. These usually occur with large para-oesophageal herniae.

(i) Flatulent dyspepsia
(ii) Fullness or distension
(iii) Shortness of breath
(iv) Tachycardia
(v) Severe upper abdominal or precordial pain with dysphagia, due to strangulation of a large para-oesophageal hernia, is rare.

d. Those due to the presence of associated conditions. In about 20–30% of cases there is associated duodenal ulceration, gallstone disease or gastric ulceration, and symptoms referable to these conditions may be indistinguishable from those of hiatus hernia.

Special tests

a. *Barium swallow and meal.* These X-rays, which are performed in the head-down position, will demonstrate the type and size of the hernia, the presence of reflux and any associated stricture formation.

b. *Oesophagoscopy.* It is important to perform an oesophagoscopy whenever a stricture is associated; then the presence of oesophagitis and reflux will be noted and a biopsy of any doubtful lesion taken. Occasionally carcinoma of the lowest oesophagus may complicate long-

standing reflux oesophagitis or occur independently and produce symptoms identical to those of hiatus hernia.

c. *Examination of the biliary tree.* Gallstones often coexist, and their presence or absence should be determined by ultrasound or cholecystography.

d. *Full blood examination.* When symptoms of anaemia are present a full blood examination is necessary to determine whether a secondary anaemia, due to chronic blood loss, is present.

e. *Gastric acid studies.* These may be of value in planning treatment, particularly if duodenal ulceration is associated.

f. *Oesophageal motility.* There is an increasing tendency to incriminate the intrinsic lower oesophageal sphincter in cases of reflux with or without the presence of a hiatus hernia. Oesophageal manometry will disclose such weakness and though not yet routine is being increasingly used. A weak sphincter is an indication for a fundoplication (see below) if conservative management fails.

TREATMENT

1. Congenital diaphragmatic herniae

In most instances, elective surgical repair of the defect and reduction of herniated viscera is undertaken by the abdominal approach. In infants who develop cardiorespiratory distress, emergency operation is necessary. The results of surgery are generally excellent.

2. Traumatic diaphragmatic hernia

In acute rupture of the diaphragm, associated injuries often take precedence over the diaphragmatic tear. A transthoracic repair of the diaphragm is often recommended and primary suture of the defect is often possible after reduction of herniated viscera.

3. Hiatus hernia

When the hernia is an incidental finding, and symptomless, then treatment is not indicated.

CONSERVATIVE
A sliding hernia associated with heartburn, regurgitation and belching is usually treated conservatively.

a. Weight reduction if overweight
b. Avoidance of stooping
c. Avoidance of constricting corsets and belts

d. Adoption of a semi-sitting position for sleep

e. Correction of constipation and chronic cough

f. Administration of alkalis or H_2 blockers when heartburn is present

g. Avoidance of gastric stimulants such as alcohol and cigarette smoking

h. Treatment of associated gallstone disease and peptic ulceration on their merits

OPERATIVE

Indications

a. Failure of conservative treatment and the persistence of reflux oesophagitis

b. Large para-oesophageal herniae which are resistant to conservative treatment and liable to obstruct or bleed

c. Presence of complications—ulceration, stricture formation, or haemorrhage

Principles of operative repair

a. Approach

(i) *Abdominal repair.* This is indicated when reflux is the main problem but when ulceration, stricture formation, or a large para-oesophageal hernia is not present. It is also indicated when an associated abdominal condition requires operation.

(ii) *Thoracic or thoraco-abdominal repair.* This is indicated when a large para-oesophageal hernia is present or when oesophageal ulceration or shortening is associated with peri-oesophagitis and fixation of the oesophagus in the mediastinum.

b. Objectives

(i) to produce a barrier to reflux at the gastro-oesophageal junction

(ii) to prevent recurrence of the previous anatomic configuration

Anti-reflux procedures

There are three types commonly used.

1. *Fundoplication (Nissen procedure)* consists of wrapping the cardia around the stomach over a large nasogastric tube; the seromuscular layer of the cardia is used and sutures are placed in the oesophagus in order to maintain the wrap-around in position.

2. *Belsey procedure* uses a transthoracic approach to construct a valvular mechanism by suturing the cardia both to the oesophagus (wrap-around 270°) and to the undersurface of the diaphragm. Allison type IV

3. *Median arcuate, posterior gastropexy (Hill repair)* consists of suturing the lesser curve of the gastro-oesophageal junction to the median arcuate ligament and preaortic fascia.

Procedures to restore anatomic configuration

The limbs of the right crus are exposed and sutured together with interrupted non-absorbable material in front of the oesophagus to create a snug tunnel, or behind the oesophagus to create a snug hole (*Allison repair*).

There are three additional procedures which may be performed alone or in combination with this simple repair and they are as follows:

a. Restoration of the acute oesophago-gastric angle, by suturing the left side of the lowest oesophagus or the adjacent diaphragm to the fundus of the stomach

b. Reconstitution of the stretched 'phreno-oesophageal' ligament when present as an impressive structure, by sutures passing between it and the anterior and lateral aspects of the oesophageal hiatus. There remains, however, considerable debate as to the anatomy of the phreno-oesophageal ligament and its importance in hiatus hernia repair.

c. Vagotomy and a drainage operation, which has real validity, particularly in those patients with associated duodenal ulceration, or an elevated preoperative acid secretion without duodenal ulceration

23

Peptic ulcer

Peptic ulcers occur at sites in the gastrointestinal tract which are exposed to acid pepsin juices and gain their name from the presumed though unproven autodigestion which occurs. They are most frequent at a junctional zone between acid-producing or acid-bathed and other mucosa, e.g. junction of antrum and body of stomach on the lesser curvature, first part of the duodenum, oesophago-gastric junction and at a stoma between stomach and small bowel.

CAUSE

In spite of a vast amount of work, not a great deal is known about cause beyond that acid is essential for the activation of pepsin that then leads to a breakdown of mucosal resistance. No acid, no ulcer still holds true.

Hyperchlorhydria. Most but not all patients with duodenal ulcer, pyloric channel ulcer (p. 150) or severe reflux oesophagitis produce more acid than normal subjects when stimulated by either gastrin analogues or via the vagus. The nature of the inbuilt defect is unknown but possibly relates to a greater sensitivity to vagal stimulation. That it is inbuilt is attested to by the young age at which ulcer symptoms begin (rare in childhood, not uncommon in the late teens and early twenties, common in the mid-twenties).

Duodeno-gastric reflux. Many patients with gastric ulcer have an incompetent pylorus and reflux of bile which produces a chronic gastric mucosal reaction which may predispose to a gastric ulcer.

Anti inflammatory drugs (e.g. acetyl salicylic acid, phenyl butazone, indomethacin) can cause ulcers in animals and are strongly associated with both gastric and duodenal ulcer in man. Whether they are truly ulcerogenic or merely potentiate other causes is a matter for debate. Steroids, which slow wound-healing rates, are also in this class but are unlikely on their own to *cause* ulcers.

Mucosal irritants—'social poisons'. Alcohol, tobacco and spicy foods have variable associations with ulcer in both stomach and duodenum. Whether there is a direct cause–effect relationship or whether the drinking–smoking syndrome is a manifestation of stress (see below) is uncertain, but there is little doubt that both agents slow ulcer healing.

Stress a. Exogenous factors such as pressure of work, mental disharmony and social disruption may precipitate ulceration in a susceptible person or make an ulcer worse if it already exists. The effect is probably mediated through the vagus. Perhaps too much has been made of the 'business man's ulcer's and most patients who present for treatment of chronic ulcer do not have such problems.

b. In acute trauma or illness 'acute erosion' may occur with the formation of one or many ulcers in stomach or duodenum. Gastrointestinal haemorrhage frequently follows. Curling's ulcer in severe burns, which was (wrongly) said to be found chiefly in the second part of the duodenum, is an example. The cause of this type of stress ulceration is unknown, but is almost certainly *not* hyperchlorhydria.

Blood groups Blood Group O is found with a higher incidence in duodenal ulcer patients, which may indicate a disorder of protective mucopolysaccharide secretion.

Excessive secretion of gastrin from an extra gastric site—Zollinger–Ellison syndrome when the source is usually an islet cell tumour of the pancreas (p. 156).

Hypercalcaemia (p. 156).

SURGICAL PATHOLOGY

ACUTE PEPTIC ULCERS

Acute ulcers are minute, most often mucosal in depth and situated anywhere in the stomach or duodenum.

148

Occasionally, either organ is extensively involved with acute ulcers (acute gastric erosions or haemorrhagic duodenitis). They are characteristic of 'stress' ulceration.

CHRONIC PEPTIC ULCERS

The relative incidence of gastric and duodenal ulcers varies greatly from community to community, presumably because of the influence of some of the factors mentioned above.

Duodenal ulcer

Duodenal ulcers have the following features:

1. Most are single and situated in the first 2–3 cm of the first part of the duodenum on its anterior or posterior wall. The exception is Zollinger–Ellison syndrome, where ulcers are often multiple and extend into second or third parts of the duodenum or even the jejunum.
2. Not infrequently two ulcers occur on opposite walls of the duodenum (kissing ulcers).
3. They are usually punched out.
4. They may be complicated by:

    a. *Penetratration*. The head of the pancreas, posterior abdominal wall and the liver may be involved.
    b. *Haemorrhage*, which will usually be the more severe the deeper the penetration.
    c. *Perforation*. Anterior duodenal ulcers may perforate into the general peritoneal cavity.
    d. *Obstruction*. Pyloric stenosis due to oedema and fibrous contracture of the duodenal wall in various proportions is always possible with any chronically unhealed ulcer.

Gastric ulcer

Gastric ulcers have the following features:

1. Most are single and situated on the lesser curvature of the stomach.
2. Those situated close to the pylorus or the cardia and those on the greater curvature should be suspected of being malignant.
3. Size varies greatly but the largest, which may occupy most of the lesser curvature, are usually benign.
4. Shape is usually round and punched out.
5. The base is often clean and smooth, and penetration through the muscularis mucosa of the stomach wall has always occurred.

COMPLICATIONS
a. *Penetration*. The wall of the stomach may be eroded

completely and penetration into neighbouring structures may result.
b. *Haemorrhage* which may be minimal when it arises from a hyperaemic mucosa or torrential if a blood vessel outside the stomach wall has been eroded by a penetrating ulcer.
c. *Perforation*. This may occur into the lesser sac, causing a peri-gastric abscess, or into the general peritoneal cavity, causing peritonitis.
d. *Obstruction*. Most often cicatricial stenosis of the stomach by a chronic gastric ulcer is not severe enough to cause obstruction. However, occasionally an 'hour-glass' deformity of the stomach may occur with unusually large ulcers.

MALIGNANT CHANGE IN GASTRIC ULCERS
There has been a long-standing controversy about whether or not a chronic gastric ulcer—like chronic inflammatory lesions elsewhere—can undergo malignant change. The answer is uncertain but opinion now suggests that the vast majority of 'malignant ulcers' are primary cancers that have been digested by the local action of acid-pepsin. It should be noted that if this is accepted it must also be realized that if acid pepsin is suppressed by, for example, H_2 blockade with cimetidine or ranitidine (p. 150), then ulceration in a malignant growth can heal. There are numerous cases on record where this has happened and in consequence 'healing' is not an indication of benignity.

CLINICAL FEATURES
ACUTE ULCERATION

The association with stress has already been mentioned. There are two clinical circumstances:

1. Typical ulcer symptoms develop in an individual because of exogenous factors. There is often rapid progression to a complication such as bleeding or perforation. If the factors causing the problem can be dealt with the ulcer will usually heal and not recur.
2. A true stress ulcer or ulcers occurs after major trauma or acute serious illness such as myocardial infarction. These ulcers are usually asymptomatic (or their symptoms are masked by the events) until they bleed (common) or perforate (rare).

GASTRIC AND DUODENAL ULCERS
Symptoms

1. *Pain*. It has always been said that it is possible to distinguish between the symptom patterns of gastric and duodenal ulcer, but this may in practice be quite dif-

ficult. Both produce 'dyspepsia'—i.e. food-related discomfort usually amounting to pain. In both the pain is epigastric in position. In duodenal ulcer it characteristically precedes a meal (hunger pain) and in gastric ulcer follows shortly after it. Relief follows vomiting (gastric ulcer) and ingestion of alkalis or milk in both types. Aggravation is said to follow spicy foods and alcohol.

2. *Vomiting* usually means pyloric or hour-glass obstruction. In both instances oedema may be the immediate cause.

3. *Weight loss* may be a feature with gastric ulceration and is due to the patient's loss of appetite because of associated gastritis. Weight loss is not usual with duodenal ulceration but weight gain may occur with the high consumption of milk.

4. *Symptoms of anaemia* if there is chronic bleeding sufficient to reduce the haemoglobin below 8 g/dl.

PYLORIC CHANNEL ULCER

This relatively uncommon ulcer occurs just proximal to the pylorus. Its features resemble duodenal ulcer rather than gastric ulcer (acid secretion is often raised) and because it is so close to the sphincter, vomiting often accompanies the pain. It is managed on the same lines as duodenal ulcer.

Signs

In all ulcers there is usually little to find. Evidence of weight loss and anaemia may be apparent.

Special tests

1. Barium meal. This is an essential requirement for any patient with a history suggestive of peptic ulceration.

Radiological features associated with duodenal ulceration include a persistently deformed duodenal cap with or without an ulcer crater and delayed emptying of the stomach over 4 hours if there is any degree of pylorospasm or stenosis present.

Radiological features associated with gastric ulceration include a constant crater usually on the lesser curvature, often associated with a notch of spasm immediately opposite on the greater curvature and distortion of the mucosal folds which approximate each other at the edges of the ulcer.

2. Fiberoptic gastroscopy. Endoscopy has been revolutionized by the development of flexible controllable glass-fibre endoscopes. With these the whole of the oesophagus, stomach and the duodenum at least to its second part can be clearly seen. It is now reasonable to say that the diagnosis in any patient with peptic ulcer is incomplete until endoscopy has been done. Further-

more, healing can best be assessed by repeat endoscopy. Finally, in gastric ulcer biopsies can be undertaken, an important move in establishing that the lesion is or is not benign.

3. Acid secretion tests. Are of little value in the diagnosis and management of peptic ulcer. They may be useful in so-called X-ray negative dyspepsia, but even here are less helpful than is endoscopy.

TREATMENT

Virtually every ulcer, whether it be gastric or duodenal, can be healed by rest in bed, vigorous antacid therapy (not just an occasional tablet or powder), prohibition of smoking and alcohol, and in the case of duodenal ulcer, by the use of a histamine H_2 receptor blocker which prevents acid production.

In gastric ulcer there are a number of agents which increase mucosal blood flow—e.g. carbenoxalone, liquorice extract—and these are effective in combination with antacids and bed rest. The problem is keeping the ulcer healed. Many gastric ulcers will stay healed but few duodenal ulcers do unless maintenance H_2 blockade is continued. The long term effects of this are not known, but reduction in acid output by drugs or surgery means bacterial colonization of the stomach. This in turn may mean the production of nitrosamines which are potentially carcinogenic. The same is of course true of operations which reduce acid output.

SURGICAL MANAGEMENT

The surgeon's role in the treatment of peptic ulcer changes rapidly with the evolution of new methods of suppressing acid secretion and changing patterns of disease in the community he serves.

Absolute indications for surgery

Perforation—see p. 153.
Massive haemorrhage—see p. 224.
Fibrous stenosis—see p. 154.
Malignant change. Duodenal ulcers are not subject to this risk. As has been stated (p. 149) gastric ulcers are usually benign or primarily malignant. Surgery is obviously needed for any malignant ulcer.

Relative indications for surgery

1. Recurrent bouts of complication such as repeated bleeding or inflammatory stenosis.

2. Relapse after medical treatment with significant problems in relation to work or social life. Since the advent of specific methods of reducing acid secretion (H_2 blockers) it has become more difficult to understand the physiology of 'unresponsive' duodenal ulcer. Probably most of it is failure of compliance and/or persistence of the use of social poisons (p. 148) which are synergistic in ulcer production.

OPERATIONS AVAILABLE

Duodenal ulcer

Surgery for uncomplicated duodenal ulcer has evolved from partial gastrectomy to highly selective vagotomy in the past 30 years but all the various operations remain in use.

Partial gastrectomy. The antrum which produces gastrin and about half of the acid secreting portion of the stomach are removed. Continuity is restored by gastrojejunal anastomosis (Fig. 23.1), which has the advantage that the residual stomach is bathed in alkaline juice. It may have the disadvantage that the atrophic gastritis which follows can lead to malignancy. The recurrence rate is low (less than 1%) but post-gastrectomy sequelae (see below) may be severe.

Vagal section. If the vagi are divided acid secretion is reduced. However, the vagus is motor to the gut and its adnexae as a whole so that certain disadvantages must follow. There may be:

1. Changes in gastro-intestinal motility and
2. Impaired emptying of the gall bladder.

Truncal vagotomy is very effective in curing duodenal ulcer provided denervation of the stomach is complete. However, it results in the pylorus failing to open and therefore in gastric stasis. Consequently, the pyloric ring must be destroyed (pyloroplasty) or bypassed (gastroenterostomy). These necessary secondary procedures also expose the patient to the risks of post gastric surgery sequelae and though the operation is safer than partial

gastrectomy, it is often associated with approximately the same incidence of unsatisfactory results.

Selective vagotomy. In this procedure only the vagal fibres to the stomach are divided. Thus, the possible effects of visceral denervation outside the stomach are avoided. However, pyloric denervation still takes place and pyloroplasty or gastroenterostomy, with their own problems, must be performed.

Highly selective vagotomy. In this operation only the nerves to the parietal cell mass are sectioned. This is done by mobilizing the lesser curvature from the antrum to the oesophagus and dividing all blood vessels and nerves. The pyloric innervation is left intact so that pyloroplasty or gastrojejunostomy are unnecessary. At the time of writing this seems the best procedure with a low rate of recurrence (less than 5%) and an equally low rate of unsatisfactory results from post gastric surgery disturbances. The operation requires some special training and skill.

Gastric ulcer

Many gastric ulcers will heal. However, a residuum do not. An unhealed ulcer has a 5–10% chance of being malignant. Though there are a number of operations available, the most satisfactory treatment is a Billroth I partial gastrectomy (Fig. 23.2).

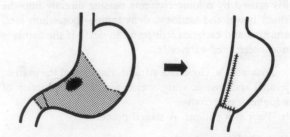

Fig. 23.2 Billroth I gastrectomy

COMPLICATIONS OF SURGICAL MANAGEMENT

EARLY

All peptic ulcer operations are subject to the complications of abdominal surgery—paralytic ileus, mechanical intestinal obstruction and breakdown of suture lines. In addition after vagotomy the stomach may occasionally be slow to empty and there may be transient dysphagia. However, it is reasonable to say that surgery is now very safe and that perhaps only one or two in a thousand patients die in the immediate post-operative period as a direct consequence of elective ulcer surgery.

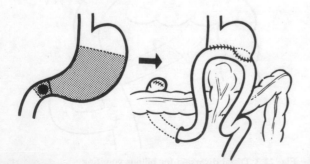

Fig. 23.1 Polya gastrectomy with Hofmeister valve

LATE

1. Anastomotic and recurrent ulceration is caused by:

    a. Inadequate resection of parietal cell mass

    b. Isolated antrum left after Polya gastrectomy and secreting gastrin at a steady rate

    c. Zollinger-Ellison syndrome (see p. 150)

    d. Incomplete vagotomy

    e. Possibly a persistent suture in the anastomosis. More usually this is merely a suture exposed as a consequence of ulceration from another cause.

Prophylaxis: adequate primary treatment.

Management is related to cause and requires investigation to ascertain the level of acid secretion or the completeness of vagotomy which can be done by stimulating the vagus to produce acid by rendering the patient hypoglycaemic with insulin. When gastrectomy has been inadequate the choice lies between permanent H_2 receptor blockade, vagotomy or a further resection and is decided on the merits of the individual case. A retained antrum is removed. Conversely recurrence after vagotomy is usually best treated by Polya gastrectomy.

2. Gastrojejunocolic fistula is now rare and occurs when a recurrent ulcer after gastrojejunal anastomosis penetrates into the colon. It should arouse the suspicion of Zollinger-Ellison syndrome.

Clinical features. Severe diarrhoea occurs due to enteritis caused by colonic contents passing directly into the small bowel and acidosis, dehydration, potassium loss, anaemia and cachexia will result in death if the fistula is not interrupted surgically.

Treatment. a. Good risk patient. Excision of the gastric, jejunal and colonic components and the construction of a higher gastrectomy.

b. Poor risk patient. A staged procedure:

Stage 1: Proximal colostomy which diverts the faecal stream from the fistula and thus stops the enteritis.

Stage 2: Excision of fistula and its visceral components and the construction of a higher gastrectomy and colonic anastomosis.

Stage 3: Closure of colostomy.

3. Post-gastric surgery symptoms and syndromes. *Late effect of ablation or bypass of the pylorus.* The stomach is a reservoir and the pylorus 'meters' food rendered iso-osmotic with plasma into the small bowel for further digestion and absorption. Consequently, ablation of gastric areas plus, as is always the case, loss or bypass of the pylorus allows the entry of hyperosmolal, large volume loads into the jejunum. Two things follow:

1. The bulk stimulates peristalsis and results in pain, rapid transit and thus occasionally diarrhoea.
2. The hyperosmolality draws fluid into the gut lumen which aggravates the bulk problem and may also reduce blood volume so creating vasomotor instability—the patient feels faint and tremulous after a meal.

These features constitute the 'dumping syndrome' which is aptly named because it does result from dumping a large volume of hypertonic liquid into the jejunum.

All sorts of methods of management have been suggested for dumping. Most cases can be prevented by an optimistic attitude that if the patient eats normally after gastric surgery there will only be a transient period of difficulty. Small meals at frequent intervals perpetuate the problem. After Polya gastrectomy—the most frequent cause of severe dumping—conversion to a Billroth I (Fig. 23.2) with the addition of an interposed jejunal loop which acts as a brake on gastric emptying is the best surgical treatment.

4. Anaemia. Partial gastrectomy and Polya reconstruction interferes with duodenal absorption of iron and a microcytic anaemia may result. More rarely, sufficient stomach has been removed to cause failure of release of intrinsic factor and thus a macrocytic anaemia. Malnutrition may contribute to both.

5. Weight loss and its complications. Particularly after partial gastrectomy when patients are unwilling to eat sufficiently, weight loss is common. Severe malnutrition is rare, but there is an increased risk of nutrition-associated diseases such as tuberculosis.

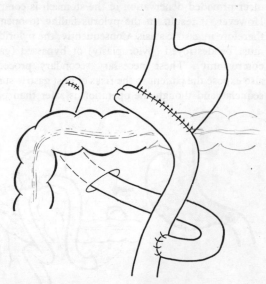

Fig. 23.3 Distal diversion for bilious vomiting

6. Bilious vomiting. Any operation which destroys or bypasses the pylorus allows bile to reach the stomach. Not only does this produce atrophic gastritis but it may also be associated with bilious vomiting. This is most likely after a Polya gastrectomy where characteristically a patient eats a meal and some 10–20 minutes later vomits bile only. In severe cases either normal anatomy should be restored usually with jejunal interposition or the bile should be diverted more distally into the intestine (Fig. 23.3).

7. Diarrhoea. Apart from the dumping syndrome, all vagotomies except highly selective ones seem to cause severe diarrhoea. Matters are made worse if cholecystectomy has been done or is subsequently done.

Though the foregoing is a formidable list, surgery for duodenal ulcer can be highly satisfactory and in particular, highly selective vagotomy is a relatively safe and innocuous procedure.

COMPLICATIONS OF PEPTIC ULCERATION

HAEMORRHAGE

The problem of upper gastro-intestinal bleeding is such a large one that it is treated separately in Chapter 31.

PERFORATION

This occurs in about 10% of all ulcers—90% of perforations are on the anterior wall of the first part of the duodenum.

Surgical pathology

Perforation occurs when digestion outruns repair, but the final event is ischaemic—the thinned out ulcer base drops out. Thus, there is little peritoneal reaction at the ulcer site and the liquid enters the free peritoneal cavity. At first the peritonitis is chemical; as time advances (12 hours plus) it becomes bacterial, presumably from escape of organisms through the bowel wall. Occasionally a small ulcer will seal against an adjacent organ or omentum so producing only local signs.

Clinical features

HISTORY

A history of ulcer may or may not be present. Any of the aggravating factors—alcohol, tobacco, stress, steroids, acetylsalicylic acid for example—may be found. Perforation may follow an acute drinking bout.

SYMPTOMS

1. Pain. Excruciating pain of sudden onset and situated in the epigastrium is the outstanding feature. Referred pain to the shoulders is common when the gastric or duodenal contents irritate the diaphragm. The pain is typically aggravated by movement such as occurs in a rapidly driven and swerving ambulance.

2. Vomiting. This is not invariably present but when it is haematemesis is occasionally associated. Persistent vomiting may occur as peritonitis becomes advanced and paralytic ileus develops.

SIGNS

1. Shock. In the initial stages this is vasovagal in type with bradycardia and hypotension from the severe pain. Gradually this merges into extracellular fluid loss and sepsis. Thus, in a patient with a recent perforation there is pallor, sweating, hypotension. Later, there are the features of hypovolaemia.

2. Peritonitis. When seen within a few hours abdominal wall tenderness, board-like rigidity and absent bowel sounds are outstanding features. When the perforation is localized, tenderness and rigidity may be confined to the epigastrium, the right hypochondrium and right iliac fossa. It is in such patients that there is a risk of confusion with (a) acute cholecystitis; (b) acute appendicitis.

When seen late there is diminishing rigidity, abdominal distension (paralytic ileus) and vomiting.

3. Diminished liver dullness. This may be present as the result of the escape of gas into the peritoneal cavity.

4. Rectal examination. In the presence of generalized peritonitis with pelvic involvement, tenderness will be elicited on digital examination. This does not occur early.

5. Respiratory embarrassment. The splinting of the diaphragm produces shallow respiration and failure to cough. Thus, there is early basal collapse. If this is severe the patient may be cyanosed.

Special tests

Plain X-ray of chest and abdomen. In about 70% of cases an erect chest film will show a raised and immobile right hemidiaphragm with free gas beneath it. Sometimes a fluid level is seen beneath the gas shadow. A serum amylase concentration should be done in any doubtful case.

Differential diagnosis

The important conditions to be considered are:

1. Acute appendicitis with spread of liquid up the right paracolic gutter

2. Acute cholecystitis
3. Acute pancreatitis

Gas under the diaphragm is one of the most important differentiating signs. Serum amylase concentrations must be interpreted with caution because the level may reach 1000 iu/l in perforated ulcer. If there is continuing doubt about the diagnosis then laparotomy should nearly always be done.

Treatment

OPERATIVE

Operation with closure of the perforation is the standard method of treatment.

Pre-operative preparation. Once the diagnosis has been established the pain is best relieved by a small dose of morphine given intravenously, the stomach is emptied with a naso-gastric tube and intravenous replacement therapy is begun. The patient is prepared for laparotomy as soon as possible.

Operation. The abdomen is opened through an upper right paramedian or midline incision and the perforation is closed with atraumatic catgut sutures assisted perhaps with a plug of omentum. Next, careful peritoneal toilet is essential and the paracolic gutters, pelvic basin and subphrenic spaces must be sucked out thoroughly, particularly if a lot of food and foul smelling peritoneal fluid is present.

Outcome. The mortality with perforated peptic ulcers depends on the delay before operation, the age and general condition of the patient and the type of ulcer which has perforated.

Perforated gastric ulcers are associated with a higher mortality than duodenal ulcers because they often occur in older people, the perforations are often larger and the peritonitis resulting is more severe because the escaping gastric content is more irritant than duodenal content.

Definitive treatment at the time of operation. The chances of recurrent ulcer symptoms after successful closure of a perforation depend on the nature of the ulcer. If it is the acute result of exogenous factors, whether these be socio-psychological or drugs and if these can be corrected, recurrent problems are unlikely. Even in patients with a chronic ulcer, long standing symptoms and a large parietal cell mass, though the chances are high (50 to 70 per cent) that in the next 10 years further trouble will occur, it is difficult if not impossible to predict in which patients this will happen. Now that blocking agents are available there should be even greater caution in suggesting that because there is a risk of recurrence, definitive treatment should be carried out at the time of perforation.

Such treatment should be reserved for:

1. When perforation occurs with haematemesis.
2. When perforation occurs with pyloric stenosis.
3. Most chronic gastric ulcers and particularly when perforation of a possibly malignant gastric ulcer occurs.
4. When simple suture and plugging of perforated duodenal ulcer is likely to cause duodenal obstruction.

The choice of a definitive operation rests with the technical problem and the surgeon's familiarity with the particular operation. Partial gastrectomy is the commonest operation but highly selective vagotomy plus any indicated local procedure on the ulcer is gaining in popularity.

NON-OPERATIVE TREATMENT OF PERFORATION

The basis of this is that many perforations are sealed to adjacent viscera at the time of operation. However, this natural propensity cannot be relied upon and non-operative treatment is usually second best. It may be used in the following circumstances:

1. When the perforation has apparently sealed off and is associated with only localized peritonitis ('forme fruste')
2. When the perforation occurred days previously and the patient appears to be in reasonable general condition
3. When expert facilities are available for repeated clinical and radiological re-appraisal
4. By contrast when operative facilities are *not* available—a ship at sea, an isolated construction camp

The method is contra-indicated:

1. When there is any doubt about the diagnosis
2. When there is a known large ulcer present
3. When there is lack of first class ability to care for the naso-gastric suction

The method entails nothing by mouth, naso-gastric suction, intravenous replacement therapy and repeated clinical and radiological assessment of the progress of the sub-diaphragmatic gas. It is abandoned if there is no marked improvement within 12 hours.

PYLORIC STENOSIS

The word pyloric is really a misnomer because fibrosis and narrowing which results from a chronic duodenal ulcer, or oedema and inflammation from an acute exacerbation, causes obstruction of the *duodenum* and not the pylorus. However, it is hallowed by time.

Surgical pathology

An ulcer is associated with inflammation and oedema. The larger or more circumferential the ulcer the more likely is this to cause obstruction. Oedema gets worse if the ulcer progresses so that an attack of pyloric stenosis may be associated with a bout of ulcer symptoms. Spasm is an unlikely cause of pyloric stenosis in most duodenal ulcers but may occur in pyloric channel ulcer.

In more long standing circumstances, fibrosis becomes an increasing part of pyloric stenosis. Occasionally in the elderly the ulcer may heal leaving only a 'cicatricial' stenosis but this is rare.

Obviously it is important to distinguisb between these different pathological states because to do so will influence management.

Clinical features

HISTORY

Nearly always there is a history of chronic duodenal ulcer.

SYMPTOMS

1. *Vomiting* is the outstanding symptom; it is typically profuse and bile free but contains partly digested and foul smelling food. The vomiting occurs at infrequent intervals and days may separate each episode.

2. *Pain* occurs only if there is an associated acute exacerbation of peptic ulceration. Often the condition is relatively painless.

3. *Constipation* is the consequence of water and electrolyte lack and starvation.

4. *Weight loss and weakness*. Again starvation is the cause. It is important to remember that a fairly high grade stenosis can exist without vomiting. The patient is anorexic and may lose weight but there is nothing to call attention to the stenosis.

SIGNS

1. The patient appears 'dehydrated'. However, much of this is weight loss which produces much the same picture of a lax skin, sunken eyes and relatively empty veins.
2. The typical appearances in the abdomen are:

   a. Fullness in the left hypochondrium
   b. Visible peristalsis passing from left to right from under the left costal margin
   c. A 'succussion splash' which is elicited by gently rocking the patient from side to side. The large quantity of liquid and gas in the stomach produces a characteristic 'sloshing' sound.

Special tests

1. *Barium meal*—shows gastric dilatation, sometimes with increased peristalsis, a narrowed pyloro-duodenal area and delayed gastric emptying.

2. *Fiberendoscopy*. The stomach contains food residue. The pyloric canal is narrow and oedematous. The endoscopist reports 'friable mucosa and difficulty in entering the pyloric ring'.

3. *The biochemical lesion*. Though in pyloric stenosis one would expect large quantities of hydrogen ion to be lost, this is not often the case. What happens is:

a. Starvation with sodium conservation and potassium loss from the kidney
b. Mild hydrogen ion loss from the stomach which in combination with (a) makes for alkalosis
c. As potassium stores are exhausted, excretion of hydrogen ion by the kidney so accelerating alkalosis
d. In very acute cases a loss of water and electrolyte that produces acute extracellular volume deficiency

Differential diagnosis

1. *Carcinoma of the pylorus*. This may be impossible to distinguish from obstruction due to duodenal ulceration until operation is undertaken. A short history is more suggestive of carcinoma.

2. *Miscellaneous causes of pyloric obstruction*. Occasionally pyloric stenosis may be produced after a pyloroplasty or after an oversewing of a perforated duodenal ulcer. Hypertrophic pyloric stenosis in the adult, a mucosal diaphragm, benign tumours, corrosive strictures, foreign bodies and supra-pyloric and sub-pyloric lymph node enlargement, are rare causes of pyloric stenosis.

Treatment

The aims are to:

1. Correct dehydration and electrolyte losses with intravenous therapy
2. Empty and wash out the stomach daily with a large bore stomach tube and saline
3. Restore nutritional status with parenteral feeding
4. Relieve the obstruction. There are two groups of patients:

   a. Those with pain (active ulcer). When inflammation and oedema are considered to be major factors precipitating obstruction, a trial with frequent milk feedings, two-hourly gastric aspirations and H_2 blockade may be attempted in the hope that the obstruction will be overcome.

b. Those without pain (chronic fibrotic stenosis). Surgery is indicated and the choice of operation will depend on the patient's general condition.

ZOLLINGER–ELLISON SYNDROME

Surgical pathology

Rarely, a peptic ulcer may be caused by ectopic gastrin production, usually in an alpha cell pancreatic adenoma but sometimes in a duodenal tumour. All such tumours have common characteristics.

1. They are histologically or histochemically distinct being of the 'amine precursor' (apudoma) type, probably derived from the neural crest.
2. Though they have the histopathological characteristics of malignancy and may metastasise to both regional nodes and the liver, they are not usually biologically malignant—that is to say, they do not destroy the patient by widespread invasion.

Clinical features

The steady drive of hypergastrinaemia produces maximum acid output from the parietal cell mass. This in turn results in aggressive peptic ulcer, often in distal sites— post-bulbar or jejunal. The ulcers tend to be progressive leading to haemorrhage or perforation. A characteristic of the syndrome is that conventional ulcer treatment fails and recurrence is early and aggressive. Secondary surgical complications such as gastrojejunocolic fistula are common and treatment becomes ever more difficult.

Diagnosis

1. Clinical features of intractable or aggressively recurrent ulceration should arouse suspicion.

2. Basal secretion is near maximal secretion because of gastrin drive. An overnight secretion study may reveal 80–100 mmol of acid as against a normal 5–10.
3. Serum gastrin concentrations are always raised but repeated determinations are needed because levels fluctuate.
4. A number of special tests are available such as anomalous responses of gastrin levels to infusion of calcium and of secretin.
5. Some patients have what appears to be Z–E syndrome but also have a raised serum calcium. Usually this is the consequence of a parathyroid adenoma and they are thus examples of the *multiple endocrine adenoma syndrome*. The hypercalcaemia should be dealt with first and may initially result in a regression of symptoms.

Management

1. Gastrin works through stimulation of the production of histamine. Thus, H_2 blockers can control the disease initially and deal with complications.
2. Theoretically, identification and removal of the gastrin producing lesion should cure the disorder. Unfortunately this is difficult because:

   a. Tumours may be small, multiple and have metastasized to the liver.
   b. Z–E syndrome can be associated with either adenomatosis in the pancreas or gastrin cell hyperplasia in the stomach.
3. Total gastrectomy is the definitive treatment because it removes the target organ. Hypergastrinaemia persists, but is now harmless.

24

Stomach

GASTRIC CANCER

Carcinoma of the stomach is relatively common, second only in frequency to carcinoma of the lung in the male and carcinoma of the breast and uterus in the female.

The condition is more frequent in Japan, Holland, Czechoslovakia and Finland than in other parts of the world.

1. Apart from Japan it appears to be on the decline throughout the Western World.
2. Other new growths are rare but sarcoma—leiomyo-sarcoma—and lymphoma occur.

PREDISPOSING FACTORS

1. Heredity. Relatives of affected people are more susceptible to the development of gastric cancer than others. There is also an increased incidence in people with blood group A.

2. Achlorhydria and pernicious anaemia. Patients with pernicious anaemia have a six times greater chance of developing gastric cancer than the general population.

3. Chronic gastritis and intestinal metaplasia. It appears that gastric cancer is likely to develop in areas of metaplastic mucosa associated with atrophic gastritis and achlorhydria. The mucosa comes to resemble intestinal mucosa with the formation of goblet cells and Paneth cells. In that gastritis is a sequel of operations for peptic ulcer that destroy the pylorus (p. 151), there is an increased incidence of cancer after Polya gastrectomy (approximately 5% after 20 years) though it is not yet clear if the same thing happens after vagotomy and drainage.

4. Benign gastric ulcer. Malignant change in benign gastric ulcer is unusual and probably occurs in less than 1% of cases. More important however is the fact that there is a 10% chance of a malignant gastric ulcer being labelled 'benign', even after careful clinical and radiological assessment.

5. Gastric polyps. About 10% of all gastric polyps are malignant when detected.

SURGICAL PATHOLOGY

Carcinoma of the stomach has its maximum incidence in the sixth decade, although no age is exempt, and the ratio of males to females is 3:2.

About 50% of tumours occur in the pre-pyloric region of the stomach, 25% on the lesser curvature and 10% at the cardia, while the remainder are evenly distributed on the greater curvature and the fundus.

Macroscopic features

1. Ulcerative
2. Polypoid or proliferative
3. Diffuse or infiltrating (leather-bottle stomach, linitis plastica)

The ulcerative type is the commonest and it is usually situated in the pre-pyloric region or the lesser curvature.

The polypoid type is the next commonest and it is usually situated in the fundus or body of the stomach.

A particular form of ulcerative cancer—'superficial spreading'—is common in Japan and is also found increasingly in other countries. The lesion remains confined to the mucosa for some time and may even heal (see p. 149).

Microscopic features

Almost all tumours are adenocarcinomas arising from mucus-secreting cells and they can be graded according to the degree of cell differentiation, lucoid changes are not uncommon.

Squamous carcinoma of the stomach is rare but it may arise from areas of metaplasia or as an extension through the cardia of an oesophageal tumour.

Spread

1. Direct. Occurs primarily by way of the subserosal, submucosal and intramuscular lymphatics of the stomach wall.

With tumours of the lower half of the stomach there is about a 50% chance of the duodenum being involved, but seldom is this beyond 3 cm from the pylorus. With tumours of the upper half of the stomach there is a similar incidence of lower oesophageal involvement, but it may be greater in extent.

Spread by direct extension through the wall of the stomach to adjacent structures (liver, pancreas, transverse colon, diaphragm, common bile duct, and greater and lesser omentum) is quite common.

Dissemination throughout the peritoneal cavity is not uncommon and ovarian implants (Krukenberg tumours) may occur.

2. Lymphatic. This is present in about 50% of all cases which come to operation. The stomach drains to the lesser and greater curvatures, in four quadrants, which correspond in area to those supplied by the right and left gastric and gastro-epiploic arteries.

Lymph flow along the course of the left gastric artery enters the superior gastric nodes; that following the right gastric artery enters the supra-pyloric nodes; that following the left gastro-epiploic artery enters the pancreatico-splenic and splenic hilar nodes, and that following the right gastro-epiploic artery enters the sub-pyloric nodes. Eventually all lymph enters the coeliac nodes about the coeliac axis (Fig. 24.1).

Although this four quadrant mode of lymphatic drainage is usual, so that areas of involvement correspond to the site of the primary, any group of lymph nodes may be involved by cancer cells from a tumour situated in any part of the stomach.

All lymph from the coeliac group of nodes drains directly into the cisterna chyli and so to the thoracic duct and at an advanced stage of malignancy the left supra-clavicular nodes may be involved (Troisier's sign).

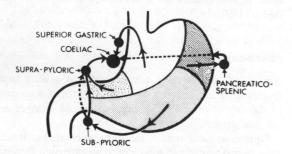

Fig. 24.1 Lymphatic drainage of the stomach

3. Blood. This may occur by way of the portal veins giving rise to metastases in the liver and occasionally to distant parts of the body.

Complications

1. Obstruction. Pyloric lesions can result in pyloric obstruction (see Chapter 23) while lesions at the cardia can cause dysphagia (see Chapter 22).

2. Perforation. Between 10 and 20% of all gastric perforations are due to carcinoma of the stomach. Perforations of gastric tumours tend to be larger than perforations of benign ulcers and the resultant peritonitis is therefore likely to be more severe.

3. Haemorrhage. Torrential haemorrhage can occur if major extra-gastric vessels are eroded by the malignant process but usually there is an insidious loss of blood causing iron deficiency anaemia.

4. Fistula formation. A gastro-colic fistula will occur if the gastric malignancy penetrates into the colon.

Prognostic factors

1. Site of tumour. Tumours at the cardia have the worst outlook. The reason may be surgical as it is difficult to estimate the extent of submucous spread up the oesophagus and so the proximal limit of the resection.

2. Macroscopic features. Linitis plastica is associated with virtually no 5-year survivals.

3. Microscopic features.
a. Poorly differentiated tumours have a grave prognosis.
b. Superficial spreading cancer has an excellent outlook—up to 60% 5-year survival.
c. Lymphocytic and plasma cell infiltration is a moderately reliable sign and the greater its intensity the better the outlook.
d. Lymph node involvement is associated with about a 10% chance of 5-year survival. In the absence of lymph node involvement there is a 40% chance of a 5-year survival.

CLINICAL FEATURES

Because initial symptoms of carcinoma of the stomach are most often vague and ill-defined, the delay before treatment is between 6 and 12 months. Considerable delay is most likely to occur with tumours situated in the body of the stomach or on the greater curvature because these are notoriously late in producing suspicious symptoms. Tumours near the pylorus, causing obstruction with vomiting, are likely to be diagnosed earlier.

Epigastric pain radiating to the back, weight loss and the development of an abdominal mass are features of advanced malignancy which are only too often present when the patient is first seen.

Modes of presentation

1. Vague dyspepsia. This is the commonest symptom and is often associated with loss of appetite and energy, a distaste for certain foods, fullness after meals, belching and sometimes an unexplained iron deficiency anaemia.

2. Pain. Pain of a gnawing type, without the regular-meal relationship which is typical of peptic ulcer, may be constant and unrelieved by food and antacids.

These are relatively early symptoms of gastric carcinoma, and when they appear for the first time in a previously healthy patient in the cancer age goup, suspicion of carcinoma of the stomach or carcinoma of the caecum should be aroused. There is always a temptation to treat dyspepsia with antacids, including H_2 receptor blockers. In an ulcerating cancer suppression of acid pepsin secretion may allow the growth to re-epithelialize so that it is wrongly assumed to have 'healed'.

3. Dysphagia. Carcinoma of the cardia may cause progressive dysphagia and regurgitation.

4. Vomiting. Carcinoma of the pre-pyloric region may be associated with progressive pyloric stenosis and vomiting, epigastric fullness, weight loss and dehydration. Even those growths that do not obstruct may be associated with vomiting presumably because peristalsis is disordered.

5. Advanced disease. Carcinoma of the stomach first presents with metastases in 25% of cases, when ascites, jaundice, hepatomegaly, enlarged supraclavicular nodes, cachexia, anaemia and an obvious abdominal mass may be outstanding features.

6. Miscellaneous. a. haematemesis; b. perforation.

Special tests

BARIUM MEAL
In expert hands this test has a 90% accuracy rate. The radiologist sees three types of lesion.

1. Ulcer
It should be remembered that most gastric ulcers are benign and therefore most of those occurring in the pre-pyloric region or lesser curvature are benign. Also very large ulcers are often benign. However some features which indicate a malignant ulcer are:

a. When an ulcer crater lies wholly within the stomach lumen, it classically sits on a plateau of cancerous tissue so that its crater appears to be within the confines of the gastric wall, unlike the niche of a benign ulcer, which projects beyond the confines of the wall.
b. Lack of convergence of mucosal folds about the ulcer. Healing of a benign ulcer is associated with scar contraction which deforms the mucosal folds and causes them to radiate from the edges of the crater.
c. Rigidity of the surrounding stomach

2. Proliferative lesion
This forms a constant filling defect in the stomach which may illustrate a 'fingerprint' pattern.

3. Infiltrating lesion
This causes rigidity and disordered mobility and loss of peristalsis. If limited in extent it is seen as a straight aperistaltic plaque, but in more advanced cases (linitis plastica) the stomach is contracted to a narrow rigid tube.

FIBEROPTIC GASTROSCOPY
Dyspeptic patients at or past the age of 40 should be endoscoped. Only by this technique is it possible to pick up the early mucosal cancer. Though radiology is accurate in the advanced lesion, it cannot have the precision of endoscopy when the cancer is confined to the superficial layers. In addition, a biopsy or brushing of a lesion for cytology is possible and, particularly when the diagnosis is 'gastric ulcer', multiple biopsies may establish the diagnosis of malignancy. Finally, endoscopy now makes it possible clearly to see the fundus—a notoriously difficult area in which to make an X-ray diagnosis.

Endoscopy can potentially be used to screen high risk groups who are asymptomatic. This is done in Japan but not to any great extent elsewhere.

GASTRIC CYTOLOGY
Cytodiagnosis is based on the knowledge that there is exfoliation of cells from all internal surfaces lined by epithelium. In addition it is known that tumour cells are exfoliated more readily and in greater numbers than cells from a normal epithelial surface.

Fluid for examination is obtained by washing out the stomach aggressively with saline, perhaps with the addition of an abrasive brush, and a skilled cytologist can differentiate between normal epithelial cells and malignant cells. It is to be remembered however that the absence of malignant cells in the gastric washings does not rule out a malignancy.

MISCELLANEOUS TESTS

1. Tests of gastric function. The absence of free hydrochloric acid in an ulcerated stomach is highly suggestive of malignancy, but it should be noted that in 50% of all gastric malignancies the gastric acid values are normal or increased.

2. Faecal occult blood. This is present in most gastric malignancies.

TREATMENT

The only form of potentially curative treatment of carcinoma of the stomach is an *en bloc* excision of the tumour, with 5 cm of macroscopically normal stomach on each side, together with the lymphatic glands draining the area.

Curative surgery

There remains some controversy as to whether a total or subtotal gastrectomy should be performed, but so long as there is an *en bloc* removal of the greater and lesser omentum, the spleen, and the lymph nodes (superior gastric, coeliac, supra- and sub-pyloric, and pancreatico-splenic), then the amount of stomach removed should be dictated by the size and position of the tumour. In other words the operation performed should be as radical an operation as a total gastrectomy, except that some stomach is retained. Alternatively a total gastrectomy may be technically easier.

An acceptable plan of curative surgery is as follows:

1. Distal tumours. For tumours of the pylorus, antrum, and lower half of the stomach, in which there is no evidence of fixation or metastases, a radical subtotal gastrectomy is performed. This includes the tumour and 5 cm. of stomach above and below, the omenta, the named lymph node collections, and the spleen (Fig. 24.2).

Continuity is preferably restored by a Billroth I (gastro-duodenal type of anastomosis) (Fig. 23.2); however, if a Polya-type reconstruction is performed, it should be of the ante-colic type.

2. Proximal tumours. For tumours of the fundus, or upper half and body of the stomach, or when tumours

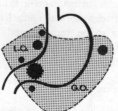

Fig. 24.2 Radical subtotal gastrectomy for distal tumours: L.O. = lesser omentum; G.O. = greater omentum

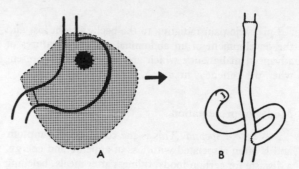

Fig. 24.3 Total gastrectomy for proximal tumours **A**. Extent of resection **B**. Reconstruction with Roux-Y oesophago-jejunal anastomosis

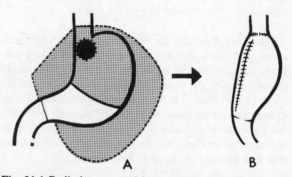

Fig. 24.4 Radical upper partial gastrectomy for cardiac tumours **A**. Extent of resection **B**. Oesophago-gastric reconstruction

are so large as to demand entire stomach removal, a total gastrectomy is performed *en bloc* with the omenta, nodes and spleen. The tail of the pancreas should also be included for posterior wall tumours.

The operation may be performed through an abdominal or thoraco-abdominal incision, and intestinal continuity is restored by either a loop or limb of small bowel (Fig. 24.3).

3. Cardiac tumours. For tumours at the cardia either a radical upper partial gastrectomy (Fig. 24.4) or a total gastrectomy is performed.

Palliative surgery

When local or distant spread of the tumour precludes a curative resection then a limited gastrectomy is preferred if the lesion is removable.

By-pass operations (gastroenterostomy or oesophago-gastric by-pass) will be effective in overcoming an obstructing tumour but benefit cannot be expected for longer than a few months.

Supportive therapy

For inoperable and incurable patients analgesics will

have to be administered frequently when pain is a problem. Currently chemo-therapeutic agents are of little proven value in advanced gastric malignancies.

SARCOMA AND LYMPHOMA

Both these tumours are rare—less than 5% of all gastric malignancies.

Sarcoma is usually a tumour of smooth muscle—a leiomyosarcoma.

Surgical pathology

Sarcoma. Because the muscle is outside the mucosa such tumours are initially submucosal and may initially grow outwards to form large pedunculated growths. If they invade the mucosa the ulceration is local and accompanied by necrosis in the tumour so that there are long tracks into the mass which produce characteristic appearances on X-ray examination.

Lymphoma. These growths are usually ulcerating masses and may occur anywhere in the stomach. Microscopically they show wide variation in cell pattern which has led to pathologists producing many different classifications to bewilder students and others.

Clinical features

Both tumours are not commonly diagnosed preoperatively though endoscopic biopsy is altering this. The presenting features are the same as for gastric cancer. Clinical examination may reveal a mass which is larger than expected from the symptoms and the patient's well being.

Treatment

The treatment is primarily surgical though a lymphoma diagnosed histopathologically by endoscopy may be treated by radiotherapy and chemotherapy. In localized leiomyosarcoma the prognosis is good but much less so is lymphoma.

RARE CONDITIONS

Menetrière's disease is a giant hypertrophy of the gastric mucosal folds of unknown cause. Presentation is by:

a. Protein losing enteropathy
b. Chronic upper gastrointestinal bleeding

Some patients can be controlled by medical means but others will require total gastrectomy.

Swallowed foreign bodies and bezoars

Children and individuals of odd disposition will often swallow undigestible foreign material. Small toys and other blunt objects can be left to pass through under X-ray control. Larger objects—which have infinite variety—may have to be removed but it is difficult to prevent recurrence. When indigestible material of animal origin (usually hair) or vegetable (skins and husks) accumulate in the stomach a bezoar results—a solid mass of the glutinous or hard material which effectively is a stomach cast. Such patients lose appetite and weight and may present with a large upper left quadrant mass the shape of the stomach. Most bezoars require surgical removal though occasionally they can be broken up or enzymatically digested.

25

Biliary and pancreatic disorders

BILIARY CALCULI AND RELATED DISORDERS

Non-malignant disease of the biliary tree is almost exclusively caused by the presence of biliary calculi.

PATHOGENESIS

1. Secretion of lithogenic bile, i.e. bile which is supersaturated with cholesterol
2. The occurrence of sepsis in the biliary tree
3. Anatomical abnormalities which predispose to stasis
4. Abnormalities of the gall bladder epithelium

Lithogenic bile

Cholesterol is 'solubilized' in bile as a 'micelle' with lecithin and bile salts. It is evident from Fig. 25.1, that only when the appropriate ratios of lecithin and bile salts are

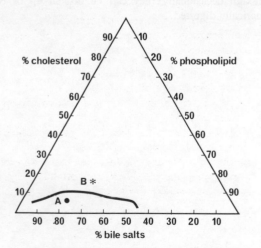

Fig. 25.1 The lipid composition of bile. The curve represents the maximum solubility of cholesterol. A. Normal composition B: 'Lithogenic' bile supersaturated with cholesterol.

present can cholesterol remain under saturated and prevented from forming crystals. It is currently thought that metabolic abnormalities in the liver predispose to the secretion of lithogenic bile. Such abnormalities may be:

1. Inborn
2. Conditioned by diet

Of the two, the second seems more likely and the 'Western' high protein, high fat diet seems the important factor. Other contributory matters are:

1. The contraceptive pill
2. Pregnancy
3. Possibly obesity
4. Low residue diet with inadequate fibre
5. Loss of the terminal ileum which interferes with the enterohepatic circulation.

Sepsis

It is likely that the liver is constantly trapping small numbers of organisms either from the portal or systemic blood. Some of these may be excreted in the bile and if they find an appropriate nidus (Cholesterol crystals, mucus, epithelial debris) will persist and proliferate. Local multiplication of organisms may then deconjugate and precipitate bile salts so that a 'mixed' stone results. Sepsis in a biliary tree which contains stones may cause bouts of:

1. Acute cholecystitis
2. Ascending cholangitis

A special form of sepsis is seen in the Far East where primary common bile duct stones (i.e. those that are associated with precipitation of bile salts and pigment rather than with cholesterol deposition) give rise to severe ascending cholangitis—so-called oriental cholangiohepatitis. Extensive damage to the liver is common. The liver fluke *Clonorchis sinensis* is frequently present in the duct (as are round worms occasionally) but its role in causation is uncertain.

Anatomical abnormalities

The biliary tree is characterized by a remarkable tendency to display anatomical variants and anomalies which incidentally make its surgery difficult and occasionally hazardous. Any cul de sac or incompletely drained branch of the tree predisposes to sepsis and stone formation.

Abnormalities of the gall bladder epithelium

It is uncertain if abnormalities of the gall bladder epithelium are primary or secondary. However, proliferation and detachment of cholesterol-laden epithelium may again form the starting point of a stone.

CLINICAL SYNDROMES

By far the greatest majority of gall stones are asymptomatic: 10–15% of all individuals over the age of 60 in Western communities have gall stones, usually in a functioning gall bladder. Stones may be found at routine investigations. If they occur in a functioning gall bladder there is no pressing indication to remove them. However, stones in a non-functioning gall bladder or in the common duct are very likely to cause trouble in the future and, other things being equal, are an indication for surgery.

Gall stones predominantly produce episodic acute or subacute syndromes characterized by pain. Contrary to popular opinion, there is no evidence to support the idea that they are associated with fatty food intolerance or 'flatulent dyspepsia'. However, an acute attack of obstruction/infection can be precipitated by a fatty meal, presumably because the release of cholecystokinin causes forcible contraction against a potential or actual obstruction.

Stones without infection cause obstructive syndromes:

1. Paraxial—no jaundice
   a. in the gall bladder neck (Hartmann's pouch) and cystic duct (common)
   b. in one of the hepatic ducts (rare)
2. Axial—jaundice
   a. in the common hepatic duct (unusual)
   b. in the common bile duct, often at its lower end (usual)

Stones with infection cause inflammatory syndromes.

1. Paraxial—acute cholecystitis
2. Axial—ascending cholangitis

Obstruction of cystic duct without sepsis leads to distension of the gall bladder. Unlike acute appendicitis the condition does not commonly progress to ischaemia and rupture of the wall. Either:

1. The condition is self limiting, the stone falling back into the fundus of the gall bladder as distension takes place, or
2. A mucocele (gall bladder distended with bile and otherwise non-functioning) forms.

The clinical syndrome is 'biliary colic'. Acute upper abdominal pain, epigastric in situation, tending to the right, sometimes radiating to the back or right shoulder. Though called colic, the pain is more characteristically of distension type—rising rapidly to a peak and then sustained relatively unchanged for some hours or even a day or two. There is reflex nausea and sometimes vomiting. Signs are unusual because there is no transmural inflammation to generate peritoneal irritation. A mucocele may be palpable as a slightly tender globular mass protruding from under the right costal margin.

Obstruction by some of the common hepatic or common bile duct without sepsis is relatively uncommon, occurring mainly in primary common duct stones. Intermittent or unrelenting jaundice with mild pain of distension type is the rule (see p 166).

Obstruction of cystic duct with sepsis—acute cholecystitis. The process does resemble acute obstructive appendicitis in many ways but again tends usually to be self-limiting. Macroscopically the gall bladder becomes inflamed on its serosal aspect; omentum and bowel may adhere and the junction of cystic duct and common hepatic may be involved in an inflammatory mass of varying density. On the internal aspect, varying degrees of mucosal ulceration take place. The sequelae may be:

1. Resolution with or without episodic recurrence
2. Progression to gangrene and perforation, usually in the fundus but occasionally at the neck because of ulceration of a stone. Perforation may be:

   a. Local with abscess formation
   b. Into the peritoneal cavity
   c. Into a neighbouring viscus—most commonly the duodenum
3. 'Chronic cholecystitis' which is a pathological rather than a clinical entity
4. Empyema of the gall bladder—an intact wall but an intraluminal abscess which can produce a varying amount of systemic disturbance

Other clinico-pathological associations of acute cholecystitis are:

1. Jaundice. The result either of:

   a. Inflammation in the angle between cystic duct and common hepatic duct

b. A more generalized infective process involving the axial biliary tree

2. Pancreatitis, which may be associated with:
   a. otherwise asymptomatic biliary tract stone
   b. an attack of acute cholecystitis (see p. 165)

3. Gall stone ileus. This follows perforation into the gastrointestinal tract with an escape of a stone which is then propelled down the small bowel to impact usually in the terminal ileum. Low small bowel obstruction then follows.

ACUTE CHOLECYSTITIS

History

Previous attacks of gall stone disease with upper abdominal pains have commonly been experienced.

Symptoms

PAIN

This is usually of sudden onset, severe in nature and situated initially centrally but thereafter beneath the right costal margin and radiating to the right to the angle of the scapula. The pain may first be colicky indicating the stage of obstruction of the cystic duct or neck of the gall bladder. Occasionally the attack stops short at this stage, while progression to acute cholecystitis is associated with more constant and throbbing pain.

VOMITING AND NAUSEA

These are common but most often mild in nature.

Signs

GENERAL

Pyrexia and tachycardia are indicative of the infective nature of the process and are invariably present.

LOCAL

1. *Tenderness* over the gall bladder is a constant sign.

2. *Guarding and rigidity* indicate involvement by the inflammatory process of the parietal peritoneum adjacent to the gall bladder. More generalized abdominal rigidity indicates that perforation has probably occurred and that the process has certainly spread beyond the limits of the gall bladder.

3. A *palpable mass* of globular proportions extending beneath the right costal margin and moving with respiration is due to either a pericholecystic collection of omentum and adjacent viscera, or an empyema.

4. *Murphy's sign*. If the patient complains of pain on taking a deep breath while a hand is placed below the right costal margin and pressed on to the gall bladder fundus, the sign is positive.

Special tests

1. *Plain X-ray*. An abdominal plain film may show radio-opaque calculi or a soft tissue mass in the region of the gall bladder. Occasionally there is evidence of small or large bowel distension. The investigation is also advisable to exclude a renal or upper ureteric calculus causing pyonephrosis, the clinical features of which may closely resemble those of acute cholecystitis.

2. *Urine and serum tests*. Tests for liver function may be indicated if jaundice is an associated feature.

Serum amylase estimations would be indicated if an acute pancreatitis was considered an alternative diagnosis. Marked elevation of the enzyme usually occurs in pancreatitis but moderate levels may be seen with cholecystitis and other abdominal conditions.

3. *Urgent intravenous cholegram*. Some surgeons like to have this for two reasons:

a. To establish the diagnosis by demonstrating that the gall bladder does not fill (occasionally false because a small proportion of normal gall bladders do not fill).
b. To demonstrate associated problems in the *axial* biliary tree such as stones.

However, this method is not universally favoured, as tomograms are usually required and the degree of resolution is often poor.

4. *Isotope excretion (HIDA) scan*. A sensitive test for demonstrating failure of the gall bladder to fill, but requires the availability of a gamma camera.

5. *Ultrasound*. This is the least expensive and least invasive test that will not only demonstrate abnormality of the gall bladder and common bile duct, but in expert hands will also give information about the liver and pancreas. For these reasons it has for many become the first line investigation for acute cholecystitis.

Differential diagnosis

EXTRA-ABDOMINAL

Myocardial infarction and acute right-sided lung conditions may offer some difficulty. Apart from obtaining a careful history and making a thorough examination, a chest X-ray and electrocardiograph may help. However, electrocardiographic abnormalities are not uncommon in elderly patients with biliary disease.

ABDOMINAL

Acute appendicitis. A high retrocaecal appendix may cause concern especially in a short thick-set person. If there is no suggestion of past gall bladder disease and there is a lack of characteristic radiation of pain then the diagnosis may only be made at operation.

Perforated duodenal ulcer. This is less often confused with cholecystitis but, if a plain abdominal film fails to indicate gas beneath the right hemi-diaphragm, a laparotomy may be required to decide the issue.

Acute pancreatitis. A constant boring pain with backache and a raised serum amylase help to differentiate this condition from cholecystitis, though the two may co-exist.

Pyonephrosis. The exclusion of this condition is important if the embarrassment of a wrongly placed incision is to be avoided.

Hepatic disease. Hepatic enlargement from viral hepatitis or cardiac failure causes a dragging pain in the right hypochondrium. Pyogenic infection (abscess) of the liver may be demonstrated by isotope liver scan or ultrasound.

Treatment of cystic duct obstruction and acute cholecystitis

Though some surgeons always operate at once in biliary colic and acute cholecystitis, non-operative management is initially indicated with either:

1. Delayed operation at the patient and surgeon's convenience as the attack resolves, or
2. Interval or postponed operation when the patient is symptom-free.

The *initial management* includes the following:

1. Intravenous fluids and nil by mouth
2. Pain relief by parenteral opiate administration, provided this is carefully controlled to avoid masking of signs
3. Antibiotics may be used in a short intensive course for 3 to 5 days but they may damp down infection rather than avoid it

Progress is judged:

1. Generally by frequent observations of pulse, blood pressure, temperature and white blood count
2. Locally by frequent palpation of the right hypochrondrium for tenderness and guarding

Urgent operation is indicated if:

1. Fever does not settle within 24 to 36 hours

2. Other systemic signs—tachycardia, leukocytosis—persist
3. Local tenderness or guarding remains unchanged or becomes worse
4. If cardiac, respiratory or combined cardio-respiratory problems are making management difficult. Acute cholecystitis is one good example where the additional demands thrown on the cardio-respiratory system by a large inflamed area, which constitutes an arterio-venous fistula, are an indication for operation if there is limited reserve. Such patients are not too ill to undergo an operation, but too ill to do without one.

The *nature of the operation* is dictated by the clinical circumstances:

1. Biliary anatomy easily visible. Patient in good general condition. Cholecystectomy and such additional procedures as are judged necessary.
2. Biliary anatomy obscured by gross local inflammation and/or patient in poor general condition. Cholecystostomy—drainage of the gall bladder—followed at a later date by cholecystectomy.

Principles of operation for calculus/inflammatory disease of the biliary tree:

1. Maximum pre-operative information. An intravenous cholegram may give prior warning of:

   a. Anomalies in the anatomy
   b. Presence of unsuspected axial stones

2. Adequate and unequivocal exposure of the anatomy of the biliary tree in *this patient*. Only by so doing can the dread complication of biliary duct damage be avoided.

3. Operative choledochography to ascertain if there is unsuspected stone or another problem in the common bile duct. A patient should not submit to cholecystectomy without the assurance that this procedure will be used.   *+ Choledochoscopy.*

4. Efficient exploration of the common duct if stones are known to be present (history, pre-operative or intra-operative X-rays, intra-operative exploration). Exploration may now include the use of the flexible choledochoscope.

The pros and cons of early operation for acute cholecystitis/cystic duct obstruction are:

Pros: 1. A certain diagnosis is made
   2. The small risk of perforation of the gall bladder is avoided
   3. Total hospitalization may be reduced
   4. Surprisingly the operation is often technically straightforward

Cons: 1. An experienced surgeon must be available
2. Pre-operative evaluation may be inadequate
3. Damage to the biliary tree is marginally more likely

PRESENTATION OF PATIENT BETWEEN ATTACKS

Perhaps the majority of patients are not admitted with an acute attack of cystic duct obstruction or of cholecystitis but are seen between attacks. The sequence of investigation is then:

1. Oral cholegram to establish:

   a. Is the diagnosis correct?
   b. Does the gall bladder function, both to concentrate and to contract?
   c. Occasionally to visualize the common duct, but this is inconsistent in an oral cholegram.

2. Intravenous cholegram to establish:

   a. Is the cystic duct obstructed?
   b. Are the axial ducts normal?

3. Ultrasound, as an alternative to X-rays, to establish:

   a. Is the diagnosis correct?
   b. Are the axial ducts normal?
   c. Are the liver and pancreas normal?

4. Operative cholegram:

   a. To establish normality of the axial tree
   b. To identify unexpected stones and/or other disease

5. Post-operative cholegram, if a T-tube has been left in after exploration of the common duct, to establish if stones or other causes of obstruction still exist.

CHOLEDOCHOLITHIASIS

Surgical pathology

Most often stones in the common bile duct have originated in the gall bladder; less commonly do they arise in the intrahepatic ducts or common bile duct—so-called primary duct stones.

Stones less than a few millimetres in diameter may be passed with or without the production of biliary colic. However larger stones may cause a ball valve obstruction in the second or third part of the common bile duct while occasionally a stone may be impacted in the lower end of the duct and result in continuous obstruction. In 10% of cases the stone becomes impacted in the ampulla and when there is a common channel of entry with the main pancreatic duct, pancreatitis may occur as the result of duct obstruction or reflux of infected bile into the pancreas.

After prolonged obstruction the common bile duct dilates and bile loses its yellow colour and becomes thick and black. Later infection may supervene with thickening of the duct wall and mucosal ulceration, and in cases of severe and prolonged obstruction, cholangitis may result in intrahepatic abscess formation.

When partial obstruction of the common bile duct occurs, ascending cholangitis can lead to biliary cirrhosis, liver failure and portal hypertension.

Clinical features

In keeping with the differentiation between axial and paraxial disorders, choledocholithiasis, which may exist with or without stones and inflammation in the gall bladder, usually presents with jaundice. Fever occurs when the bile is infected. The triad of right upper quadrant pain, shaking chills and jaundice is characteristic of duct stones and was first described by Charcot. These three features do not always co-exist.

SYMPTOMS *Charcot's triad.*

1. Pain occurs in 90% of patients. It is usually colicky in nature and situated in the right hypochondrium and it often radiates through to the back.

2. Jaundice is present in 50% of patients and it is always present if a stone is causing complete obstruction. Jaundice is nearly always preceded by biliary colic and when a ball valve type of obstruction exists, the jaundice will tend to fluctuate from day to day; it will also be associated with pruritis, dark urine and pale stools.

3. Fever is present in 30% of patients and rigors often occur. The fever is intermittent in type occurring every few days with exacerbation of pain and jaundice. The organism involved is usually *E. coli* and occasionally the cholangitis is so severe that septicaemia with shock, vomiting and dehydration results.

SIGNS

1. General. Fever and weight loss will occur if jaundice has been present for a prolonged period.

2. Local. Tenderness in the right hypochondrium.

3. Mass in the right upper quadrant.

SPECIAL TESTS

1. Urinary urobilinogen may be absent, indicating total duct obstruction, while fluctuating levels suggest intermittent obstruction.

2. Serum bilirubin is elevated.

3. Serum alkaline phosphatase is usually raised. Other liver function tests, including serum transaminase estimations, may indicate associated liver cell damage.

4. Blood cultures and white cell counts are important when cholangitis is suspected.

5. Plain X-ray of the gall bladder area will visualize radio-opaque stones in 10% of cases.

6. Ultrasound may demonstrate dilatation of, and/or stones in, the axial ducts.

7. Percutaneous transhepatic cholegram (PTC) or endoscopic retrograde cholangio-pancreaticogram (ERCP) will show the degree of dilatation and site of stones (p. 182)

8. Oral and intravenous cholegrams are of no value in the presence of jaundice.

Differential diagnosis

Episodes of pain, fever and jaundice are typical of choledocholithiasis. However, in the absence of pain and fever other causes of cholestatic jaundice must be considered and the appropriate investigations pursued (see p. 78)

Treatment

The initial management of acute symptomatic choledocholithiasis is non-operative with:

1. Fluid and electrolyte replacement
2. Antibiotics
3. Frequent general and abdominal examination.

Urgent operation is indicated in the same circumstances as in acute cholecystitis with the occasional addition of persisting or increasing jaundice.

Definitive operation is *always* indicated and involves:

1. Removal of gall bladder and its contained stones
2. Adequate duct exploration if necessary by the transduodenal route
3. Duct drainage to decompress the liver with T-tube, transduodenal sphincteroplasty or choledochoduodenostomy.

Post-operative management includes restriction of oral feeding and intravenous replacement therapy until coordinated bowel sounds have returned and until small volumes of fluids given by mouth are tolerated.

Bile from the tube in the common bile duct is collected into some convenient container. The tube is not removed for 8–9 days by which time the following state of affairs should exist:

1. The patient's general condition is satisfactory and jaundice has subsided.

2. Bile drainage is lessening in amount and it is a golden yellow colour.
3. The urine and stools are normally coloured.
4. A *post-operative choledochogram* performed by injecting contrast medium into the T-tube in the common bile duct shows that there are no filling defects and there is a free flow into the duodenum. An alternative less precise method is to clamp the T-tube for increasing periods and if this does not result in abdominal pain or increasing discomfort then it is assumed that bile must be flowing into the duodenum.

ACALCULUS ACUTE CHOLECYSTITIS

Acalculus acute cholecystitis takes two forms:

1. An acute infection which punctuates the course of another bacterial illness and which has the same organism responsible. For example, a considerable number of instances have been described in patients with long standing open wounds. The commonest organism has been *Streptococcus viridans*. Patchy gangrene and early perforation are not uncommon.

2. Anaerobic cholecystitis with gas formation—'emphysematous cholecystitis'. A much rarer disease characterized by a fulminant course and fatal outcome unless the gangrenous gall bladder that ensues can be quickly removed.

In addition to these two forms of patient there has been described a small group of sufferers in whom typical biliary colic occurs, but conventional radiology fails to show stones. There are probably two causes:

1. Small stones or cholesterol crystals are present, but are not seen and are often passed.
2. There is true gall bladder dyskinesia—i.e. the gall bladder responds to normal stimuli such as the duodenal release of cholecystokinin by incoordinate contraction. There is some evidence to support this. Patients with radiologically negative 'biliary colic' should be submitted to a provocation test (preferably carried out with radiological control) with intravenous cholecystokinin. If the agent reproduces the pain then cholecystectomy is likely to produce a good result. For patients who do not have this syndrome a conservative policy is initially justified. Some of them will develop stones; others may get better with dietary adjustment, particularly bran.

BILIARY DUCT STRICTURE

Duct stricture is almost exclusively the result of surgical trauma. The causes are:

1. Failure to appreciate biliary tract anatomy
2. Anatomy that just cannot be unravelled at surgery
3. Over-enthusiastic surgery for acute disease which leads operators to plunge into the right upper quadrant as distinct from opting for a cholecystostomy
4. Haemorrhage with blind clamping

There are other rare causes of axial strictures:

1. Localized malignant disease
2. Sclerosing cholangitis—an entity that may be related to the following:
   a. 'True' inflammatory disease
   b. Malignancy

Both of these are occasionally associated with ulcerative colitis.

Clinical features

SURGICALLY INDUCED
Bile duct trauma may present as follows:

1. At operation—some 15%
2. Early post-operative

   a. A persistent discharge of large amounts of bile through a wound or a drainage tube indicates some loss of continuity or at best a lateral hole
   b. Rapidly developing obstructive jaundice implies a ligated axial duct (usually the common hepatic)

3. Late post-operative—intermittent or progressive jaundice, often associated with cholangitis

MALIGNANT AND SCLEROSING CHOLANGITIS
The mode of presentation is nearly always progressive obstructive jaundice. In sclerosing cholangitis there may be associated evidence of infection.

Management of stricture

Cause is all important:
1. Traumatic stricture—the damaged area must be bypassed. There was formerly a vogue for reconstruction of the axial ducts. However, nearly everyone would now agree that in most traumatic strictures a new communication should be made between healthy duct and healthy intestine. Therefore some form of choledochoenterostomy is appropriate. The usual one will be choledochojejunostomy Roux-en-Y (Fig. 25.2).
2. Malignant stricture. Very occasionally a malignant stricture can be resected. Cure is unlikely but palliation is good. Otherwise proximal decompression is used. Percutaneous insertion of an 'endo-prosthesis' as an internal bypass, under X-ray control, is now available giving palliation without surgery

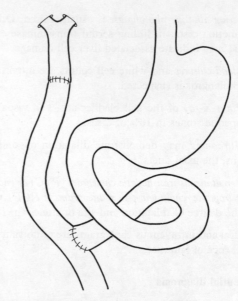

Fig. 25.2 Choledocho-jejunostomy Roux-en-Y

3. There remains the vexed problem of *non-malignant sclerosing cholangitis*. Some doubt the existence of such a 'benign' condition. However, it probably is a real and progressive entity. The surgeon has a small role to bypass or dilate strictures. However, the disease tends to be progressive, involving all radicals of the biliary system, and is unresponsive to cortico-steroids or immunosuppression.

COMPLICATIONS OF BILIARY SURGERY

Cholecystectomy is one of the commonest intra-abdominal operations and the outcome is usually satisfactory. When complications do occur, they are usually the result of technical errors. It must be appreciated that not only may the anatomy of the region vary (see Figs.

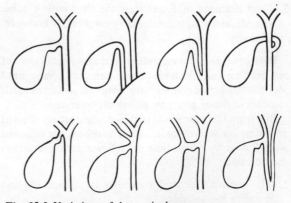

Fig. 25.3 Variations of the cystic duct

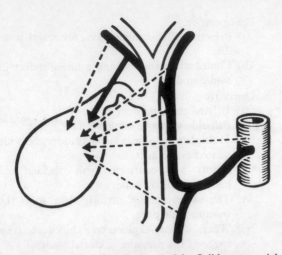

Fig. 25.4 Variations of cystic artery origin. Solid arrow = right hepatic (commonest). Broken arrows (above downwards) = distal right hepatic; left hepatic; common hepatic; aorta or superior mesenteric; gastroduodenal.

25.3 and 25.4) but its visualization may be very difficult because of gross inflammatory changes.

Operations on the gall bladder or bile ducts should not be undertaken by those who are unskilled in this type of surgery.

Classification

1. Duct system
2. Vascular
3. Visceral
4. Post-cholecystectomy syndrome

1. Duct system

BILE LEAKAGE
Small collections of bile about the gall bladder area are not uncommon after cholecystectomy or common bile duct exploration. More profuse leakage may result from a slipped ligature on the cystic duct, damage to the right hepatic or common bile duct or from the choledochotomy site. A not infrequent cause is the too early removal of a drain tube placed in the region of the gall bladder bed after cholecystectomy and exploration of the common bile duct.

The low surface tension of bile predisposes to its escape which may manifest itself in the following ways:

1. External biliary fistula is associated with profuse discharge of bile from the abdominal incision or the drain tube placed to the region of the gall bladder bed but provided there is no obstruction to the common bile duct then gradual lessening of discharge and spontaneous res-

olution will occur. In the meantime the skin about the fistulous opening must be protected from excoriation by the use of aluminium paste, zinc cream or by means of continuous low pressure suction.

Correction of electrolyte losses will be essential and can usually be done by mouth.

An external fistula which does not close spontaneously within 3–4 weeks will probably require operative intervention. Occasionally the injection of radio-opaque contrast medium along the fistula will outline a missed stone in the common bile duct.

2. Biliary peritonitis. Normal bile is a mild irritant and the extent of the inflammatory response will depend upon the amount of intraperitoneal outpouring and also upon the degree of infection which may be associated.

With a profuse extravasation of infected bile into the general peritoneal cavity there may occur a rapid onset of abdominal pain, vomiting, distension and shock, followed by paralytic ileus. Abdominal wall rigidity may be absent or only slight. The mortality rate from this complication is about 50% and, after resuscitation, operation must be performed to drain the collection. It is also important to try to define the exact site of leakage and close the defect but this is sometimes impossible.

Less frequently bile may leak slowly into the peritoneal cavity without causing shock or features of peritonitis. In such cases there may be a slowly increasing abdominal distension. Nevertheless, the end result will be fatal unless the leakage is stopped or directed to the exterior.

T-TUBE PROBLEMS
A T-tube may be:

1. *Blocked*
2. *Kinked* in the common bile duct, in the peritoneal cavity, in the abdominal wall or between skin and collecting device
3. *Too long* and therefore able to pass through the ampulla into the duodenum. Obstruction to the main pancreatic duct can occur and cause pancreatitis.
4. *Too short*, fall out of the common duct and allow bile to collect in the peritoneal cavity
5. *Pulled out too early* and allow the leakage of bile from common bile duct

STRICTURE
See p. 167

2. Vascular

1. The right hepatic artery, when it runs close to the cystic duct, may be ligated in mistake for the cystic artery. This may lead to liver necrosis and death of the patient.

2. Portal vein trauma may occur during a difficult dissection in the region of the common duct. Tears will be recognized at the time of operation and repaired.

3. Visceral

1. The liver may be lacerated, particulary in the region of the gall bladder bed. Deep through-and-through sutures usually required to control haemorrhage.

2. Duodenal fistula formation may occur after a transduodenal exploration or following the division of dense adhesions between the gall bladder and duodenum during a cholecystectomy. Protection of the skin while spontaneous closure occurs will be necessary.

4. Post-cholecystectomy syndrome

This is a persistence or recurrence of symptoms which are indistinguishable from those for which cholecystectomy was performed.

Removal of the gall bladder and of axial stores will cure 95% of patients with calculus disease. Some persistent symptoms occur in approximately 10% of patients who have had a cholecystectomy for gall stones and in 50% of those in whom no gall stones were found.

Investigation of residual pain includes exclusion of retained common bile duct stones by intravenous cholegram or ERCP. Evidence for chronic pancreatitis may be obtained. Treatment is often unsatisfactory and relies on accurate diagnosis.

CAUSES

1. **Wrong diagnosis.** Other abdominal conditions may produce symptoms which appear indistinguishable from those due to cholelithiasis.

A careful history is essential and it is always advisable to have a full gastrointestinal investigation when the cholecystogram is normal. One should always suspect some other diagnosis when stones are not found at operation. The temptation to take out the gall bladder for mild and atypical symptoms just because it is known to contain stones should also be resisted.

2. **Residual and reformed stones in the common bile duct.** 5% of patients have stones in the common bile duct with no clinical features suggesting their presence, and even after careful exploration of the common bile duct there is a 5% chance of a stone or stones being overlooked. Only occasionally do stones reform in the common bile duct.

The possible causes for missed stones are:

1. Inadequate anaesthetic, exposure or illumination.
2. Failure to appreciate the standard indications for exploration of the common bile duct which are:

a. Pre-operative
   (i) Presence of abdominal pain, fever and jaundice
   (ii) Choledochogram showing a filling defect in common duct
b. Operative
   (i) Dilated common duct
   (ii) Palpable stones in common duct
   (iii) Multiple small stones in gall bladder and wide dilated cystic duct
   (iv) Empty and contracted gall bladder and history of biliary colic
   (v) The aspirations of 'muddy' bile from the common bile duct
   (vi) When a pre-exploration choledochogram suggests the presence of ductal stones

3. Inadequate exploration of the common duct

Modes of presentation of missed or reformed stones
1. *Early.* The patient experiences abdominal pain when the tube draining the common duct is clamped off. Alternatively a post-operative T-tube choledochogram will show a persistent filling defect in the duct. If the stones are less than a few millimetres in diameter there is a fair chance that they will be passed, otherwise re-operation is indicated. Newer techniques now becoming available permit.

a. Dissolution, *in situ* with bile acids
b. Non-operative removal with a radiologically guided catheter along the T-tube track
c. Removal by sphincterotomy through the fiberoptic duodenoscope

2. *Late.* The usual features of choledocholithiasis with recurrent pain, jaundice and fever become apparent. Operation is indicated.

4. **Pancreatitis.** This is not infrequently an association of gall stone disease. It may be precipitated by operation on the sphincter of Oddi.

5. **Cystic duct stump syndrome.** When the cystic duct is not ligated flush with the common bile duct during a cholecystectomy it is claimed that a diverticulum may form in which infection and stone formation can occur. However, the reality of this is doubtful and the ascription of symptoms to a duct stump followed by its removal rarely makes the patient better.

PANCREATIC DISORDERS

ACUTE PANCREATITIS

Acute pancreatitis usually results from varying degrees of autodigestion of the pancreas by its escaped enzymes.

The aetiology of the condition remains somewhat obscure but it has more than a casual relationship with biliary tract disease and alcoholism.

Aetiological factors

1. Biliary tract disease. Obstruction of the common bile duct as the result of gall stones, spasm or stenosis of the sphincter of Oddi, oedema of the duodenal papilla or the ampulla of Vater, and tumours of the lowest end of the common bile duct may all be associated with pancreatitis. In these situations it is postulated that reflux of bile, in particular infected bile, into the pancreatic duct may initiate pancreatitis, especially when there is a common channel of entry of the pancreatic and common ducts into the duodenum.

Acute pancreatitis is associated with gall stones in 30 to 40% of cases in most reported series and in some it has been placed as high as 90%. However, common channel obstruction is not the prime cause of pancreatitis, although about 80% of people have this anatomical arrangement.

2. Alcohol. Excessive alcohol intake is associated with pancreatitis in about 25% of patients in Australia; in the United Kingdom the relationship is a little less frequent. The nature of this association is unknown, though the production of a gastro-duodenitis with duodenal papilla oedema has been mentioned. Vomiting with increased pancreatic duct pressures and increasing secretion of pancreatic enzymes have also been considered as causative processes in association with alcoholism.

Biliary tract disorders and alcohol can be subsumed under the same heading in McCutcheon's concept of *duodenal reflux* of activated enzymes consequent upon poor function of the sphincter.

3. Atherosclerosis. Pancreatitis is rare in children but common in the fifth and sixth decades in patients with generalized arterial disease. Many of these have associated thrombotic or embolic disease and it has been suggested that an ischaemic organ, can release trypsin and other enzymes which initiate pancreatitis.

4. Pancreatic duct obstruction. Obstruction to the duct of Wirsung by pancreatic calculi, tumours or duct metaplasia is a rare cause for pancreatitis and accounts for less than 5% of cases in most reported series.

5. Trauma. The pancreas may be damaged during upper abdominal operations and pancreatitis may occur and account for 5–10% of cases. External abdominal violence, particularly crush injuries, can result in contusion, laceration or even division of the pancreas and the development of pancreatitis.

6. Idiopathic. In about 20–30% of cases there is no evidence of a definitive causative factor. Some patients in this group may be suffering from undetected arterial thrombotic or embolic disease.

7. Miscellaneous. Haematogenous infection of the pancreas including mumps, allergic phenomena, metabolic disturbances in association with liver disease, hyperparathyroidism and hyperlipaemia with obesity are known associated factors. A number of drugs have been implicated, including steroids.

Surgical pathology

The changes seen in acute pancreatitis vary according to the severity of the attack. Oedema, exudation, haemorrhage, suppuration and necrosis may occur alone or in combination. In the mildest cases oedema of the pancreas will occur with minimal symptoms and signs; pancreatic haemorrhage and necrosis may be associated with profound shock from blood loss and ECF loss, because of exudation of fluid retroperitoneally and into other tissues, i.e. loss of ECF into the 'third space' (see p. 16), all as a consequence of increased capillary and cellular permeability.

Severe haemorrhagic pancreatitis is likely to be followed by necrosis which also effects adjacent tissues. The result is a large retroperitoneal phlegmon which, if infected, leads to abscess formation, septicaemia and often secondary haemorrhage from an eroded artery or false aneurysm.

Fat necrosis, a common accompaniment of acute pancreatitis, is due to the combination with calcium of fatty acids liberated from hydrolized fat, and is seen as white flakes in the omenta, mesocolon and mesentery; occasionally it may be metastatic and appear in subcutaneous tissues and periarticular fat as the result of the action of circulating lipase.

A pseudocyst forms when a pancreatic duct is breached and digestive enzymes egress into the abdominal cavity. Over a period of 2–3 weeks the fluid is walled off by fibrous tissue. They are usually sited in the lesser sac. The term 'pseudocyst' is used as the 'cyst' does not have an epithelial lining.

Mortality and prognosis

The death rate from acute severe pancreatitis varies between 6 and 20%. A patient who survives the attack, has a 20% chance of complete resolution, a 40% chance of relapsing and a 10% chance of developing chronic disease.

The causes of death in acute pancreatitis include the following:

1. Hypovolaemic shock
2. Electrolyte disturbances

3. Toxaemia
4. Renal failure
5. Respiratory failure resulting from collapse, consolidation or effusion

EARLY PROGNOSIS

Early assessment of the severity of an attack is not only an indication of prognosis but will also identify those patients more likely to develop the complications listed above and therefore those patients that may benefit from aggressive conservative treatment or early surgery.

A system of prognostic signs was shown by Ranson to predict outcome and may be used on admission to hospital and again after 48 hours of treatment. The bad prognostic signs are as follows:

1. On admission
a. Age: greater than 55 years
b. Blood glucose: greater than 11 mmol/l
c. Blood leukocyte count: greater than 16 000 per μl
d. Serum LDH: greater than 70 iu/l
e. Serum AST: greater than 60 iu/l

2. At 48 hours
a. Serum calcium: below 2 mmol/l
b. Blood urea: an increase of 10 mmol/l
c. Haematocrit: a fall of over 10%
d. Base excess: less than −4   *CUBEHOF*
e. Arterial Po2: below 8kPa (60 mmHg)
f. Estimated fluid sequestrated: over 6l

The presence of three or more of these signs at either time of assessement is associated with a greater incidence of haemorrhagic pancreatitis and death.

Other signs that may be of prognostic value are an increase of plasma fibrinogen and the presence of an elevated serum methaemalbumin level (see below). The absolute value of the serum amylase does not correlate with the severity of the attack.

LATE PROGNOSIS

1. The cause of pancreatitis. In cases where biliary tract disease can be surgically eradicated, the ultimate prognosis is excellent.
2. When alcoholism is a factor and can be successfully controlled, the outlook is also good.
3. In the idiopathic group, provided pancreatic duct carcinoma can be excluded, many will settle with the passage of time.

Clinical features

The clinical features of acute pancreatitis vary considerably because this is a disease with an unpredictable sequence of pathological changes. Not infrequently a diagnosis is impossible without laparotomy.

SYMPTOMS

1. Pain. This is invariably present but its severity is related to the degree of peritoneal irritation caused by haemorrhage and liberated pancreatic enzymes.

It is usually of sudden onset, intense, continuous and situated in the upper abdomen. Radiation to the back and the flanks is associated with spread of blood, enzymes or an effusion to the retroperitoneal space. The severity and location of the pain is rarely diagnostic, but often suggests the diagnosis.

Patients with pancreatic pain often assume bizarre positions while those with a perforated viscus are afraid to move.

2. Vomiting. Continuous retching is common and it may be prolonged and faeculent in nature as the disease progresses and becomes associated with paralytic ileus.

SIGNS

General

1. Shock. When pancreatitis is severe and associated with loss of blood and tissue fluid from the circulation, shock will be apparent. The patient is pale, and sweating with an elevated pulse rate, and lowered blood pressure. Cyanosis and dyspnoea may be accompaniments.

2. Fever. This is occasionally present.

3. Jaundice. This may be present in the early stages if there is associated bile duct disease, or later if the inflammatory process causes oedema and obstruction.

Local

1. Peritonitis. Local or general abdominal wall rigidity and rebound tenderness are usually present but less in degree than when due to a perforated peptic ulcer. Rigidity may in fact be absent.

2. Paralytic ileus. Abdominal distension, vomiting and absent bowel sounds indicate ileus.

3. Abdominal mass. This may become apparent days later and is due to pseudocyst, palpable omentum or pancreatic abscess formation.

4. Abdominal discolouration. Extravasion of blood from haemorrhagic pancreatitis to the peri-umbilical region is a rare occurrence, but when it does occur umbilical discolouration may be seen (Cullen's sign). Similarly, discolouration in the flanks has been described (Grey Turner's sign).

Special tests

1. Plain X-ray of chest and abdomen. This is invariably performed, not as a diagnostic test but to exclude the presence of free gas which has originated from a perforated peptic ulcer. Occasionally radio-opaque gall stones, a gas-filled right colon or a distended loop of small bowel (sentinel loop) may be seen. A left basal pleural effusion is not uncommon. Lung field mottling is a bad sign.

2. Serum amylase. Most laboratories now use the Phadebas tablet method for estimating serum amylase levels the normal range being 70–300 iu/l. A value of 1000 iu/l or greater is diagnostic of acute pancreatitis.

The serum amylase peak is reached within 48 hours but the magnitude of the rise is not a guide to the severity of the attack. Similarly, the rate of fall gives no indication of the rate of resolution of the disease.

Serum amylase levels may also be raised in cases of perforated peptic ulceration, acute cholecystitis and bowel obstruction but the levels reached are usually not as high as those found with acute pancreatitis.

3. Other blood tests. In order to make an early assessment of the severity of the attack the following tests are recommended: full blood count and haematocrit, blood glucose, blood urea, serum calcium, liver function tests and arterial blood gases.

Differential diagnosis

The diagnosis of acute pancreatitis may be difficult or impossible without laparotomy.

1. In severe cases of pancreatitis, coronary occlusion may cause confusion, particularly when epigastric pain is severe. However, abdominal rigidity is unusual with cardiac disease and an electrocardiograph may show ischaemic heart changes.
2. In less severe cases, a perforated peptic ulcer may be difficult or impossible to exclude. The presence of free gas beneath the right hemidiaphragm on X-ray examination is a most helpful sign of perforation.
3. In milder cases of pancreatitis, acute cholecystitis will require consideration. The situation and radiation of pain of cholecystitis and low serum amylase levels may give a clue.

Treatment

Patients with acute pancreatitis fall into one of three groups.

1. WHEN DIAGNOSIS CERTAIN

Treatment is conservative in the first instance.

The treatment may be described as the 'R' regimen and includes the following:

a. *Rest the patient.* Pethidine, 100 mg, is given by injection four-hourly.

b. *Rest the pancreas.* Nil by mouth. Parenteral fluid and electrolytes.

Anticholinergic drugs used to suppress pancreatic secretion and spasm of the sphincter of Oddi, have not proved to be of sufficient value to warrant their routine use.

c. *Rest the bowel.* Gastric suction is indicated in the presence of abdominal distension due to paralytic ileus.
d. *Resuscitation.* This is an essential requirement in the presence of hypovolaemia, when replacement therapy with blood, plasma expanders, saline and dextrose solution will be indicated.
e. *Resist enzymatic activity.* The kallikrein inhibitor Trasylol, which has a biological half life of 150 minutes, is active against trypsin and chymotrypsin, but has no effect against pancreatic amylase or lipase. A final judgement of its value in acute pancreatitis has not yet been made but it would appear that it must be used early in the disease and given in high doses as a continuous infusion to be of any value. Doses of the order of 500 000 to 800 000 units several times per day for 4–5 days are indicated.

Therapeutic peritoneal lavage may be a help in severe cases to remove pancreatic enzymes. Careful monitoring of fluid balance is indicated.

f. *Resist infection.* Septic complications and intra-abdominal abscess formation may occur and broad spectrum antibiotics may be given, although there is no evidence that they reduce the mortality or morbidity.
g. *Repeated examinations.* Frequent assessment of the progress of general and local features is mandatory and particular attention is paid to fluid balance and the progress of abdominal signs. The development of a mass will indicate an abscess, a necrotic mass, fat necrosis or a pseudocyst which may require operative intervention.
h. *Repeated serum estimations.* Daily estimation of the serum calcium is of more value than serum amylase levels, as it indicates the severity of the disease. A fall of serum calcium below 2.00 mmol/l indicates severe disease and levels below 1.5 mmol/l indicate a grave prognosis. 10% calcium gluconate is given as often as is required in the presence of hypocalcaemia.

Frequent white cell counts are valuable, particularly when there is persistent elevation or resurgence of the temperature indicating continuing activity or a developing complication.

More sophisticated are estimations of serum fibrinogen and methaemalbumin. A persistently elevated serum fibrinogen level, especially after 2 weeks, indicates either persistently active disease or the onset of some complication. The presence of methaemalbumin in the serum indicates an underlying haemorrhagic pancreatitis.

Serum magnesium levels may fall in acute pancreatitis at which time 25% magnesium sulphate can be given.

i. *Respiratory support*. Oxygen or assisted respiration for pulmonary complications.

j. *Renal output*. Careful monitoring of urinary output, to be greater than 25 ml/h, is needed and an indwelling catheter is needed if the attack is severe. A CVP line is an advantage to maintain a positive central venous pressure and to monitor fluid administration and diuretic therapy.

2. WHEN DIAGNOSIS UNCERTAIN

Whenever the diagnosis is in doubt peritoneal lavage is first indicated. If doubt continues a laparotomy must be done. In the past, operation in the presence of acute pancreatitis has been condemned but it is now apparent that operation does not influence the overall morbidity or mortality and it can be undertaken in the doubtful case provided fluid replacement is well advanced. The dangers of misdiagnosis with persistent conservative treatment are greater than those of a properly conducted laparotomy.

At operation the following may be performed:

a. Abscesses and necrotic collections are drained.
b. Gall stones, if present, may be removed if pancreatic necrosis or suppuration is not present. Whether this entails a cholecystectomy or cholecystostomy depends on the degree of local inflammation and the experience of the surgeon.
c. The common bile duct should be explored and external biliary drainage instituted if the patient is jaundiced but it is not justifiable to perform a sphincterotomy.
d. Special attention is paid to closure of the abdominal wall. Digestion of catgut sutures by pancreatic enzymes may lead to a burst abdomen and the use of non-absorbable suture material is essential.

3. WHEN COMPLICATIONS BECOME APPARENT

a. 'Toxic patient'. When the patient continues to remain unwell with a persistently elevated temperature and white cell count in association with a falling haemoglobin and serum calcium levels, then persistently active or complicated disease is present and operation is indicated. In the past it has been a common surgical error to operate too late in this secondary or septic phase of acute pancreatitis. At operation necrotic masses are removed and any abscess collection is drained.

b. Abdominal mass. This is nearly always present in a toxic patient. The mass may be due to fat necrosis, pseudocyst or abscess. Exploratory laparotomy is indicated and debridement and drainage is performed.

Pseudocyst may also present in the non-toxic patient and are best sought by ultrasound. If the pseudocyst does not resolve then drainage into the stomach—cyst–gastrostomy—or the small bowel—cyst–jejunostomy Roux–en–Y—may be required.

c. Persistently high gastric aspirations. After severe pancreatitis with prolonged paralytic ileus, duodenal obstruction may develop after 3–4 weeks as the result of extrinsic pressure from the inflammatory mass in the head end of the pancreas. Management is conservative.

d. Jaundice. This is uncommon but may be the result of pancreatic oedema or a stone obstructing the distal common bile duct. Ultrasound or PTC may resolve the problem and early surgery is indicated if biliary calculi are implicated.

AFTERMATH

Once recovery from acute pancreatitis has occurred, the biliary tract is investigated radiologically and any abnormality detected is treated on its merits.

Patients are advised to abstain from alcohol when this is considered to be a factor.

RELAPSING AND CHRONIC PANCREATITIS

The classification of pancreatitis of the non-acute type is confusing. The recommendations made at the Marseilles Symposium on Chronic Pancreatitis were based on *clinical* criteria and are as follows:

1. *Acute pancreatitis*. An attack of oedematous pancreatitis with complete resolution.
2. *Acute relapsing pancreatitis*. Recurrent attacks of oedematous pancreatitis with normal pancreatic function between attacks.
3. *Chronic pancreatitis*. Constant pain associated with pancreatic dysfunction, either exocrine and/or endocrine.
4. *Chronic relapsing pancreatitis*. Recurrent attacks of pain with associated pancreatic dysfunction.

Chronic pancreatitis may be further classified into localized, diffuse and diffuse with calcification.

Overlap between these categories occurs.

Aetiological factors

These are the same as for acute pancreatitis, where biliary tract disease and excessive alcohol intake are sometimes associated.

Surgical pathology

After repeated attacks of pancreatitis, the pancreas becomes atrophic and fibrotic; the pancreatic duct shows varying degrees of obstruction frequently at multiple sites along its length, proximal to which duct dilatation occurs with the formation of 'lakes' or cyst-like cavities. Eventually calcification and calculus formation occur with loss of parenchyma and associated with this is a corresponding deterioration in endocrine function. Occasionally pseudocysts or abscesses develop while progressive pancreatic fibrosis may possibly lead to obstruction of the common bile duct, portal vein or duodenum.

Clinical features

As the natural history and pathological changes are variable so are the clinical features.

1. Pain. Upper abdominal pain, which may be precipitated by alcoholic or dietary indiscretions, is the commonest symptom.

2. Backache. Severe and intractable backache, which proves resistant to various forms of therapy, is a common symptom.

3. Pancreatic failure. Gradual weight loss, anorexia, anaemia, steatorrhoea and diabetes occur in the most severe cases leading to malnutrition and death.

4. Jaundice. Obstructive jaundice is an unusual complication of chronic pancreatitis and may be difficult to distinguish from jaundice due to carcinoma of the head of the pancreas.

SPECIAL TESTS
Except in those cases where pancreatic failure is obvious, pancreatitis most often presents a diagnostic challenge, and because there is no one reliable test, the diagnosis is often made only at laparotomy.

The following tests may prove helpful:

1. Cholecystogram and choledochogram. Biliary tract disease must always be suspected.

2. Plain X-ray of the abdomen. This will demonstrate pancreatic calcification if present.

3. Pancreatic function tests. The degree of permanent damage to the pancreas may be assessed by the following:

a. Reduced serum amylase levels after secretin stimulation
b. Increased faecal fat
c. Reduced glucose tolerance
d. Reduced electrolyte and enzyme content of duodenal juice after stimulation with secretin or pancreozymin

4. Endoscopic retrograde cholangio-pancreatography. This technique of passing an endoscope to the second part of the duodenum and then cannulating both the common bile duct and the pancreatic duct has become increasingly reliable.

E.R.C.P. may demonstrate calculi in the common bile duct or abnormalities of the pancreatic ducts. Demonstration of the type of duct abnormality allows planning of operative treatment. Dilatation of the pancreatic duct with the so-called 'chain of lakes' appearance may be amenable to a Puestow's operation (see below) whereas extensive narrowing may be better treated by pancreatic resection. Similar information may be obtained by operative pancreatography.

The congenital anomaly of *pancreatic divisum* occurs when the ventral and dorsal buds of the pancreas fail to coalesce. Relapsing pancreatitis is common in this condition and ERCP may demonstrate an abnormal ventral duct (of Santorini).

5. Angiography. Coeliac angiography may demonstrate a space-occupying lesion and help to distinguish chronic pancreatitis from carcinoma.

6. Pancreatic scanning. This is unreliable and has largely been abandoned.

7. Pancreatic biopsy. Ultrasound or CT scan guided needle biopsy is proving to be useful in obtaining representative specimens for microscopic study (see p. 177).

DIFFERENTIAL DIAGNOSIS
In the presence of jaundice, carcinoma of the head of the pancreas or ampulla of Vater will have to be excluded and the following may be helpful features.

a. Pain. If present with carcinoma of the pancreatic head it is usually a vague epigastric discomfort and of insidious onset. It may radiate to the back. Pain is less common with ampullary carcinoma.

b. Jaundice. This appears early and is usually progressive with carcinoma of the pancreatic head; with ampullary carcinoma it may be intermittent.

c. Palpable gall bladder. This sign is present in about 40% of cases of carcinoma of ampulla or pancreatic head but is absent in pancreatitis.

d. Weight loss. Progressive and marked weight loss usually occurs with pancreatitis and pancreatic head carcinoma. In cases of ampullary carcinoma little or no weight loss occurs.

e. Melaena stools. This is common with ampullary carcinoma, rare with pancreatic head carcinoma, and does not occur in pancreatitis.

f. Barium meal. This may illustrate widening of the duodenal curve in pancreatic head lesions ('inverted 3 sign').

TREATMENT

Correct predisposing factors
It is most important to eliminate any possible predisposing factor which may perpetuate pancreatitis. If gall stone disease is apparent it must be corrected. Stenosis of the sphincter of Oddi, as indicated by choledochography or by exploration of the common duct at the time of operation, should be relieved by sphincteroplasty.

Conservative
1. Alcohol should be forbidden and a low fat, high protein and high carbohydrate diet advocated.
2. Pancreatic ferments such as pancreozymin may be added to the diet.
3. Hypoglycaemic agents may be indicated if diabetes mellitus is present.
4. Coexistent anaemia is treated by oral iron.
5. Relief of abdominal pain is provided by mild analgesics.

Failure of conservative treatment is apparent if invalidism occurs as the result of severe and persistent pain or progressive pancreatic failure. In such circumstances drug dependency is likely and in the alcoholic this produces a vicious cycle that is difficult to break.

Operative
The results of operative treatment for pancreatitis are often disappointing but when the operation performed is individualized according to the nature of the pathological changes in the pancreas and its duct system then good long term results can be expected in 65% of patients. There are varied approaches to the problem which can be classified as follows:

1. Diversion of bile. A sphincteroplasty may be indicated if reflux of bile up a common channel or obstruction at the sphincter of Oddi is considered an important aetiological factor and good results may be expected in relapsing pancreatitis not associated with gross and irreversible changes such as pancreatic duct strictures and calcification.
A cholecystoduodenostomy may be required in the rare cases of pancreatitis associated with recurrent jaundice.

2. Relief of pancreatic duct obstruction. Catheterization or direct puncture of the main duct of Wirsung and the injection of a radio-opaque dye may produce a pancreaticogram with valuable information about the duct system.

When major duct obstruction is confined to the pancreatic head, in the absence of pancreatic calculi, sphincteroplasty and retrograde pancreatic duct dilatation may prove beneficial.
When duct dilatation is widespread throughout the gland or when it is attended by multiple strictured sites and calculi then the main pancreatic duct may be opened along the major part of its length and anastomosed to a defunctioned loop of small bowel (Puestow's operation); alternatively a retrograde pancreatico-gastrostomy can be performed by excising the tail of the pancreas and anastomosing a dilated pancreatic duct and cut surface of the remaining pancreas to the posterior wall of the stomach.

3. Excision of portion of the pancreas. Subtotal or total pancreatectomy are operations attended by a considerable morbidity and mortality and they are reserved for cases of severe and intolerable pain where there is diffuse parenchymal damage without duct dilatation. A 95% resection, which avoids the necessity of removing the duodenum and common bile duct, may give as good results as a total removal and is associated with a lower mortality and morbidity.

4. Relief of pain. Operations such as splanchnicectomy and sympathectomy have no effect on the progress of pancreatitis and their ineffectiveness in relieving pain does not encourage their further use.

CARCINOMA OF THE PANCREAS

Predisposing factors

In most developed countries the incidence of carcinoma of the pancreas is increasing, with a twofold increase in the last 25 years. It occurs with increased frequency in smokers and diabetics. The peak incidence is in the fifth and sixth decades.

Surgical pathology

Ductal adenocarcinoma accounts for 80% of cases, two-thirds of which are located in the head of the gland. Islet cell tumours, secreting insulin, gastrin or rarely glucagon, and cystadenocarcinoma account for the remaining malignancies. Most ductal carcinomas are poorly differentiated, spread early into contiguous structures and metastasize to regional lymph nodes and the liver.

Spread may be:
1. *Local*, leading to

   a. Common bile duct obstruction and jaundice
   b. Invasion of the duodenum, stomach or small intestine
   c. Direct invasion of portal vein or superior mesenteric vessels, or coeliac plexus

2. *Lymphatic* to coeliac, para-aortic and even supra-clavicular nodes
3. *Blood*, via the portal vein to the liver
4. *Peritoneal and omental*, causing ascites

Periampullary carcinoma is a special form of pancreatic carcinoma in that it is biologically less aggressive and presents early with jaundice and/or melaena and may exist in three forms:

a. A small lesion of the distal pancreatic duct
b. Carcinoma of the lower common bile duct
c. Duodenal carcinoma

Clinical features

Because of the retroperitoneal site of the pancreas and as the symptoms are usually vague, delay in presentation and diagnosis is common. There is no reliable screening test and the at risk population is poorly defined. All too often the patient presents with features of advanced disease; weight loss, back pain and an epigastic mass.

MODES OF PRESENTATION
1. *Weight loss* is commonest, occurring in 70–90% of cases
2. *Pain* is more often epigastric than lumbar and may be relieved by sitting forward
3. *Jaundice* is the presenting feature in 75% of patients with tumours in the head of the pancreas and may be associated with a non-tender palpable gall bladder (Courvoisier's law states that a palpable gall bladder in obstructive jaundice implies that the gall bladder is normal and therefore the cause is not stones.). Pain may precede the jaundice but the latter is usually unrelenting and associated with severe pruritis.
4. *Steatorrhoea* is uncommon, but when combined with a bleeding periampullary lesion the classic 'silver' stools are seen.
5. *Diabetes mellitus* of sudden onset in middle age with no family history may be associated with a pancreatic carcinoma.
6. *Thrombophlebitis migrans* (Trousseau's sign) may also occur with other malignancies and is characterized by spontaneous thrombosis of peripheral veins that appears only to resolve and recur elsewhere.
7. *Acute pancreatitis* due to pancreatic duct obstruction by tumour is an occasional presenting feature.

Special tests

1. *Barium studies*. Double contrast barium meal with hypotonic duodenography may show a filling defect or early mucosal abnormalities of the duodenum suggestive of invasion by tumour.

2. *Fiberoptic endoscopy and ERCP*. A periampullary lesion may be seen, duodenal aspirates can be taken for cytology and ERCP demonstration of the pancreatic duct may show obstruction or distortion.

3. *Ultrasound* is the non-invasive investigation of choice in the jaundiced patient, will show intrahepatic duct dilatation and may show a mass in the pancreas.

4. *CT scan* gives better resolution of space occupying lesions of the pancreas and is used as an adjunct to ultrasound.

5. *Angiography* may show encasement or distortion of vessels by a tumour mass and less often 'tumour circulation'. It is not now greatly used.

6. *Histology and cytology*. Differentiation of cancer from pancreatitis is not always easy, and ultimately the diagnosis rests on obtaining histological or cytological proof. This may be achieved:

Pre-operatively by
a. Duodenal aspiration
b. ERCP
c. Fine needle aspiration of tumour under ultrasound or CT control

Intra-operatively by
a. Fine needle aspiration cytology
b. Transduodenal needle biopsy
c. Wedge incisional biopsy

Treatment

Most patients have overt or occult spread at the time of presentation and the overall 5-year survival is only 2%; therefore treatment is essentially palliative. Invasive and non-invasive tests are often rigorously pursued in an attempt to make a diagnosis, to stage the disease and sometimes to avoid an operation.

Curative resection. This is occasionally possible for peri-ampullary carcinoma as the 5-year survival after radical surgery in this subgroup is 40%. Total pancreatectomy for localized ductal carcinoma has promising results in selected patients without evidence of distal disease.

Palliative surgery. The high operative mortality of pancreatic resection combined with the advanced nature of the majority of cases has made bypass procedures the first option of surgical treatment. Common duct obstruction may be bypassed by cholecystjejunostomy, if the gall bladder is dilated, or high choledochojejunostomy, if the gall bladder is involved. Gastrojejunostomy is often added because of the likelihood of duodenal obstruction as the tumour grows. Injection of the coeliac plexus with alcohol to relieve pain may be performed at the time of surgery or percutaneously, but works only in expert hands.

Radiotherapy and chemotherapy. Neither form of treatment has to date prolonged survival. Combination chemotherapy may become more effective in the future.

Insulinoma

The majority, 80% of these tumours are benign. Insulinomas arise from the beta cells of the pancreatic islets and consequently secrete insulin. The classic diagnostic triad (Whipple's) is: hypoglycaemic symptoms produced by fasting; documented hypoglycaemia; and relief of symptoms by intravenous glucose. The diagnosis is confirmed by measuring circulating immunoreactive insulin and by the failure of insulin suppression by fasting.

Pre-operative localization of the tumour is vital because identification at surgery is notoriously difficult. A combination of angiography, CT scan and selective venous sampling by percutaneous catheterisation of the splenic vein via the liver makes localization more definite but does not always succeed. Surgical resection is the treatment of choice and this applies also to metastases, even when the disease is incurable. The alternative is suppression of insulin with diazoxide which can give a fairly prolonged period of relief.

JAUNDICE

Jaundice is a yellow staining of the body tissues produced by an excess of circulating bilirubin. Normal serum bilirubin concentration is 5–19 mmol/l and jaundice is detected clinically when the level rises above 40 mmol/l. It is most evident in tissues which have a high elastic tissue content (skin, sclera and blood vessels).

SURGICAL PHYSIOLOGY AND PATHOLOGY

Bilirubin is formed from haem, a compound of iron and protoporphyrin and about 85% of that produced daily comes from the breakdown of haem from mature red cells in the reticulo-endothelial system. The actual mechanism involved is still unknown. The remaining 15% is derived from marrow compounds incorporated into red cell precursors which have not been released into the circulation and from haem compounds in the liver which have not been incorporated into red cells. In increased haemolytic states there is a release of haem from red cells which have a shortened life span and an increased production of bilirubin which causes acholuric jaundice. Following its release, unconjugated bilirubin, which is insoluble in water, is transported attached to plasma proteins to the liver cell.

In the cell, lipid-soluble bilirubin is conjugated into water-soluble bilirubin glucuronide. Defective uptake or conjugation of bilirubin can occur in such conditions as Gilbert's disease and Crigler-Najjar's disease, with the result that unconjugated bilirubin appears in excess in the blood but not in the urine because, it is water insoluble.

The transport of conjugated bilirubin from the liver cells into the bile ducts and bowel is probably an active mechanism but the controlling influences are unknown. Disturbances of the flow of bile lead to stagnation and retention of conjugated bilirubin (cholestasis) which may occur in the intra-hepatic biliary tree (intra-hepatic cholestasis) or in the extra-hepatic biliary tree (extra-hepatic cholestasis).

Bacterial deconjugation of bilirubin occurs mainly in the colon to form stercobilinogen, which is partly reabsorbed into the circulation and re-excreted by the liver or the kidneys (urobilinogen) and partly excreted in the faeces in an oxidized form (stercobilin) (Fig. 25.5).

CLASSIFICATION OF JAUNDICE

The standard classification of jaundice into pre-hepatic, resulting from excessive red cell destruction; hepatic, due to liver damage; and post-hepatic (obstructive or 'surgical'), due to obstruction of the biliary tree, is inadequate for two reasons:

1. Obstruction (cholestasis) can occur without any evidence of a lesion requiring surgical correction, e.g. intra-hepatic cholestasis due to drugs and early primary biliary cirrhosis.
2. Little indication is given of the site of the disturbance of bilirubin metabolism.

In addition, classifications which ascribe diseases to particular types of jaundice are too rigid: a patient with viral hepatitis may have considerable cholestasis and a patient with obstruction of a large duct may go on to develop a degree of hepatocyte insufficiency which interferes with bilirubin conjugation or manifests itself in terms of increased levels of intracellular enzymes in the blood. Thus, separation of causes of jaundice in an individual patient may be difficult or impossible. What should always be borne in mind is that the diagnosis required is one that permits *action* of the appropriate kind—be this surgical or non surgical (Fig 25.5).

1. Increased bilirubin load

Jaundice due to excess of unconjugated bilirubin.

HAEMOLYTIC JAUNDICE
a. Hereditary spherocytosis
b. Hereditary non-spherocytic anaemias
c. Sickle cell disease

d. Thalassaemia
e. Paroxysmal nocturnal haemoglobinuria
f. Acquired haemolytic anaemia
g. Incompatible blood transfusion
h. Severe sepsis
i. Drugs

2. Disturbed bilirubin uptake and conjugation of bilirubin

Jaundice due to excess of unconjugated serum bilirubin.
a. Viral hepatitis
b. Hepatotoxins
c. Cirrhosis
d. Gilbert's familial non-haemolytic hyperbilirubinaemia
e. Familial neonatal hyperbilirubinaemia
f. Crigler-Najjar's familial non-haemolytic jaundice

3. Disturbed bilirubin excretion (Cholestasis)

Jaundice due to excess of conjugated serum bilirubin.

INTRA-HEPATIC CHOLESTATIS (without mechanical obstruction)
a. Cirrhosis
b. Viral hepatitis
c. Drugs, e.g., chlorpromazine, methyl testosterone
d. Dubin–Johnson's familial conjugated hyperbilirubinaemia
e. Primary biliary cirrhosis (chronic, non-suppurative, destructive cholangitis)
f. Parenteral or enteral feeding with synthetic nutrients.

EXTRA-HEPATIC CHOLESTASIS (obstructive or 'surgical' jaundice with mechanical obstruction of common bile duct)
1. *Inside duct*—gall stones
   foreign body, e.g. broken T-tube
   parasites (hydatid; liver fluke; round worms)
2. *In duct wall*—congenital atresia
   traumatic stricture
   sclerosing cholangitis
   tumour of bile duct

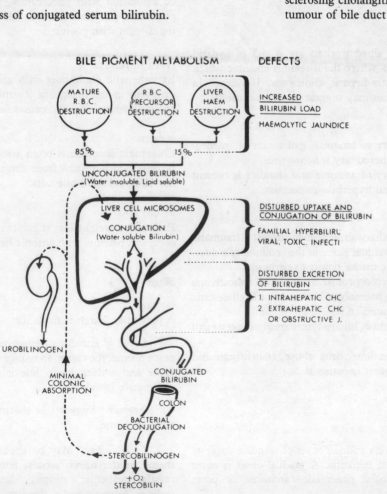

Fig. 25.5 Bile pigment metabolism and associated disorders

3. *Outside duct*—carcinoma of head of pancreas
carcinoma of ampulla of Vater
pancreatitis
porta hepatis metastases
chronic duodenal ulcer

COMMONER CAUSES OF EXTRA-HEPATIC CHOLESTASIS
1. Gall stones
2. Carcinoma of the pancreas
3. Porta hepatis metastases

DIAGNOSIS OF CAUSE OF JAUNDICE

The surgeon is mainly concerned with extra-hepatic cholestasis, though occasionally he is called upon to perform a splenectomy for hereditary spherocytosis.

The diagnosis is established from a consideration of the usual triad of history, examination and special tests.

History

Occupation
Sheep farmers or allied workers are at risk of hydatid infestation in areas where the disease is endemic which may result in extra-hepatic cholestasis. Residence in developing countries may suggest an exotic cause.

Family history
1. A family history of anaemia, gall stones or splenectomy suggests hereditary spherocytosis.
2. A family history of anaemia and jaundice is present in the congenital hyperbilirubinaemias.

Personal history
1. Past difficult biliary surgery may suggest a traumatic stricture or a residual stone in the common bile duct.
2. Heavy alcoholic intake points to cirrhosis.
3. Drugs such as chlorpromazine or methyl testosterone may indicate a haemolytic or intrahepatic cholestatic cause for the jaundice.
4. Intermittent pain of biliary type strongly suggests gall stones.
5. History of injections, drug abuse, transfusions and tatoos may suggest hepatitis B.

Symptoms

JAUNDICE
Onset. A relatively sudden onset of jaundice suggests gall stones or viral hepatitis. A gradual onset is more likely with cirrhosis, pancreatic carcinoma or porta hepatis metastases.

Progression. Remorseless and progressive jaundice is typical of malignant obstruction. Fluctuating jaundice is likely with a stone in the common bile duct, carcinoma of the duodenal papilla (often called the ampulla of Vater), or repeated haemolytic episodes.

PAIN
Absent. Painless jaundice may occur in viral hepatitis, though a dragging subcostal ache is common, the consequence of hepatic enlargement. In older people, painless but fluctuating jaundice suggests intermittent obstruction by gall stones or a necrosing ampullary carcinoma. Painless but progressive jaundice is usually due to malignant obstruction of the common bile duct.

Present. Painful jaundice strongly suggests gall stones or pancreatic disease. Colicky right subcostal pain radiating beneath the costal margin to the shoulder blade suggests biliary colic.

Moderate boring pain passing through to the back can be associated with pancreatitis, pancreatic tumour or possible a penetrating duodenal ulcer. There is sometimes relief with posture.

FEVER AND CHILLS
Extra-hepatic cholestasis with cholangitis (which happens only in non malignant obstruction or with a tumour of the Vaterian ampulla) causes fever and chills.

PRURITIS
Cholestatic jaundice is often associated with persistent pruritis which results from the irritation of cutaneous nerves by retained bile salts.

WEIGHT LOSS
Progressive weight loss suggests malignancy but it also occurs in patients with chronic hepato-cellular damage.

Signs

GENERAL
A particular search is made for:

1. Depth of jaundice. Lemon-yellow colour may suggest a haemolytic cause, an orange colour a hepatocellular cause and a deep green hue is usual with prolonged obstructive jaundice.

2. Anaemia. Suggests a haemolytic, malignant or cirrhotic cause.

3. Liver failure. May be apparent with palmar erythema, spider naevi, ascites, fetor hepaticus, gynaecomastia, testicular atrophy, finger clubbing, ankle oedema, bruising and a 'flapping' tremor.

4. *Supra clavicular lymph node enlargement*. Suggests metastatic carcinoma.

5. *Skin*. Scratches and xanthomata are seen in chronic cholestasis.

6. *Pyrexia*, caused by

a. Cholangitis
b. Viraemia and hepatic involvement, e.g. infectious mononucleosis
c. Septicaemia and haemolysis
d. Hepatic abscess

LOCAL (ABDOMINAL)

1. *Scars*. May indicate previous surgery on the biliary tree.

2. *Caput medusa*. Dilated peri-umbilical veins indicate portal hypertension and cirrhosis.

3. *Sites of tenderness*. Tenderness over the gall bladder indicates biliary inflammation.

4. *Gall bladder*. A palpable gall bladder in the presence of jaundice means that the jaundice is unlikely to be due to a gall stone (Courvoisiers' law). In these circumstances, carcinoma of the head of the pancreas must be suspected.

5. *Liver*. A palpable hard nodular liver of large proportions suggests metastatic malignancy, while a small nodular liver indicates cirrhosis. A slightly enlarged smooth liver suggests chronic cholestasis. If the liver is tender, viral hepatitis must be considered.

6. *Spleen*. Splenomegaly may be evident in congenital haemolytic anaemia or portal hypertension.

7. *Abdominal mass*. A hard and irregular abdominal mass suggests malignancy.

8. *Ascites*. This may be due either to abdominal malignancy or liver failure.

9. *Rectal examination*. An essential requirement. It will indicate the colour of the stools and it may reveal the presence of a primary malignancy or of metastatic deposits in the pouch of Douglas.

Investigations

PRELIMINARY TESTS

Urine
1. Absent urobilinogen indicates obstruction to the common bile duct.
2. Excess urobilinogen occurs in haemolytic jaundice and sometimes in liver damage.

3. Absent bilirubin indicates haemolytic jaundice.
4. Excess bilirubin is present in obstructive jaundice.

Faeces
1. Absence of bile pigment indicates biliary obstruction at any level.
2. Excess of bile pigment indicates haemolytic jaundice.
3. A positive occult blood test indicates ampullary carcinoma, bleeding oesophageal varices (cirrhosis) or an alimentary carcinoma.

Blood
1. A raised serum bilirubin level confirms the presence of jaundice and also gives some indication of its severity. However, it is unusual for the bilirubin to rise linearly and in obstruction it often 'peaks out' to a plateau.
2. Serum alkaline phosphatase over 100 iu/l is indicative of cholestasis if bone disease is absent.
3. Serum albumin and globulin levels are reversed in chronic hepatocellular damage.
4. Serum transaminase levels are above normal in viral hepatitis.
5. Prothrombin time. Normal in haemolytic jaundice; prolonged but correctable with vitamin K in cholestatic jaundice, provided there remains some functioning liver tissue; will be prolonged and not correctable in advanced hepatocellular disease.
6. Haematology. Spherocytosis, red cell fragility, reticulocytosis and a positive Coomb's test will establish a haemolytic cause.
7. Immunology. Auto-antibodies may be elevated, in primary biliary cirrhosis, especially anti-mitochondria immunoglobulin, and in other connective tissue diseases that involve the liver.

SPECIAL TESTS

Parenchymal disease suspected
When biochemical studies clearly delineate a parenchymal origin of the jaundice, then the plan is:

a. *Scintilation liver scan*, to delineate the pattern of hepatic involvement
b. *Coagulation profile*
c. *Liver biopsy* to provide tissue for histological and immunofluorescent analysis

Obstructive jaundice suspected

Ultrasound scan is the first step to establish the presence of dilated intrahepatic ducts implying extra-hepatic obstruction. In expert hands ultrasound will also given detailed information concerning the gall bladder, the common bile duct, the pancreas and the parenchyma of the liver.

CT scan may give better resolution than ultrasound, particularly in:

a. demonstrating pancreatic lesions
b. obese patients
c. patients with excess bowel gas shadows

1. Dilated intrahepatic ducts

Percutaneous transhepatic cholangiography (PTC) is the test of choice. The coagulation profile is checked and the procedure covered by parenteral antibiotics. A fine, pliable needle is inserted under local anaesthetic into the liver, a duct entered and contrast medium injected.

Should decompression of the biliary tree be desired pre-operatively then a fine-bore catheter may be left in the ducts to allow continuous drainage. The benefits of pre-operative drainage are yet to be proven. Similarly, if an unresectable malignancy compressing the ducts is suspected then the percutaneous insertion of an endo-prosthesis may avoid an operation but the long-term results and incidence of cholangitis are not yet known.

PTC is ideal for demonstrating the anatomy above an extra-hepatic obstruction which is most relevant to the surgeon.

2. Non-dilated ducts

Endoscopic retrograde cholangio-pancreatography (ERCP) is the test of choice. Using a side-viewing fiberoptic endoscope the duodenal papilla is cannulated and contrast medium injected into either the common bile duct or pancreatic duct or both. Simultaneous endoscopic sphincterotomy and removal of common duct stones may be performed.

ERCP is ideal for demonstrating the anatomy distal to an extra-hepatic obstruction.

Both PTC and ERCP are effective techniques and the choice, for either situation of duct dilatation, depends upon the expertise available.

SURGICAL TREATMENT OF JAUNDICE

Clearly this will relate to the cause, and the various procedures have been outlined in the previous sections of this chapter. Pre-operative preparation is vital.

Pre-operative preparation

The almost universal availability of ultrasound or CT scan has simplified the management of obstructive jaun-

dice and it is a rare occurence when exploratory laparotomy is used as the definitive investigation for a patient with suspected extra-hepatic obstruction.

Laparotomy on a patient who does *not* have extra-hepatic obstruction is very harmful.

Laparotomy in patients *with* extra-hepatic biliary obstruction carries three special risks:

1. Hypocoagulability because of prothrombin deficiency which is corrected by vitamin K administration in the days preceding surgery.

2. Renal failure post-operatively. The exact cause is uncertain but it is probably a combination of:

a. Increased bile pigment load on the tubule
b. Increased post-operative distal tubular re-absorption of water because of the secretion of antidiuretic hormone
c. Perhaps most important, failure of the liver to trap enteric nephrotoxins derived from bowel organisms.

The condition is prevented by pre-operative bowel preparation and diuretic therapy is used intra- and post-operatively either with mannitol (osmotic diuresis) or frusemide (loop diuretic). Mannitol is usually given at the time of induction in a dose of 100 ml of 10% mannitol and the infusion continued for 24 hours at a sufficient rate to give a urine output of 1 ml/min or more.

3. Sepsis. Stasis of bile, with or without calculi or other foreign bodies, will predispose to bacterial colonization and overgrowth. A combination of biliary sepsis and renal failure is usually fatal. Antibiotic prophylaxis is therefore given with an antibiotic to deal with coliforms.

Common findings and operative procedures

1. Liver. Enlarged and smooth with hepatitis, small and fibrotic with cirrhosis and hard and irregular with secondary malignancy.

2. Gall bladder. Small and fibrotic with chronic cholecystitis, cholelithiasis and choledocholithiasis, distended and thin-walled with carcinoma of the peri-ampullary region, collapsed and empty with obstruction of the common hepatic duct and normal with hepatitis.

3. Common bile duct. Dilated and thickened with choledocholithiasis or pancreatitis, dilated thin-walled and appearing bluish and transparent with peri-ampullary carcinoma, though the diagnosis will usually have been established.

Operative choledochography may be indicated, particularly when the duct is of abnormal calibre. Intra-hepatic obstruction due to stones, carcinoma or hydatid disease, may thus be revealed. However, if the intra-hepatic ducts are normal, the abdomen is closed after a liver biopsy.

Cure is usually possible in stones, traumatic stricture and a variety of miscellaneous conditions. The exception is sclerosing cholangitis, a progressive inflammatory process which spreads to involve the intra-hepatic biliary tree and which is very difficult to distinguish from infiltrating slowly growing carcinoma of the common bile duct (see p. 168).

4. Pancreas. Usually hard and irregular throughout most of its length with chronic pancreatitis. An irregular mass in the head indicates carcinoma, but sometimes it is impossible to distinguish between carcinoma and pancreatitis, even after careful mobilization and palpation of the head of the pancreas. A pancreaticogram will be of assistance if it demonstrates duct abnormalities consistent with pancreatitis or a uniformly dilated duct system proximal to an obstructing carcinoma.

26

Intestinal obstruction

There are many ways of classifying intestinal obstruction: by the site of the obstruction in relation to the bowel wall—in the lumen, in the wall, outside the wall; by the surgical pathology—simple or strangulation; by the site—large or small bowel; high or low. All have something to contribute to our understanding but the most useful is an understanding of surgical pathology.

SURGICAL PATHOLOGY

Obstruction may be either: *mechanical* in which there is a bowel capable of contracting normally or excessively proximal to a local site of obstruction; or *paralytic* in which contraction ceases, usually diffusely throughout the greater part of the bowel.

MECHANICAL OBSTRUCTION

There are three main types.

1. Simple occlusion

The bowel above the obstruction distends as the result of a raised intraluminal pressure from increased secretion of fluid and the accumulation of gas by air-swallowing, and as a consequence, to a lesser extent, of fermentation. At first the bowel above the obstruction shows increased peristalsis but this becomes unco-ordinated and later may cease if the obstruction is not overcome.

Increased secretion of fluid into the obstructed bowel is associated with decreased re-absorption and these losses, together with those from vomiting, deprive the patient of electrolytes and water. The higher the level of obstruction the more severe are the fluid and electrolyte losses; the worst effects are seen with high small bowel obstruction while the least effects are seen with large bowel obstruction. The picture is that of acute, extra-cellular volume deficiency (p. 10).

The arterial supply of the bowel is jeopardized as the intraluminal tension rises above the capillary pressure. Then mucosal ulceration, gangrene and subsequent perforation of the bowel wall will occur.

Bacteria multiply in the lumen proximal to an obstruction. This is not of great concern unless perforation or surgical damage occurs, when a severe peritonitis will result.

2. Closed loop obstruction

This begins as a special variety of simple occlusion in which the pathological processes are accelerated. Both ends of a loop are obstructed: closed loop obstruction can occur with torsion of the small bowel, obstructed external hernia, colonic obstruction with a competent ileocaecal valve or volvulus of the sigmoid colon. In these cases there is a rapid rise in intraluminal tension and gangrene or perforation can develop more quickly. In such cases the contents of the bowel are always infected.

3. Strangulation

This is usually the end result of a closed loop obstruction when the major arterial supply to the affected bowel has been occluded, causing gangrene over a considerable area; a special variety is a superior mesenteric artery thrombosis or embolism, in which many feet of bowel may become gangrenous.

PARALYTIC OBSTRUCTION (ILEUS)

Paralytic obstruction (paralytic ileus) occurs: when there is excessive sympathetic efferent discharge, as in the first 24 post-operative hours after abdominal surgery or perhaps after a lumbar spine fracture or large retroperitoneal haematoma; when there is diffuse peritoneal irritation—blood or pus. It is sometimes induced by drugs which act on the autonomic nervous system

MANAGEMENT OF MECHANICAL OBSTRUCTION

The following questions must be answered:

1. Is it obstruction, and if so, at what level?
2. Is strangulation present?
3. Is dehydration (extracellular volume deficiency) present?
4. What is the cause?
5. What is the treatment for the individual case?

1. Is it obstruction, and if so, at what level?

The question is answered by considering the clinical features.

SYMPTOMS

The cardinal features of bowel obstruction are pain, vomiting and constipation.

Pain is usually colicky in nature but will become continuous if perforation or strangulation is present. Pain may be absent in paralytic ileus.

Vomiting is early in high small bowel obstruction, late in low small bowel obstruction and delayed or absent in large bowel obstruction. Characteristically in small bowel obstruction the vomitus is initially clear, becomes discoloured and finally faeculent—dark and foul-smelling.

Constipation is early with large bowel obstruction and is absolute in complete obstruction but there may be an initial motion at the onset of obstruction. This may be blood-stained in a mesenteric occlusion, volvulus or intussusception.

The patient may have a subjective sensation of abdominal distension.

SIGNS

General signs may reveal evidence of dehydration and/or strangulation—see below.

The local signs in the abdomen are:

On inspection
a. Scars from previous operations
b. Distensions, which tends to be central in small bowel obstruction and peripheral in large bowel obstruction
c. Visible peristalsis in a thin abdomen
d. Irreducible swellings at external hernial orifices

On palpation:
a. Abdominal mass which may suggest carcinoma, or strangulated bowel

b. Rigidity and rebound tenderness which indicates peritoneal irritation
c. Obstructed herniae

On percussion
Resonance because of gas filled bowel

On auscultation
a. Metallic clicks and pressure is raised if much gas is present in the bowel
b. Gurgling borborygmi if gas and fluid are present in the bowel
c. Silence if generalized peritonitis or paralytic ileus is present

On rectal examination
a. Impacted faeces
b. Rectal tumour
c. Blood on finger which may be present with mesenteric artery occlusions, intussusception or volvulus

These clinical features are nearly always sufficient to permit a working diagnosis of mechanical intestinal obstruction to be made. Supplementary or confirmatory tests are:

Sigmoidoscopy. In large bowel obstruction sigmoidoscopy may reveal a carcinoma, sigmoid volvulus or inflammatory stricture. In sigmoid volvulus the procedure can be therapeutic.

Plain X-ray of the abdomen, supine and erect, for distended and fluid filled coils of bowel. A closed loop obstruction may not contain gas and a low ileal obstruction may not show fluid levels.

Contrast X-rays. In doubtful cases gastrografin orally or thin barium rectally may outline the level of obstruction. However, what is more important, the latter may reveal a normal colon in a suspected large bowel obstruction.

2. Is strangulation present?

There are no cardinal signs of strangulation. However the presence of marked shock, fever and tachycardia together with all or some of the following would be strongly suggestive:

a. Abdominal wall rigidity
b. Abdominal wall rebound tenderness
c. Tense, hard and irreducible external hernia
d. Metabolic acidosis when clinical intestinal obstruction is diagnosed.

3. Is dehydration present?

Examination must include a general assessment of the patient's condition and state of hydration (i.e. does the patient look well, relatively well, sick or very ill). In small bowel obstruction particularly, persistent vomiting may result in dehydration the features of which are:

a. Tachycardia
b. Hypotension
c. Dry skin
d. Dry mouth
e. Poor tissue turgor
f. Small volume of concentrated urine

4. What is the cause?

a. Previous abdominal operation and features of small bowel obstruction suggest adhesions as the cause. The attacks may have been recurrent and managed non-operatively. Nevertheless the present attack may involve strangulation so that great caution is needed in these cases.
b. Large bowel obstruction and a history of constipation, perhaps with intermittent mucus or bloody diarrhoea, suggest carcinoma of the colon. Diverticulitis of the colon is a much less common cause.
c. No previous abdominal operation and symptoms of small bowel obstruction suggest either an obstructed external hernia or an uncommon cause such as a congenital band, gall stone ileus, internal hernia or mesenteric occlusion.

Treatment

In general, once bowel obstruction has been diagnosed, the treatment is operation, although there may be a delay while the severely dehydrated patient receives intravenous therapy. When strangulation is strongly suspected because of clinical signs and metabolic acidosis the time taken for preoperative replacement therapy must be as short as possible.

Operation for bowel obstruction are contra-indicated in the following circumstances:

1. Paralytic ileus (see below p. 187)
2. Impacted faeces, when disimpaction by digital manipulation is all that is required
3. Volvulus of the sigmoid colon provided that the twisted loop of bowel can be negotiated with a rectal tube passed under vision through a sigmoidoscope. Then resection of the sigmoid loop may be deferred to a later date.
4. When there have been many previous explorations for adhesions and there is confidence that strangulation is *not* present

PRE-OPERATIVE PREPARATION

If obstruction is detected early and there are no signs of dehydration then special preoperative preparation is not necessary apart from starting naso-gastric suction and intravenous therapy. A large gastric tube may be passed and the stomach emptied immediately before surgery. Alternatively, if it proves difficult or impossible to persuade the patient to swallow a tube, then anaesthesia can be induced while pressure is applied to the cricoid cartilage, which will prevent regurgitation from the oesophagus.

If obstruction is detected later, for example 24 hours after the onset of symptoms when signs of dehydration are present, then the following will be required:

a. *Naso-gastric suction*. The stomach must be emptied so that the risk of inhalation of vomit is minimized. This also reduces the fluid which has collected in the small bowel. Suction may be performed intermittently or continuously but continuous suction is preferred.

b. *Intravenous therapy*. Correction of water and electrolyte losses must be effectively performed within a few hours. Adults who are dehydrated require about four litres of fluid while those who are hypotensive from reduction of extracellular volume may need up to six or eight litres. Nearly all of this should be given as normal saline or Hartmann's solution.

c. *Monitoring*. A central venous line for measuring pressure may be useful in debilitated or elderly patients so as particularly to prevent too rapid or over-resuscitation.

OPERATION

This may entail removing the cause e.g. division of adhesions, reduction of a hernia, resection of a gangrenous loop, excision of an obstructing carcinoma, proximal decompression by colostomy as in left sided colon lesions or bypass by anastomosis of proximal obstructed to distal unobstructed bowel. In addition it is usual to empty the distended bowel by either direct aspiration or by milking its contents back to the stomach whence they can be removed by nasogastric suction. These manoeuvres allow the abdomen to be more easily closed.

POST-OPERATIVE CARE

Nasogastric or gastrostomy decompression is continued as is intravenous therapy until bowel function has recovered as shown by normal bowel sounds, small aspirates and/or the movement of a colostomy.

NON-OPERATIVE TREATMENT

Simple occlusion caused by adhesions may be managed non-operatively provided that strangulation is certainly not present. The common circumstances in which non-operative treatment is considered are:

a. Immediately (2–10 days) after an operation when abdominal re-entry may be hazardous
b. In patients with multiple prior attacks of adhesive obstruction
c. When physical circumstances are unfavourable (compare peptic ulcer p. 154)
d. Rarely in a patient thought "too ill" for an operation.

The principles are to institute nasogastric suction and intravenous therapy, the latter first for replacement and then for maintenance. If the obstruction persists parenteral nutrition will have to be used. Indications of success are: progressive resolution in abdominal distension; decline in nasogastric suction volume; return of bowel sounds to normal; and passage of flatus per rectum. Failure is indicated by persistent pain, increasing distension and the development of local signs. Particularly in the post-operative patient there should be no hesitation in switching from a non-operative to an operative policy.

MANAGEMENT OF PARALYTIC ILEUS

Predisposing factors

Paralysis of bowel movements is common in the first 24 hours after abdominal operations, but may be prolonged if generalised peritonitis was present or if considerable rough handling of the bowel occurred. Under these conditions the features of a small bowel obstruction become apparent. Other causes have already been mentioned.

Clinical features

SYMPTOMS
1. Vomiting of large volumes of gastric contents
2. Distended abdomen
3. No flatus or faeces passed

SIGNS
1. Central abdominal distension
2. Central abdominal tympany
3. Absent bowel sounds
4. Tachycardia, hypotension

SPECIAL TESTS
Plain X-ray of the abdomen will demonstrate distended coils of bowel containing fluid levels, but these tend to be grouped at the same levels rather than staggered as in mechanical obstruction.

Treatment

Prophylaxis. Peritoneal toilet and gentle handling of bowel at a time of original operation. Restriction of oral feeding and gastric aspiration is routine post-operative care after many abdominal operations and this usually prevents paralytic ileus from developing.

Treatment. This is always conservative and consists of intravenous replacement therapy and nasogastric suction, either continuously or intermittently, until the paralysis subsides, co-ordinated bowel sounds return and flatus has been passed. The use of parenteral nutrition has made prolonged conservative management much easier.

POST-OPERATIVE MECHANICAL OBSTRUCTION

Though paralytic ileus is the common cause of intestinal obstruction in the first week after operation, the possibility of mechanical obstruction must be considered after day three. Thereafter, it can occur at any time up to at least 40 years.

Surgical pathology

1. Strangulation through holes and cul-de-sacs left at operation
2. Volvulus of an attached loop of gut
3. Adhesions. There are two types:

   a. *Fibrinous*: delicate webs of exudate which glue the serosal surfaces of bowel together. They occur within the first few days of operation, particularly after an operation for peritonitis and usually resolve spontaneously.
   b. *Fibrous*: dense, organized, strong vascular bands between coils of bowel or between the bowel and the abdominal wall. There appears to be little evidence that peritonitis itself causes these adhesions; more likely, they are outgrowths of blood vessels from adjacent tissues which act as vascular grafts into areas of poor blood supply.

Clinical features

1. Fibrinous adhesions: early post-operative 'windy' pains and occasionally vomiting
2. Fibrous adhesions

   a. Small bowel obstruction with abdominal pain, vomiting, distension, constipation and dilated coils of fluid filled bowel on X-ray
   b. Strangulating obstruction with the above features in association with muscle guarding and rigidity

Treatment

Prophylaxis. Careful operative technique, avoiding the production of ischaemia and raw surfaces on the bowel.

Treatment

1. *Fibrinous adhesions*. These are treated conservatively as they will break down or be reabsorbed.
2. *Fibrous adhesions*. These require operation and relief of obstruction (see p. 186). In general, there is more of a danger in not operating in the early post-operative period than in operating.

PSEUDO-OBSTRUCTION

This is a poor term (in that the patient *is* obstructed) for a condition halfway between mechanical and paralytic obstruction. The essential defect is not fully understood but appears to be disco-ordinate contractions of the large bowel as a consequence of either inappropriate neural input or a disordered metabolic environment. Common causes are:

a. Hypoxia
b. Anaemia
c. Retroperitoneal haematoma or malignant infiltration
d. Potassium deficiency with hypokalaemia

Clinical features

The patient is often elderly and it has in the past been a common trap to admit an old patient to hospital with intestinal obstruction and, having failed to recognize pseudo-obstruction, to operate, with disastrous results. Both the history and the physical findings suggest large bowel obstruction. On radiological examination, however, gaseous distension is diffuse and there is no 'cut off' such as is likely to be seen in colonic cancer.

Special investigations

When there is doubt, sigmoidoscopy and urgent barium enema should be done.

Treatment

If the diagnosis is made without laparotomy (as it should be), then the treatment is conservative with attention to the cause, nasogastric suction and intravenous therapy.

27

Inflammatory bowel disease

The gastrointestinal tract can be affected by specific inflammatory disorders such as actinomycosis, amoebiasis, or tuberculosis. The incidence of these is low in 'developed' Western communities but still high where public health measures are rudimentary. With free movement of people around the world, amoebiasis in particular must be considered in patients who present with acute bleeding or diarrhoea.

However, more often bowel inflammation which affects surgical practice is caused by conditions of uncertain aetiology in which there is no specific infective organism present and these conditions, together with those following ischaemia, have been collected under the heading of 'non-specific inflammation of the colon'.

Deep X-ray therapy for pelvic malignancy may cause irradiation proctitis with inflammation, ulceration and stricture formation in the absence of a specific infective organism but its precipitating factor is so obvious that it is not included here for discussion.

Therefore the conditions which will be considered in this Chapter are:

1. Diverticular disease
2. Ulcerative colitis
3. Crohn's disease
4. Ischaemic colitis
5. Amoebiasis
6. Pseudomembranous colitis
7. Chemical colitis.

DIVERTICULAR DISEASE

Aetiological considerations

A diverticulum of the colon is a herniation of the bowel mucosa through the bowel wall, which occurs at a potentially weak spot where the bowel is pierced by blood vessels near the taeniae coli (Fig. 27.1). Most often there are many diverticula, situated in the sigmoid and descending colon and less frequently in the more proximal parts of the colon.

Raised intraluminal pressure which may occur with

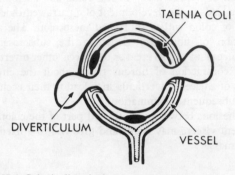

Fig. 27.1 Colonic diverticula

constipation has been suggested as an aetiological factor but there is no real evidence for this concept. There is however considerable evidence that abnormal muscle contraction of the colon may lead to development of pulsion diverticula. The aetiological concept now most favoured is that segmental contraction, in some way the result of a low bulk Western diet, creates high pressure zones in which pulsion diverticula then develop.

Inflammation of a diverticulum results in diverticulitis and this probably occurs when faecal material becomes inspissated and retained in the sac. There is no evidence to suggest that a specific organism is an aetiological factor.

Surgical pathology

Most often diverticula appear initially within a segment of the sigmoid colon but later the process may spread to involve other segments. It is also apparent that many patients show little clinical or radiological evidence of inflammation. This is why the term diverticular disease is more generally applicable than 'diverticulitis'.

When inflammatory changes supervene there are three basic pathological types.

ACUTE DIVERTICULITIS
Retention of faecal material in a thin-walled pouch ini-

tiates a non-specific acute inflammatory response. The response may be localized to a solitary diverticulum or spread to involve the adjacent mesentery, appendices epiploicae, the bowel wall and the adjacent peritoneum. Occasionally the inflammatory process may spread to involve other diverticula in a segment of bowel.

CHRONIC DIVERTICULITIS

Repeated attacks of acute inflammation are associated with fibrous tissue proliferation and the accumulation of fat in the submucosa and subserosa of the colon, the appendices epiploicae and the mesentery. Gradually contraction of fibrous tissue in the colon and surrounding tissues leads to the development of a narrowed rigid segment of colon with a shortened mesocolon. The accumulation of fibro-fatty tissue in the subserosa and submucosa may be so great as to conceal other diverticula while contraction of fibrous tissue about the circular necks of adjacent diverticula may lead to their occlusion and subsequent inflammation.

Adhesions between the affected part of the colon and adjacent viscera may occur and give rise to a fixed and rigid mass.

COMPLICATED DIVERTICULITIS

1. Abscess formation. Ulceration and perforation of an inflamed diverticulum can lead to a well localized pericolic abscess containing thick and foul-smelling pus. The abscess is surrounded by adjacent viscera, adhesions and the greater omentum and may present as a mass in the left iliac fossa, in the pelvis or occasionally in the groin.

2. Diffuse peritonitis. An inflamed diverticulum will, on rare occasions, perforate freely into the peritoneal cavity causing a generalized faecal peritonitis.

A peri-colic abscess may rupture into the peritoneal cavity when the natural powers for localizing intra-abdominal infection are inadequate (as in the debilitated, the aged and possibly in those receiving steroid therapy). More commonly however there is an intense and widespread peritoneal reaction to a severe acute diverticulitis without the presence of purulent or faecal fluid in the peritoneal cavity.

3. Obstruction. A thickened, narrowed, distorted and rigid segment of the colon may precipitate a large bowel obstruction. However complete large bowel obstruction is very rare.

Small bowel obstruction may also complicate diverticulitis. It will present either as a paralytic ileus consequent upon an acute and severe attack of diverticulitis or perforation, or as a mechanical obstruction from fibrous adhesions which have developed after previous attacks.

4. Fistula formation. An external fistula (colocutaneous fistula) is rare, but it may develop if a peri-colic abscess points and discharges on to the surface, or when operation and drainage of a peri-colic abscess has been performed.

Internal fistula formation occurs when a peri-colic abscess points and discharges spontaneously into an adjacent and adherent viscus. The organ most commonly involved is the bladder—a vesico-colic fistula. Vaginal, uterine and tubal fistulae are less common.

5. Haemorrhage. Blood loss per rectum can take place with diverticulitis. Severe and continued haemorrhage is rare but undoubtedly occurs. The source is usually an ulcerated vessel traversing the neck of a diverticulum.

Clinical features

Approximately 75% of patients are over 50 years of age. The sexes are equally affected and in 60% of cases the sigmoid colon is primarily involved.

MODES OF PRESENTATION

Acute diverticulitis
1. *Pain*, which is situated in the left iliac fossa and is colicky or dragging in nature
2. *An elevated temperature* and pulse rate
3. *Local tenderness* which is present in the left iliac fossa
4. *A mass* in the left iliac fossa and palpable on abdominal and/or rectal examination
5. *Mucus per rectum*
6. *Leucocytosis* and a raised sedimentation rate

Chronic diverticulitis
1. *Recurrent pain* in the left iliac fossa over many months or years
2. *Irregular bowel habit*, particularly constipation and bouts of diarrhoea
3. *The passage of blood per rectum* occasionally
4. *Sigmoidoscopy* usually reveals no abnormality. Occasionally an oedematous mucosa and rigidity in the region of the recto-sigmoid junction may be evident. Pain may be evoked by angling the tip of the instrument. Flexible sigmoidoscopy may permit the orifices of diverticula to be seen.
5. *Barium enema* is most often diagnostic. Narrowing of the colon over several centimetres may be associated with a classical 'saw tooth' appearance due to oedema and spasm. Open mouthed diverticula are clearly seen between attacks of inflammation and in long-standing cases narrowing and rigidity of the colon can be demonstrated. The mucosal surface is intact but the appearances are sometimes difficult to distinguish from those of carcinoma.

Complicated diverticulitis

1. *Generalized peritonitis.* Sudden onset of lower abdominal pain which becomes severe and continuous and is associated with vomiting, tachycardia, elevated temperature, board-like abdominal rigidity and absent bowel sounds.
2. *Peri-colic abscess.* Most often follows an attack of acute diverticulitis and causes marked local tenderness and guarding in the left iliac fossa. A mass of variable proportions is palpable in the left iliac fossa or in the pelvis on rectal examination and there are systemic signs of contained pus.
3. *Large bowel obstruction.* A past history of recurrent attacks of acute diverticulitis or of irregular bowel habit with a present history of colicky abdominal pain, constipation and abdominal distension is an uncommon mode of presentation. Rectal examination and sigmoidoscopy reveal an empty bowel.
4. *Vesico-colic fistula.* This should be suspected in a patient with a past history of chronic diverticulitis and a present history of dysuria. Frequency and 'scalding', haematuria, pneumaturia or faecaluria occur when the fistula is established. Microscopy of the urine shows pus, faecal debris and intestinal organisms and cystoscopy shows cystitis and occasionally the fistulous opening. Sigmoidoscopy usually reveals very little and barium enema illustrates a narrowed area of chronic diverticulitis in close proximity to the bladder.
5. *Massive bleeding* from an eroded vessel in the neck of a diverticulum may bring the patient into hospital in shock from blood loss. The bleeding is nearly always bright red.

DIFFERENTIAL DIAGNOSIS

Acute diverticulitis

Consideration may have to be given to acute salpingitis and acute appendicitis (see Chapter 28). There is not usually any danger in carrying out a barium enema which can be very helpful.

Chronic diverticulitis

This can be difficult or impossible to distinguish from carcinoma of the colon. The two conditions occur in the same age group, produce similar symptoms and give rise to the same complications. They may also occur together. When sigmoidoscopy and barium enema fail to clarify the situation, laparotomy is indicated.

Complicated diverticulitis

1. Other causes of general peritonitis—appendicitis, perforated ulcer.
2. *Peri-colic abscess.* It may be impossible to exclude carcinoma of the colon as the cause of a peri-colic abscess until the diseased segment has been excised.

3. *Large bowel obstruction.* When this is due to other causes it will usually be revealed by findings at operation. However on occasions the distinction between carcinoma and diverticulitis is impossible until the affected part has been excised and subjected to microscopy.
4. *Vesico-colic fistula.* Other causes of vesico-colic fistula, which include carcinoma of the colon, carcinoma of the bladder, Crohn's disease and post-irradiation necrosis, may have to be considered.

Treatment

ACUTE DIVERTICULITIS

When the diagnosis is certain, treatment is conservative and includes rest in bed and a fluid diet. It is doubtful whether antibiotics are of any value.

When the diagnosis is uncertain and acute gynaecological conditions or 'pelvic' appendicitis cannot be excluded, operation may be indicated to establish the diagnosis.

Once the acute phase has settled with or without operation, a barium enema is performed, if it has not already been done, to note the extent of the disease and the presence or absence of any other abnormality.

CHRONIC DIVERTICULITIS

Conservative management of chronic diverticulitis entails keeping the motions soft and regular. It is now generally agreed that a high fibre intake produced by the consumption of bran is very useful.

Surgery is indicated under the following conditions:

1. Doubtful diagnosis, when carcinoma cannot be excluded
2. Recurrent or chronic invalidism when the patient's livelihood is threatened

The operation performed is usually a segmental resection of the affected part of the colon and an end-to-end anastomosis. The operation is preceded by the usual bowel preparation (see Chapter 29).

COMPLICATED DIVERTICULITIS

Generalized peritonitis. Operation is essential after a short period of resuscitation. The procedure involves peritoneal toilet and either the placement of a drain tube to the region of the perforated colon, with or without a transverse colostomy, or, if it is possible, resection, usually without reconstruction, of the affected segment of colon.

Formal resection of the diseased segment of colon is indicated at a later date if a transverse colostomy has been performed. Formal closure of the colostomy is required if an exteriorization operation has been performed.

Peri-colic abscess. Operation and evacuation of the collection of pus is essential. Then either the placement of a drain tube into the abscess cavity, or if it is possible, resection of the affected segment of the colon, is performed. There would appear to be no advantage in adding a transverse colostomy.

Formal resection of the diseased segment of colon is indicated at a later date if a barium enema failed to exclude a malignancy or if a post-drainage faecal fistula failed to close spontaneously.

Large bowel obstruction. Complete obstruction is rarely seen. Sometimes it can be overcome by a single enema; if not, colostomy is indicated and 2–3 weeks later a resection of the diseased segment is performed, with or without concomitant closure of the colostomy. However the latter is probably most safely performed several weeks later.

Vesico-colic fistula. Resection of the affected portion of the colon with anastomosis and closure of the opening in the bladder is preferable as a one-stage operation. The alternative is to perform an initial colostomy and follow this weeks or months later with a resection and anastomosis of the colon and closure of the bladder opening. At a third operation 2–3 weeks later, the colostomy is closed.

Massive haemorrhage. Rarely is operation necessary for continued rectal haemorrhage due to diverticulitis. When it is, great difficulty can be experienced in isolating the bleeding site. A subtotal colectomy may have to be done.

ULCERATIVE COLITIS (Ulcerative procto-colitis)

This is a disease of unknown cause characterized by non-specific and diffuse inflammatory changes of the mucosa of the rectum and the large bowel.

Included under the heading of ulcerative colitis are 'proctitis' and 'procto-sigmoiditis'.

Possible aetiological factors which have been considered included the following.

1. Infection. There is no evidence that bacteria, parasites or viruses are causative factors. They may however play a part as secondary invaders and influence the severity and chronicity of the disease.

2. Allergy. An allergic response in the colon to an allergen, particularly in a hypersensitive individual, has not been substantiated with the possible exception of a response which may occur to milk antigens.

3. Autoimmunity. Autoantibodies to colonic mucosal protein have been demonstrated in about 15–20% of patients with ulcerative colitis but experimental evidence available has failed to show whether these antibodies are a cause or an effect of the pathological changes in the colon.

4. Psychogenic. There is little evidence that psychiatric disorders have anything to do with the onset of ulcerative colitis but many psychiatric factors can prolong or aggravate the condition.

Surgical pathology

The disease is mucosal and affects the entire colon and rectum but it is usually more severe in the left half of the colon. Significant changes may remain localized to the rectum for many years.

Although the name suggests that ulceration is an outstanding feature, this is not so. The mucosal inflammatory process is primarily an exudative and hyperaemic type and ulceration is not a universal accompaniment.

MACROSCOPIC

The salient features are:

1. *Serosa.* There is no serositis except in rare fulminating causes when full-thickness involvement, with or without perforation, occurs.
2. *Length of colon.* Involved bowel is always shortened and this is most obvious in the sigmoid region.
3. *Mucosa.* This is reddened, oedematous, granular and friable, and affecting the distal colon initially before spreading proximally. Ulceration when present, is usually pin-point and shallow but wide areas of mucosa can be lost.
4. *Pseudopolyps* (inflammatory polyps). In long-standing cases surviving islands of mucosa are inflamed and oedematous, so appearing to be polypoid.

MICROSCOPIC

The salient features are:

1. Inflammatory cellular infiltration of the mucosa and the submucosa
2. Crypt abscesses (within crypts of Lieberkühn) which point and discharge into the submucosa allowing the mucosa to slough off and leave ulcers
3. Relative lack of fibrous tissue reaction
4. Metaplasia, cellular atypia and frank adenocarcinoma, the incidence of which rises steeply after 10 years of the disease
5. Transmural inflammation only in severe or fulminating types of the disease

Complications

Local complications include:

1. *Perforation of the colon*, which is more likely to occur in severe first attacks of colitis and is sometimes overlooked in patients receiving apparently beneficial steroid therapy and is often preceded by dilatation of the colon—so called *toxic megacolon*
2. *Ano-rectal suppuration, fissures and fistulae*—much commoner in Crohn's disease
3. *Stricture*, which may be due to carcinoma formation submucous fibrosis or muscular hypertrophy
4. *Carcinoma* (see Chapter 29).
5. *Haemorrhage*, which is not usually severe but can lead to anaemia

General complications include:

1. *Skin lesions*: erythema nodosum, pyoderma granulosum and leg ulceration
2. *Joint lesions:* arthritis and ankylosing spondylitis
3. *Eye lesions*: corneal ulceration and iritis
4. *Liver lesions:* cirrhosis and fatty infiltrations

+ sclerosing cholangitis

Clinical features

This condition occurs with maximum incidence between 20 and 30 years but is becoming more common in the elderly. The sexes are equally affected and the disease is typically a relapsing one of varying severity in which the outstanding features are mucous diarrhoea and abdominal discomfort or pain.

MODES OF PRESENTATION

Mild ulcerative colitis
The patient's general health is not disturbed and vomiting, fever and weight loss are not present during the attack which may last for days or weeks.

1. *Diarrhoea*. Approximately four to six loose bowel actions per day containing blood and mucus occur.
2. *Abdominal discomfort* is usual.
3. *Tenderness* over the affected colon can usually be elicited.
4. *Sigmoidoscopy*. The mucosa is red and granular with loss of the vascular pattern and there may be a little haemorrhage when it is lightly touched (contact bleeding). Superficial pin-points ulcers may or may not be present. A biopsy shows either nonspecific inflammation or the characteristic crypt abcesses.
5. *Barium enema*. This may be normal or show abnormal or absent haustration, loss of colonic distensibility and fine serration of the bowel mucosa.

Acute and severe ulcerative colitis
1. *Diarrhoea*. Up to 20–40 bowel actions per day with considerable loss of fluid, blood and mucus accompanied by tenesmus and colicky pain

2. Signs of *large bowel distension* or *peritonitis* or both
3. *General features*: acute extracellular volume deficiency, fever, tachycardia, anaemia
4. *Rectal examination and sigmoidoscopy*. Blood, pus, mucus, profuse contact haemorrhage, mucosal oedema, loss of mucosal blood vessel pattern and inflammatory polyps.
5. *Barium enema*. Features which indicate severe colitis with a poor prognosis are decreased bowel wall tone, ulceration, a finely serrated contour and polyposis.

Recurrent and chronic ulcerative colitis
Has the features already described in varying amounts and characterized by relapse and remission over the years.

Complicated ulcerative colitis

1. *Peritonitis*. Perforation of the colon may occur, particularly in acute or fulminating colitis in which the whole colon is involved. Then severe abdominal pain, distension and abdominal wall rigidity will be outstanding signs. In patients receiving steroid therapy signs may be masked and rigidity absent thus making the diagnosis difficult. There is no proof however that steroids induce perforation.
2. *Ano-rectal suppuration, fissures and fistulae*. Perianal or ischio-rectal abscesses, when thought to be due to local infection, will fail to subside after apparently adequate treatment. Fissures often occur at unusual positions. The occurrence of perianal suppuration more commonly means that Crohn's disease is present.
3. *Massive haemorrhage*. This is rare and most often it will settle spontaneously with supportive therapy.

TREATMENT

Medical treatment

There is no truly specific therapy for ulcerative colitis and treatment is based largely on supportive therapy and steroids aimed at:

1. Terminating the acute attack
2. Preventing further attacks.

TERMINATING THE ACUTE ATTACK
Mild attacks can be treated on an out-patient basis but severe attacks must be regarded as a medical emergency and admission to hospital is required.

General measures
 1. *Rest the patient*. This must include adequate sleep,

sedation and tranquilization. Psychotherapy may be of value in some cases.

2. *Rest the colon*. Intravenous feeding is required in the severely ill patient. Later a fluid diet and still later a low-residue, high calorie, high vitamin, high protein diet will be indicated. Antispasmodics (propantheline, Lomotil tabs) may also be prescribed.

3. *Relieve the diarrhoea*. Lomotil tabs, codeine phosphate tabs or methylcellulose granules are useful.

4. *Replacement therapy*. This is especially required in severe cases and includes blood transfusion and correction of dehydration, and protein and potassium losses.

5. *Resist infection*. Antibiotics are not recommended unless the patient is acutely ill with fever, pus is present in the stools, there is a specific pathogen such as a *Salmonella* which can complicate ulcerative colitis, or surgery is contemplated.

Special agents

These are used alone or in combination. The latter is particularly desirable in severe forms of colitis.

1. *Corticosteroids*. All patients who do not respond rapidly to simple supportive measures should be given corticosteroids. They are also indicated in those cases of colitis associated with general complications such as eye or joint lesions.

Corticosteroids are contra-indicated in the presence of diabetes, chronic peptic ulceration, or acute fulminating colitis in association with toxic dilatation of the colon.

Corticosteroids never cure the disease and they probably increase the risk of infection, particularly in the peri-anal region, but they have a most beneficial symptomatic effect if the disease is of recent onset and confined to the mucosa.

Corticosteroids are administered by:

a. *Injection*—hydrocortisone, 300 mg daily, intravenously or intramuscularly for severe attacks
b. *Orally*—prednisolone 20–40 mg a day for mild attacks. Maintenance dose 10–15 mg daily
c. *Rectal drip*—hydrocortisone hemisuccinate 100 mg in 100–200 ml of saline
d. *Retention enema*—prednisone-21-phosphate 20 mg administered daily for mild colitis in which the disease predominantly affects the distal colon
e. *Suppositories*—prednisone-21-phosphate, 5 mg inserted night and morning for mild colitis or proctitis

2. *Salazopyrine* (compound of sulphapyridine and salicylic acid)

The mode of action of this drug is unknown but it has about a 50% chance of producing a remission. Plain or enteric-coated tablets are given (1 g 4–6 times a day).

About 10% of patients suffer from nausea, vomiting and allergies but it is rare for leucopenia or other blood dyscrasias to occur.

Male infertility is now a recognized side-effect, but the oligospermia is usually reversible.

3. *Immunosuppressive agents*. The place of such agents as azathioprine (Imuran) and 6-mercaptopurine in the treatment of ulcerative colitis is not yet established. Though these drugs suppress immune reactions and limit lymphocytic proliferation in response to antigenic stimuli they do have the serious diadvantage of unpredictable bone marrow depression causing anaemia, leucopenia and thrombocytopenia, and they cannot therefore be recommended as part of routine treatment.

PREVENTING FURTHER ATTACKS

About half of the patients will remain well for one year whether maintenance therapy is prescribed or not.

Salazopyrine, 0.5 g four times a day, is probably beneficial in reducing the relapse rate but it is still prone to produce side effects.

There is no evidence that small doses of steroids will prevent relapses and large doses of steroids given over long periods are associated with a high incidence of side-effects.

Surgical treatment

RELATIVE INDICATIONS

1. *Chronic invalidism*. Patients in whom severe colitis over a few years has resulted in chronic ill health with persistent anaemia and weight loss.
2. *Relapsing colitis* in association with *total or near total involvement* of the large bowel. Further attacks are most likely to be severe and life-threatening, particularly in the elderly.
3. *Relapsing colitis of 10 years duration* or more when associated with total or near total involvement. The risk of carcinoma developing is greatest in this group.

    It has been suggested, but not widely confirmed, that regular biopsies of the rectal mucosa at multiple sites are advisable for these patients. The detection of premalignant changes (atypical mucosa, glands and cells) indicates that the whole colonic mucosa is potentially malignant and that colectomy is required.
4. The presence of *complications*, both local and systemic.

ABSOLUTE INDICATIONS

1. Failure to respond in fulminant colitis plus:

    a. Toxic megacolon
    b. Perforation

    Surgery should not be long delayed in the fulminant case.

2. Massive bleeding unresponsive to transfusion
3. Cancer as a complication of the disease

OPERATIONS AVAILABLE

1. A diverting or split ileostomy was originally used to 'rest' the bowel but went out of favour. It has recently been revived and has a small place.
2. Proctocolectomy with either permanent ileostomy or ileal pouch (Koch pouch); the latter is emptied daily
3. Total colectomy and ileostomy and subsequent excision of the rectum or ileorectal anastomosis
4. Total colectomy and ileorectal anastomosis with or without mucosal proctectomy and ileal reservoir (Park's pouch)
5. Total proctocolectomy, performed in one or two stages, and a permanent ileostomy is still the operation favoured by most surgeons.

Total colectomy and ileorectal anastomosis has, however, considerable appeal as the rectum is retained and a permanent ileostomy is avoided. The disadvantages of the procedure are persistent loose bowel actions, a slight risk of carcinoma developing in the rectal stump and the possible development of fistulae and abscesses as the result of persistent disease in the rectum.

The new Park procedure is still under test: a complete removal of the bowel is undertaken with anastomosis of the ileum to the anal margin. Usually a reservoir is made in the ileum. Such patients can be wholly continent.

PRE-OPERATIVE PREPARATION

Apart from the usual preparation of a patient for major surgery two special matters should be noted:

1. Ileostomy preparation. The patient is informed about the nature of the future stoma and whenever possible guidance and reassurance should be given by others with such a stoma. The ileostomy site is planned so that its appliance will not encroach on abdominal scars or bony prominences.

2. Steroid preparation. Any patient who has received corticosteroids within the previous year should be given hydrocortisone 100 mg by injection before and during surgery and this therapy should be continued 8-hourly for a few days post-operatively. These measures are designed to avoid possible acute adrenal insufficiency.

CROHN'S DISEASE (regional enteritis, ileo-colitis, transmural colitis)

Aetiological considerations

This condition was first described as a clinical entity by Crohn and his colleagues in 1932 though, as with most diseases, it was recognized as an entity earlier. It is of unknown cause, characterized by a discontinuous full-thickness inflammation anywhere in the gastrointestinal tract.

Possible aetiological factors which have been consioered include the following:

1. An *infective agent* which has been diligently sought but never found.
2. *Allergy and autoimmunity.* Many of the microscopic features in Crohn's disease, viz. oedema and infiltration of the bowel wall with lymphocytes, plasma cells, eosinophils, and giant cells, suggest an allergic type of reaction. Tissue oedema and lymphoid hyperplasia are early characteristic features of the disease and this is most marked in the submucosa and accompanied by hyperaemia and lymphangiectasis. Such changes could be secondary to an allergen, but detailed immunological studies have so far failed to reveal anything specific. It is more likely that the disease is one of a group in which there is ineffective white cell action leading on to granuloma formation mainly involving macrophages.
3. It is to be noted that Crohn's disease commonly occurs in the Western world rather than in developing countries.

Surgical pathology

Though Crohn's disease may occur anywhere, the two common sites are the ileocaecal angle, where a variable length of terminal ileum and the adjacent caecum and ascending colon are involved, and the large bowel, which is usually involved throughout its length. Particularly in large bowel disease a prodromal feature may be persistent intractable peri-anal suppuration. Unlike ulcerative colitis, which is predominantly a mucosal disease, Crohn's disease is segmental and *transmural*. The characteristic features are a chronic infiltrative inflammatory process which frequently causes the involved segment to become attached to adjacent structures with the formation of internal fistulae. Narrowing by fibrous tissue is common, so that a stricture in the large bowel afflicted by inflammatory disease nearly always means Crohn's (other comparisons and contrasts between colonic Crohn's and ulcerative colitis are summarized in Table 27.1). Microscopically, the diagnostic feature is the occurrence of *granulomas*—focal collections of chronic inflammatory cells usually surrounding an area of amorphous debris and containing giant cells.

Clinical features

The age, incidence and sex distribution are similar to ulcerative colitis.

Table 27.1 Differentiation of Crohn's disease and ulcerative colitis

Macroscopic features	Ulcerative colitis	Crohn's disease of colon
Distribution in colon	Continuous throughout	Discontinuous (segmental)
Ileal involvement	Rare if ever	30% and may be extensive
Rectal involvement	Always	50%
Serosa	Normal	Granular or fibrous
Ileo-caecal valve	Normal or dilated	Often narrowed or thickened
Mucosa of bowel	Granular or ulcerated or continuous	Cobblestoned, fissured (cracked), patchy ulceration
Pseudopolyps	Usual	Unusual
Internal fistulae	None	80% (when colon involved)
Anal lesions	25%	75% (when colon involved)
Extent of inflammation	Mucosal and submuscosal	Transmural (full thickness)
Sarcoid foci (granulomas)	Absent	75%
Full-thickness fissuring	Absent	Common
Fibrosis	Absent or minimal	Present
Lymphoedema and Lymphoid hyperplasia	Absent	Present
Mesenteric nodes	Reactive hyperaemia	'Sarcoid' foci 25%

MODES OF PRESENTATION

Acute regional ileitis
Most commonly the features are indistinguishable from those of acute appendicitis, when colicky abdominal pains, right iliac fossa tenderness and an elevated temperature predominate. The diagnosis is then determined at operation. Some such patients have acute infection with *Yersinia pseudotuberculi* and care should be taken to exclude this condition by serological studies before labelling a patient with acute ileitis as having Crohn's disease.

Chronic regional enteritis
Ulceration and fibrosis at the ileocaecal angle produce a clinical syndrome of ill-health, anaemia from gastro-intestinal bleeding, colicky abdominal pain and diarrhoea. Subacute or acute intestinal obstruction may supervene. A mass is often palpable—usually loops of small bowel encased in a mass of granulation tissue and, if there is perforation, pus. In this presentation a barium follow-through examination shows distortion and narrowing of the distal ileum (string sign) and sometimes an irregular caecum which can also be outlined by a barium enema. The differential diagnosis is between ileocaecal tuberculosis (rare in the West but still common elsewhere) and, in older patients, carcinoma of the caecum.

Crohn's disease of the colon
1. Diarrhoea. This is most often intermittent and rarely are there more than four to five loose semi-solid bowel actions per day. Blood in the motions is not common unless there is extensive colonic involvement.

2. Abdominal pain. This is a common accompaniment and is usually colicky in nature, but continuous or throbbing pain occurs if peri-colic inflammation is present.

3. Weight loss with lassitude and malaise is common.

4. Perianal suppuration. Recurrent and multiple: fissures, abscesses and fistulae are common.

5. Sigmoidoscopy The mucosa is normal in about 50% of cases; in others there are patchy reddened or granular areas between areas of normal-looking mucosa. Contact bleeding is uncommon. A deep biopsy usually shows the characteristic histopathology. Radiological changes are discontinuous and separated by skip areas of normal bowel wall. Fissuring and the cobblestone effect are classical signs. Fistula formation between the colon and the small bowel (entero-colic fistula) may also be seen.

DIFFERENTIAL DIAGNOSIS
Ulcerative colitis is most often easily diagnosed on the sigmoidoscopic and radiological findings. The distinction between ulcerative colitis and Crohn's disease may be difficult when the sigmoidoscopic, radiological and pathological differences previously outlined are not clear.

Occasionally, other causes of diarrhoea may need to be considered, particularly amoebiasis and tuberculosis.

Treatment

ACUTE REGIONAL ILEITIS
Operation is most often mandatory as it is impossible to distinguish this condition from acute appendicitis.

At operation, once the condition has been diagnosed, nothing further should be done, though it is now generally accepted that it is safe to remove the appendix.

CHRONIC REGIONAL ENTERITIS

Resection of the involved bowel is required for obstruction, fistula or perforation with abscess formation. Anastomosis must be done through healthy bowel if leakage is to be avoided.

CROHN'S COLITIS

There is no specific treatment and whatever is done the relapse rate is high.

Medical treatment

This follows the same line as that of ulcerative colitis (p. 193), though there is not much evidence that corticosteroids are useful. Salazopyrin is, however, thought to be valuable.

Surgical treatment

Experience indicates that Crohn's colitis is not very responsive to medical treatment and 80–90% of cases ultimately require surgery. Because of this, many surgeons now consider that earlier intervention is indicated while the disease is confined to the colon and not complicated by internal fistulae and abscesses.

If the entire colon is involved proctocolectomy and ileostomy has proved satisfactory, while colectomy and ileo-rectal anastomosis is occasionally indicated if the rectum is normal.

Ileal pouch and reservoir procedures are not recommended in Crohn's disease, though each case has to be judged on its merits.

ISCHAEMIC COLITIS

Aetiological considerations

An inflammatory response in the colon following an ischaemic episode due to occlusion or narrowing of the inferior mesenteric artery by atheroma, aneurysm formation, or after aortic reconstruction. The severity of the reaction will depend on the extent and duration of the ischaemia, the bacterial flora present in the bowel at the time and the adequacy of the collateral circulation by way of the marginal artery and its connection to the superior mesenteric artery and its middle colic branch. Occasionally a similar condition occurs without obvious major vessel obstruction.

Surgical pathology

When the circulation through the inferior mesenteric artery or its arcadal communications is impaired, various segmental changes may occur in the colon, particularly in the region of the splenic flexure. These changes have been classified as follows:

Ischaemic colitis with gangrene follows a period of pro-found vascular insufficiency due to a thrombotic or embolic episode in an atherosclerotic vessel. It can also occur after aortic reconstructive surgery when major colic vessels are occluded.

The condition has two phases:

1. Infarction of the colon causing varying degrees of mucosal gangrene, oedema and haemorrhage and intravascular platelet thrombi.
2. Secondary invasion with organisms which are able to accelerate the gangrenous process under anaerobic conditions and cause necrosis of the entire bowel wall. This stage may be difficult to distinguish from fulminating ulcerative colitis. A similar event takes place in amoebic colitis (see below p. 198)

Transient ischaemic colitis. This is the mildest form of ischaemia. Mucosal ulceration with transmural inflammation of the colon resolves as an adequate collateral circulation is developed.

Ischaemic stricture of the colon. Incomplete recovery from ischaemia can lead to a full thickness inflammation of the colon with fibrosis and fusiform stricture formation. Microscopically the strictured areas show fibroblastic proliferation, atrophy and haemosiderin-laden macrophages—quite different from those of ulcerative colitis and Crohn's disease.

Clinical features

Occlusion of the inferior mesenteric artery may be symptomless.

The majority of patients are in their sixth decade and it is usual for evidence of atherosclerosis to be present at other sites (brain, heart, kidney, lower limb).

MODES OF PRESENTATION

Ischaemic colitis with gangrene
The following are usually present:

1. *Acute left-sided abdominanal pain*
2. *Abdominal tenderness*, rigidity, distension
3. *Bloody diarrhoea*
4. *Shock and toxaemia* depending on the length of gut involved and speed and severity of gangrene
5. *Sigmoidoscopy.* This may reveal blood in the bowel lumen, but the rectum and lowest sigmoid are usually normal in appearance.
6. *Plain X-ray of the abdomen.*—toxic dilatation of the colon

Transient ischaemic colitis
The following are usually present:

1. *Transient abdominal pain* of sudden onset
2. *Rectal bleeding* which subsides within a few days

3. *Diarrhoea* which subsides within a few days
4. *Sigmoidoscopy*. Usually reveals no abnormality; the rectum is always spared and the lowest sigmoid is usually normal. Flexible sigmoidoscopy or colonoscopy may reveal more proximal non-specific inflammation.
5. *Barium enema*. The abnormal segment is of variable length and is most usual at the splenic flexure or the upper part of the sigmoid colon. Here the normal haustral pattern may be lost and rounded filling defects and crescentic irregularities ('thumb printing') may be present in a sacculated or narrowed segment.
6. *Aortography and selective mesenteric arteriography*. In expert hands these specialized techniques may demonstrate occlusion of the inferior mesenteric artery or a diminished arterial supply to the region of the splenic flexure.

Ischaemic stricture of the colon
The following are usually present:

1. *Symptoms of subacute or acute large bowel obstruction*
2. *Sigmoidoscopy*. This is normal.
3. *Barium enema*. A short fusiform or long tubular narrowing of the colon occurs.
4. *Laparotomy*. This will be indicated when acute large bowel obstruction is present or when the radiological features cannot be distinguished from those of carcinoma.

Treatment

ISCHAEMIC COLITIS WITH GANGRENE
The patient presents an acute abdominal emergency, and laparotomy is essential after a short period of resuscitation.

At operation excision of the necrotic bowel is obligatory and reconstruction is deferred to a later date.

ISCHAEMIC STRICTURE
Operation is advisable to establish the diagnosis firmly and it is imperative if acute large bowel obstruction is present.

In the non-obstructive case resection of the strictured area by a generous margin is indicated.

TRANSIENT ISCHAEMIC COLITIS
Occasionally laparotomy is indicated when other causes for rectal haemorrhage cannot be excluded by other means.

AMOEBIASIS

Though often thought of as a tropical disease, amoebiasis is found wherever carriers in the community are associated with poor sanitation.

Surgical pathology

The organism is *Entamoeba histolytica* which can survive as a cyst either in the colon from whence it is shed or in water or on the ground that it enters. Infection is by oral ingestion and often from uncooked green foods manured with human excreta.

The disease takes four forms:

1. Acute superficial colitis with shaggy confluent ulcers involving all of the colon. In contrast to early acute ulcerative colitis the ulcers are frequently large enough to be visible to the naked eye. Deep penetration is rare and perforation quite uncommon. The disease may become chronic and intermittent.

2. Transmural colitis in which the disease, as the name implies, spreads through the full thickness of the bowel wall. The predominant pathological lesion is invasion of the medium-sized arteries at the mesenteric border. Full-thickness necrosis with perforation may then result, or fibrosis with local strictures.

3. Localized intestinal disease. Occasionally an amoebic cellulitis affects only a short length of gut and gives rise to an inflammatory mass. This 'amoeboma' may be confused with cancer or with other forms of inflammatory disease.

4. Amoebic hepatitis. The amoebae enter the portal venous system and set up an acute inflammatory process, usually more marked in the right lobe. The inflammation is diffuse and pus soon forms to give rise to an amoebic abscess. Characteristically the abscess does not have a thick granulation tissue or fibrous wall so that, if the underlying condition can be treated and the pus removed by aspiration, formal drainage is not required.

Clinical features

INTESTINAL DISEASE
Acute bloody diarrhoea with watery mucus is characteristic. Pain is unusual. Systemic disturbance with a high fever is common. Progress to toxic dilation is relatively unusual but then the patient complains of abdominal pain and distension and more severe systemic upset.

On examination there may be little to find in the abdomen except in the fulminant case when the appearances are as in toxic megacolon. Peritonitis is present when perforation has occurred.

Sigmoidoscopy shows:

1. Blood and mucus
2. Diffuse inflammation
3. Shallow ulcers

In amoeboma there is usually a history of diarrhoea and blood. The mass does not have any specific features.

At sigmoidoscopy a distal amoeboma may be very difficult to distinguish from a carcinoma.

AMOEBIC HEPATITIS

Intestinal symptoms may or may not precede the onset of fever, right upper quadrant pain, mild jaundice and sometimes shoulder tip pain. An abscess can rupture through the diaphragm and give rise to chest signs. In late disease broncho-pleural fistula with purulent sputum may ensue.

Examination shows:

1. Icterus
2. Tenderness in the right upper quadrant
3. Palpable liver, usually smooth and tender

Confirming the diagnosis

1. Warm stage examination of a stool passed within the previous 10 minutes may show motile amoebae but this is less reliable than:
2. Histopathological examination of a rectal biopsy which has been fixed in formalin.
3. A specific complement fixation test is available but usually some days elapse before a report can be obtained.
4. In amoebic hepatitis
   a. Chest X-ray may show pleural effusion
   b. Liver scintiscan or ultrasound may demonstrate a filling defect
   c. Needle aspiration may produce 'anchovy sauce' pus

Treatment

COLITIS

All former methods of treatment have given way to the use of metronidazole 800 mg orally three times a day for 5–10 days. In urgent cases or where oral administration is difficult, suppositories can in theory produce high blood levels, but may be expelled. Intravenous metronidazole is now available for the severe case. If the acute symptoms do not subside over 2–3 days with metronidazole there is a risk of perforation which carries a high mortality. Urgent investigation by selective arteriography can be used to define those patients in whom vascular occlusion has occurred and operation to resect the compromised area is vital.

AMOEBIC HEPATITIS

Aspiration should be undertaken if a significant abscess (estimated at 200 ml or more of pus) is thought to exist. However, smaller collections will usually resolve.

PSEUDOMEMBRANOUS COLITIS

The disorder is referred to on p. 22. Though often associated with a surgical procedure, it can follow the administration of antibiotics in a non-surgical context. Particular agents which seem to be associated with the disease are clindamycin and lincomycin. The cause is super infection with *Clostridium difficile* and the effects of its toxin.

Surgical pathology

There is superficial mucosal inflammation with very marked oedema and a grey-brown membrane. Under the microscope the oedema is confirmed and focal ulceration may be seen.

Clinical features

Acute watery diarrhoea, not often bloody, with toxic features and water and electrolyte depletion. Clinical examination is non-specific, but the diagnosis can be made on sigmoidoscopy, biopsy, and stool culture to isolate *C. difficile* and its toxin.

Management

1. Withdraw causative agents.
2. Replace water and electrolyte loss.
3. Administer antibiotics against *C. difficile*—the current choices are vancomycin or metronidazole.
4. Rarely, resect the colon when the condition progresses to toxic dilatation.

CHEMICAL COLITIS

In parts of the world where it is common practice to administer 'therapeutic' enemas occasionally astringent or toxic materials (e.g. battery acid) come in contact with the colorectal mucosa. The effect is often to produce a severe colitis of non-specific type with sloughing of the mucosa. Blood loss can be significant and perforation may occur. It is clearly important to make the differential diagnosis from other causes of colitis: it may be difficult to do so because a history is rarely forthcoming and the appearances are non-specific. Thus the diagnosis is usually by exclusion.

Treatment is expectant with local steroids. Surgery may be required for complications—haemorrhage, perforation or later stricture.

28

Acute appendicitis and other causes of acute abdominal pain

One person in six or seven develops appendicitis at some time, so that this condition is the commonest abdominal surgical emergency. Appendicitis is a 'disease of civilization'—and relatively uncommon in developing rural communities.

SURGICAL ANATOMY

The appendix is attached at the point of convergence of the three taeniae coli of the caecum on its postero-medial wall. The mesoappendix is a peritoneal fold containing a variable amount of fat and the appendicular artery which arises from the posterior caecal branch of the ileocolic artery.

The appendix, like the hands of a clock, may be long or short and may occupy any position radially from its base; however it is commonly situated behind the caecum (retrocaecal) or on the psoas major muscle near or hanging over the pelvic brim (pelvic) and rarely in other positions (pre-ileal, post-ileal, para-caecal).

SURGICAL PATHOLOGY

PREDISPOSING FACTORS

There are two major factors:

1. Obstructive agents

   a. Foreign bodies
      (i) Animal—threadworms, round worms
      (ii) Vegetable—seeds, date stones, etc
      (iii) 'Mineral'—faecoliths (commonest cause)
   b. Submucous lymphoid tissue—most abundant in childhood and adolescence and may cause obstruction of the appendix lumen

2. Infective agents

There is often a mixed infection which may gain access

to the wall of the appendix through an area of epithelial erosion caused by pressure of an obstructing agent. The organisms involved include *E. coli*, *Streptococcus faecalis*, *Bacteroides* sp. and other intestinal commensals.

TYPES OF ACUTE APPENDICITIS

There are three clinico-pathological types of appendicitis, in each of which obstructive and infective factors play a part:

1. Acute appendicitis
2. Acute appendicitis with an inflammatory mass
3. Acute appendicitis with generalized peritonitis

1. Acute appendicitis

Organisms enter the wall of the appendix and lodge in the submucosa where they proliferate rapidly or slowly depending upon their virulence to involve eventually the full thickness of the wall causing it to become swollen, reddened and turgid.

The rate of acceleration of the inflammatory process is increased in the presence of obstruction of the lumen of the appendix. 'Catarrhal appendicitis' and 'diffuse appendicitis' are terms sometimes used to describe mild and moderate degrees of inflammation of the appendix.

2. Acute appendicitis with an inflammatory mass

In the presence of obstruction together with severe infection the appendix becomes distended with pus which causes an increase in intraluminal pressure. If the process is allowed to proceed, venous occlusion, further oedema and later arterial occlusion result in gangrene of part of the wall of the appendix. This appears commonly close to the tip of the appendix or at the site of frank obstruction where presumably the precarious blood supply at the former site and pressure necrosis at the latter, play a part. Perforation follows and infected material is rapidly localized by the defence mechanisms, in particular the greater omentum and coils of small bowel, and a mass results, part of which may be a collection of pus.

3. Acute appendicitis with generalized peritonitis

With severe degrees of obstruction and infection in patients with poor powers of localization (the young and the old), perforation of the appendix allows infected material to disperse widely in the peritoneal cavity, causing an intense peritoneal reaction with outpouring of fluid which is initially clear but which rapidly becomes purulent. The serosal surfaces of the bowel become injected and flaked with clotted lymph.

CLINICAL FEATURES

Acute appendicitis

SYMPTOMS

1. Pain. Abdominal pain may vary considerably in type and situation. It is classically initially peri-umbilical — the result of appendicular obstruction — followed by movement to the right iliac fossa within a few hours where it becomes persistent. However, it may start in the right iliac fossa. The onset is usually sudden, particularly if there is a high degree of obstruction to the lumen of the appendix but there may be a preceding 12–24-hour period of nausea and of vague abdominal discomfort. The pain may be colicky in nature if a significant degree of obstruction is present or continuous, nagging, or 'toothache like'.

2. Vomiting. This may be early and repeated if obstruction to the appendix is present. Otherwise it is not an outstanding feature.

3. Diarrhoea. This is more likely in the presence of an inflamed 'pelvic' appendix irritating the rectal wall or a retroileal appendix irritating terminal small bowel.

4. Urinary symptoms. Frequency or dysuria may also occur with an inflamed 'pelvic' appendix.

SIGNS

General
The patient may look unwell and have a coated tongue and foul breath. Pyrexia and tachycardia are indicative of an infective process but their absence does not exclude appendicitis.

Local
1. Tenderness of a localized and persistent nature is the most important abdominal observation. It is situated over the appendix, at some place in the right iliac fossa; this may be at McBurney's point (the junction of the

middle and outer thirds of a line from umbilicus to anterior superior iliac spine).

2. Rigidity of the abdominal muscles overlying the right iliac fossa indicates involvement of the underlying peritoneum. The sign may be absent in early, 'retro-caecal' or 'pelvic' appendicitis.

3. Rectal examination. Tenderness on the right side indicates involvement of the pelvic peritoneum by the inflammatory process. This may be the only sign with a 'pelvic' appendicitis.

Special
Many tests have been described to determine the presence or absence of local peritonitis. None is reliable. They are included here because examiners like them! Some of these are:

1. Rovsing's sign. Deep pressure in the left iliac fossa may cause pain in the right iliac fossa. However there is no evidence to confirm the thought that pain is produced by distension of the caecum with gases forced into it from the left colon.

2. Blumberg's sign. Deep pressure in the left iliac fossa may be associated with pain in the right iliac fossa when the hand is suddenly released. This 'crossed' or 'rebound' tenderness is said to be strongly suggestive of local peritonitis.

3. Cope's sign. Flexion and internal rotation of the right hip may cause pain if the obturator internus muscle is in close relation to an inflamed 'pelvic' appendix.

4. Psoas sign. Extension of the right hip may cause pain if the psoas muscles is in close relation to a 'retro-caecal' or 'pelvic' appendix.

5. Straight leg raising sign. With digital pressure over the tender spot in the abdomen, elevation of the right leg may cause increased pain. This is suggestive of a 'retro-caecal' appendicitis.

6. Testicular retraction in the male on palpation in the R.I.F. Said to indicate an unperforated appendix.

LABORATORY AND OTHER INVESTIGATIONS
1. Abdominal X-rays are not helpful
2. The leukocyte count in peripheral blood is often raised, particularly a neutrophilia
3. The urine should always be examined by ward test and by microscopy in a doubtful case

DIFFERENTIAL DIAGNOSIS
Usually there is little difficulty in diagnosing acute appendicitis. However, one must remember other possibilities, particularly in the female. These conditions may be divided into the following:

Extra-abdominal

Right basal pneumonia and diaphragmatic pleurisy may be associated with abdominal symptoms but the presence of respiratory symptoms and specific signs in the chest should cause little difficulty with the diagnosis.

Abdominal

Almost any abdominal condition can mimic acute appendicitis. Some of these are:

Mesenteric adenitis. Approximately 5% of all operations performed for suspected acute appendicitis discover mesenteric adenitis. The presence of enlarged pink and fleshy lymph nodes in the mesentery of the terminal ileum associated with a normal appendix are the characteristic features. In all cases the appendix should be removed to avoid future confusion when confronted with an appendicectomy scar and right iliac fossa pains.

Mesenteric adenitis usually occurs in children and may be suspected when there is a history of recent sore throat together with a high fever, attacks of pain with complete relief between attacks, a tender spot medial to and above McBurney's point, shifting tenderness and little or no muscle guarding. Under these conditions it may be permissible to observe the patient, particularly if the abdominal signs are minimal in degree. However, if there is any doubt, operation is indicated.

Pyelitis. Right-sided abdominal and loin pain associated with rigors and urinary symptoms is suggestive of a urinary tract infection. The absence of abdominal rigidity and the presence of pus in the urine indicate the diagnosis.

Ureteric colic. A calculus in the right ureter may cause confusion but the radiation of the pain along the line of the ureter and the presence of blood in the urine should eliminate any doubt. Sometimes a plain X-ray of the abdomen will indicate the stone.

Gastroenteritis. Diarrhoea, vomiting, central abdominal pain, and fever, without local tenderness or rigidity over the appendix region suggests gastroenteritis.

Non-specific ileitis may cause a similar picture and *Yersinia* or *Campylobacter* sp. may be identified.

Meckel's diverticulitis. In this rare condition the clinical picture is very similar to appendicitis. Meckel's diverticulum and its disorders are discussed below.

Acute cholecystitis. Right upper abdominal pain associated with acute cholecystitis may be confused with high 'retrocaecal' appendicitis (see also Chapter 25).

Diverticulitis. Acute diverticulitis of the sigmoid colon may be confused with 'pelvic' appendicitis (see also Chapter 27).

Gynaecological conditions. Pelvic inflammatory disease, which includes salpingitis, pyosalpinx, tuboovarian abscess and parametritis, is the most common non-pregnancy-associated condition to exclude when considering appendicitis as the cause of abdominal pain in women of the reproductive age group. This condition is particularly common in large city hospitals where promiscuity and prostitution are frequent predisposing factors. Pelvic examination of women who may have appendicitis is therefore mandatory. Torsion of a Fallopian tube, torsion, haemorrhage or rupture of an ovarian tumour and endometriosis may have to be considered. Pain of sudden onset in the right iliac fossa, on the day a period begins, may be caused by the rupture of or minor haemorrhage from a corpus luteal cyst.

During early pregnancy, abortion, retroverted and impacted uterus, degeneration of uterine fibroids and ectopic pregnancy, may require consideration.

During late pregnancy, labour, abruptio placentae, ruptured uterus, fulminating pre-eclampsia and rectus sheath haematoma may require consideration.

Women often develop recurrent acute or subacute RIF pain particularly in their teens and twenties. Frequently no cause is found. Appendicectomy should be avoided because it does no good. Laparoscopy to reassure both patient and surgeon is being increasingly used in such circumstances.

Acute appendicitis with an inflammatory mass

SYMPTOMS

These are similar to those of acute appendicitis, but pain is often more severe, entirely right-sided and present for 2–3 days. In addition the patient feels ill and nauseated.

SIGNS

In addition to those already described there may be:

1. A tender mass, sometimes not well defined, in the right iliac fossa; after 5 or 6 days there is usually little rigidity, and the mass is more easily felt
2. A tender extension of the mass into the pelvis on rectal examination

DIFFERENTIAL DIAGNOSIS

An appendix mass may be confused with other masses in the right iliac fossa such as:

Carcinoma of the caecum. A history of large bowel symptoms, anaemia and weight loss may give a clue but the diagnosis may not be apparent until operation. A perforated carcinoma of the caecum with pericaecal abscess formation will be indistinguishable from an appendiceal abscess until operation.

Carcinoma of the left side of colon. With obstruction to the left colon, the caecum will be distended in the presence of a competent ileocaecal valve and present as a compressible and tympanitic mass in the right iliac fossa.

Rarely, the caecal wall becomes attenuated or even gangrenous and appendicitis is even more accurately mimicked.

Empyema of the gall bladder. Pain in the right hypochondrium radiating to the back, together with a tender globular mass projecting from beneath the costal margin and moving on respiration, indicates an empyema.

Renal mass. A right perinephric abscess should be suspected if loin pain and tenderness are associated with rigors and a possible distant staphylococcal focus.

Hydronephrosis may present as a uniform mass in the loin which moves on respiration. It may be associated with a classical band of colonic resonance anteriorly.

Miscellaneous. Ovarian cyst, fibroid uterus, psoas abscess, Crohn's disease and ileo-caecal tuberculosis may need to be considered on occasions.

Acute appendicitis with generalized peritonitis

CLINICAL FEATURES

These often follow severe obstructive appendicitis with increasingly severe colicky abdominal pains and vomiting.

There are three stages of peritonitis:

1. Stage of shock
a. Patient is pale, sweating and anxious
b. Pulse rate is elevated
c. Blood pressure is lowered
d. Temperature may be subnormal
e. Respirations are rapid and shallow
f. Pronounced local tenderness is present in the right iliac fossa

2. Stage of peritoneal reaction
Shock has improved and the following become apparent:

a. Severe local tenderness in the right iliac fossa
b. Rebound tenderness
c. 'Board-like' rigidity
d. Marked rectal tenderness

3. Stage of frank peritonitis
Rigidity is less but paralytic ileus becomes apparent with the following features:

a. Abdominal distension
b. Absent bowel sounds
c. Faecal vomitus and later dehydration with 'Hippocratic facies' (hollow cheeks, sunken eye balls, circles round eyes and 'pinched' expression)

DIFFERENTIAL DIAGNOSIS

Extra-abdominal
Myocardial infarction with basal pneumonia.

Abdominal
Inflammation, colic, perforation, strangulation, torsion, haemorrhage, vascular occlusion, tabes dorsalis or acute porphyria may present with severe abdominal pain, vomiting, shock and board-like rigidity.

The commoner conditions requiring consideration are:

Perforated peptic ulcer. A past history of dyspepsia or epigastric pain after meals, together with abdominal signs most marked in the upper abdomen and a plain X-ray showing gas beneath the right hemi-diaphragm, are diagnostic features. The distinction may be difficult if, as is not uncommon, the initial spread from the perforated ulcer is down the right paracolic gutter.

Perforated diverticulitis of the colon. A past history of attacks of left iliac fossa pain and constipation, in conjunction with abdominal signs most marked in the left iliac fossa indicate a likely colonic origin. Yet it must be remembered that when inflammation from a perforated 'pelvic' appendicitis spreads upwards, it does so most often on the *left* side.

Acute pancreatitis. The presence of severe abdominal pain passing through to the back and causing the patient to roll about, in addition to a past history of a heavy alcohol intake, should arouse suspicion. A negative abdominal X-ray together with an elevated serum amylase will usually establish the diagnosis of pancreatitis but in a doubtful case a laparotomy is occasionally indicated.

Ruptured ectopic pregnancy. This diagnosis must be considered in a woman whose period is overdue and in whom there is haemorrhagic shock with signs of pelvic peritoneal irritation. The latter is evidenced by extreme pain when the cervix is moved.

Superior mesenteric artery occlusion. Thrombosis or embolism in the superior mesenteric artery may cause infarction of part of the small bowel and pain, severe shock and peritonitis follow. This condition usually occurs after the fifth decade in patients with generalized atherosclerosis or atrial fibrillation. The features of an associated small bowel obstruction, blood loss through the rectum and a 'boggy' abdominal mass should leave no doubt as to the diagnosis.

Perforated acute cholecystitis. A confident diagnosis of this unusual condition can usually be made from an appreciation of the symptoms and signs of gall bladder disease. Pain situated beneath the right costal margin and radiating to between the shoulder blades together with features of peritonitis are usually diagnostic. Sometimes radio-opaque gall stones are demonstrated on X-ray. A high 'retrocaecal' or 'sub-hepatic' appendix may, however, cause confusion on occasions.

TREATMENT

Acute appendicitis

Once appendicitis has been diagnosed the treatment is appendicectomy. Where the diagnosis is in doubt, especially in young women, it may be very useful to carry out laparoscopy to help establish a diagnosis.

Acute appendicitis with an inflammatory mass

The early stage is a mass comprising the inflamed appendix and surrounding coils of bowel and greater omentum; later a frank abscess may form or the mass may resolve without pus formation.

There are two schools of thought on the treatment of acute appendicitis with an inflammatory mass and these are as follows:

CONSERVATIVE SCHOOL

This is not a popular method and should never be used in the young or the elderly because of the poor powers of localization of infection which exist in these patients; in addition, it should not be used if a definite diagnosis cannot be made.

The method entails the following:

1. Semi upright position (in bed)
2. Fluids by mouth or intravenously if necessary
3. Four-hourly, or more frequent, observation of the pulse rate and twice daily record of the temperature
4. Palpating the abdominal mass regularly and marking its limits on the skin surface daily
5. Chemotherapy. The use of a broad spectrum antibiotic and metronidazole may possible aid resolution of an appendical mass but it will not alter a frank appendiceal abscess though it may suppress the systemic signs.
6. Analgesics and purgatives are forbidden.

With this regimen, the following may happen:

Resolution. The patient recovers and the mass subsides in about 80% of cases.

Deterioration. Elevation of the pulse rate, increased pain, tenderness, muscle guarding and size of the mass indicate failure, and operation becomes essential. This probably occurs in 10% of cases and at operation a generalized peritonitis may be found.

Abscess formation. Rectal or vaginal examination may reveal a fluctuant mass indicating that the abscess should

be drained at these sites. Very rarely the abscess may point suprapubically and require drainage from this direction.

No change. In a small percentage of cases the inflammatory mass remains unchanged for days or even weeks and the decision as to what should be done may be difficult. The possibility of a wrong diagnosis and the presence of some other condition such as Crohn's disease or caecal carcinoma usually indicates that operation should be carried out.

Appendicectomy should be performed three to six months later in those patients in whom resolution occurred or simple drainage of an appendical abscess was performed.

The advantages of the conservative method of treatment are:

1. A difficult and perhaps dangerous operation in an infected field is avoided.
2. An elective appendicectomy can be performed months later when the patient's general condition has improved and when technical difficulties are no longer a hazard.

The disadvantages of the conservative method of treatment are:

1. It should not be employed in young or elderly patients
2. General peritonitis may result during the 'watching' period
3. There remains uncertainty of diagnosis on some occasions
4. There is a necessity for a second admission to hospital at a later date for appendicectomy

OPERATIVE SCHOOL

This is the usual method of treatment. At operation one of two procedures will be carried out:

1. Appendicectomy and drainage of an abscess cavity is usually possible
2. Drainage alone, when for technical reasons it is decided that appendicectomy may involve excessive hazards; an elective appendicectomy would then be performed 3–6 months later

The advantages of the operative approach are:

1. A certain diagnosis is made
2. A second admission to hospital can usually be avoided
3. A shorter stay in hospital results

The disadvantages are:

1. Manipulation through a mass or an abscess to remove the appendix may cause dissemination of infected material, haemorrhage or a faecal fistula.
2. Post-operative complications such as wound infection

and residual abscess are more frequent than after an elective appendicectomy.

Acute appendicitis with generalized peritonitis

The treatment is operative after a short period of resuscitation.

Pre-operative gastric suction, intravenous replacement therapy, analgesics and antibiotics are administered.

At operation peritoneal toilet is performed when generalized peritonitis is present and whenever possible the appendix is removed and a drain tube placed to the site of the appendix bed.

In all generalized peritonitis it is common practice to carry out intraoperative peritoneal lavage with saline and an antibiotic.

Wound complications are reduced by perioperative antibiotics, by a short course of metronidazole (to treat anaerobes) and by leaving the wound open.

MECKEL'S DIVERTICULUM

The surgical problems of this persistence of the vitello-intestinal duct are considered here because it is frequently encountered in relation to acute appendicitis.

Incidence

It is said that 3% of individuals have some form of persistent Meckel's diverticulum. However, clinical problems are very much less common.

Types of problem

1. Persistence of umbilical connection

a. An open duct—very rare; present at birth and causing an ileal fistula. Requires surgical closure.

b. An umbilical sinus without an opening into the ileum. Also rare—there is umbilical discharge of watery blood-stained material also usually from birth. Treatment is excision.

c. A vitello-intestinal cyst. Closure of both ends may produce a midline sub-umbilical cyst at any age but commonly in infancy or childhood. Usually asymptomatic but easily removed.

d. The attachment of the diverticulum or a cord from its apex to the umbilicus provides a fixed point around which torsion may occur, so producing volvulus and acute intestinal obstruction. Alternatively herniation of small bowel through the gap between the attachment and the abdominal wall may take place with the same effects. Can occur at any age. The presentation is acute intestinal obstruction.

2. Acute inflammation

A narrow mouthed diverticulum can become inflamed, usually because of retained content. The condition is clinico-pathologically and clinically virtually identical to acute appendicitis. Treatment, as for the latter condition, is surgical.

3. Consequences of heterotopic gastric mucosa

For a reason that is far from clear Meckel's diverticulum may contain acid–pepsin-secreting gastric mucosa. In consequence a peptic ulcer may form in the adjacent small bowel mucosa either of the diverticulum or the adjacent ileum. Bleeding or perforation may occur, though the former is much more common.

a. Bleeding has been described at any age but is commonest before the age of 20. There are usually episodes of bright red or slightly altered blood being passed per rectum. Often the haemorrhage is haemodynamically significant. No cause is found on conventional investigation by barium enema. The gastric mucosa in a diverticulum can be outlined with radio-labelled technetium and the diverticulum itself visualised with the same material when bleeding is occurring. Treatment is by excision.

b. Perforation. Presents in the same manner as perforated appendix or Meckel's diverticulitis.

29

Large bowel tumours

CLASSIFICATION

Rare tumours
Polyps of the colon and rectum
Large bowel cancer

RARE TUMOURS

Lipomas and fibromas are sometimes found in the sub-mucosa and may cause intussusception. Dermoid cysts occur in the rectal wall, usually posteriorly and more commonly in the post anal space.

POLYPS OF THE COLON AND RECTUM

Neoplastic polyps

Three types of growth pattern are recognized, but all are essentially the same pathological process, namely neo-plasia of the intestinal epithelium.

1. Tubular adenoma may be sessile but is usually pedunculated and typically it is small and spherical with a smooth surface which is broken up into lobules by inter-communicating clefts. When it is small (0.5 cm) and the same colour as the surrounding mucosa, it is usually benign but when large carcinomatous change should be suspected. There is some evidence, however, to suggest that the malignant potential of adenomatous polyps is not as great as that of the villous adenoma.

Microscopically adenomatous polyps show a well marked acinar pattern with a stroma of variable vascu-larity.

2. Villous adenoma. These occur almost exclusively in the rectum and lower sigmoid colon and the majority are therefore accessible to the finger or sigmoidoscope.

Typically villous tumours are large and sessile with a shaggy surface appearance made up of thousands of finger-like processes. However sometimes small pedun-culated tumours have a typically villous growth pattern as well.

206

There is appreciable risk of a villous tumour becoming malignant and while palpation reveals a soft and slippery growth when it is completely benign, the slightest sug-gestion of induration raises the suspicion of malignancy and biopsy is therefore essential.

Villous tumours characteristically produce a profuse mucous diarrhoea but occasionally it may be blood-stained. Potassium may be lost in significant quantities.

3. Tubulo-villous adenoma are often large and sessile tumours with a mixed surface configuration in which some parts appear tubular and others villous. Malignant change is well recognized.

Familial polyposis (polyposis coli) is a rare form of intestinal polyposis in which multiple adenomatous polyps (both sessile and pedunculated), form in the rec-tum and colon and have a high propensity for malignant change (see below, p. 208).

Hamartomatous polyps

These may be defined as non-neoplastic polyps composed of an abnormal mixture of normal tissues; they are really malformations and include:

1. Juvenile polyps which are rare, occur most often in children but occasionally in adults. They are prone to prolapse through the rectum or cause intussusception, or to infarct and to fall off their stalks causing rectal haemorrhage.

Microscopically they consist of epithelial tubules lined by mucus-secreting cells embedded in loose areolar con-nective tissue. There is no increased epithelial activity nor tendency to neoplastic change.

Associated congenital abnormalities such as cardiac defects, malrotation of the gut, and hydrocephalus are present in about one-third of cases.

It is probable that juvenile polyposis results from some modification of the function of the gene responsible for producing familial polyposis.

2. Peutz-Jeghers syndrome. The essential features of this rare syndrome are gastrointestinal polyposis, mucocutaneous pigmentation and Mendelian-dominant inheritance.

The polyps usually appear during childhood in the small bowel where they may cause intussusception but they may affect the colon and rectum and result in rectal haemorrhage. They are not adenomata and are probably not pre-cancerous, their appearance suggesting malformation.

Microscopically a tree-like malformation of the muscularis mucosae is seen to be covered by normal mucosa.

TREATMENT OF POLYPS

SOLITARY POLYPS

The first requirement is to determine whether an apparently solitary polyp is in fact part of a multiple polyposis, or whether it is associated with a carcinoma elsewhere in the large bowel. Therefore a meticulous examination of the entire large bowel is essential. Barium enema, of the double contrast type, is mandatory and colonoscopy should be used where it is available.

Solitary polyps are treated in the following way:

1. Within reach of the sigmoidoscope

Pedunculated polyps. It may be possible to deliver the polyp through the anus where it can be ligated and excised; alternatively it may be twisted off or excised with a diathermy loop.

Sessile polyps below the peritoneal reflection of the rectum. These are either twisted off with alligator forceps or removed with a diathermy loop.

Villous tumours. If the tumour is entirely soft and situated in the lower rectum it may be removed with diathermy or ligated and excised.

If the tumour is indurated or extensively involving the rectum, then an abdomino-perineal excision or an anterior resection of the rectum will be indicated depending on its position.

2. Beyond reach of the sigmoidoscope and sessile polyps above the peritoneal reflection of the rectum

Until recently polyps beyond the reach of the sigmoidoscope (15 cm or so from the anal verge) could only be removed by laparotomy. As this is a major undertaking not without risk and as a single polyp is in many ways a trivial lesion (except for the risk of malignancy), it was customary to recommend excision only for lesions in excess of 1 cm in diameter. Below this size, the risk of invasive cancer being present is less than 1% and it was thought preferable to keep such patients under review.

Now the situation has been greatly altered by the availability of fiberoptic endoscopy. Nearly all polyps can be reached and snared by a skilled colonoscopist.

3. Subsequent treatment

Following total excision of a polyp careful pathological examination is necessary and further treatment will be indicated under the following conditions:

a. *Invasive carcinoma of high malignancy.* Radical excisional surgery is then necessary.

b. *Invasive carcinoma of average or low grade malignancy.* Pedunculated polyps without total involvement of the stalk are kept under observation.

Pedunculated polyps with total involvement of the stalk, or sessile polyps, are treated by radical excisional surgery unless the patient's poor general health is a greater hazard than the risk of recurrent carcinoma.

MULTIPLE POLYPS

Familial polyposis

This condition is associated with a 100% chance of the development of large bowel cancer, and theoretically the only logical treatment is total procto-colectomy with a permanent ileostomy. However, 20 years of experience at St Mark's Hospital, London, indicates that the operation of choice is a colectomy with an ileo-rectal anastomosis. In only two of 72 patients in the St Mark's series had carcinoma developed in the retained rectal stump.

A policy of careful and regular follow-up, with removal or destruction of any rectal stump polyps, is performed. It is of interest to note that in some cases there is a tendency for the rectal polyps to regress, or spontaneously disappear, after colectomy.

Hamartomatous polyps

Juvenile polyps and the Peutz-Jeghers syndrome are non-malignant conditions but treatment is often difficult because polyps continue to develop throughout the gastrointestinal tract in adult life.

LARGE BOWEL CANCER

The large bowel is a common site for carcinoma and in the majority of cases the tumour affects the left side and rectum. The reported incidence of multiple primary carcinomas, either simultaneous or at different times, varies in different series. It has been placed as high as 10%.

PREDISPOSING FACTORS

There are three known predisposing factors:

1. Benign tumours

Neoplastic polyps (tubular, tubulo-villous or villous adenoma), whether sessile or pedunculated, are generally accepted as being pre-cancerous lesions. There seems little doubt that patients with several polyps in the bowel have an increased risk of developing carcinoma and polyps are not infrequently found adjacent to a cancer.

2. Familial polyposis

This is an hereditary disease which is transmitted as a Mendelian dominant and affects the sexes equally. Multiple adenomatous polyps are not present at birth but form at about puberty. Though the polyps may extend throughout the large bowel, there are always polyps visible on sigmoidoscopy. If the condition remains untreated, there is a 100% risk of large bowel cancer developing between 20 and 40 years of age. Colonic polyposis may be associated with skin tumours—so-called Gardner's syndrome.

3. Ulcerative colitis

Carcinoma develops more frequently in a colon affected by ulcerative colitis than in a normal colon and the chances of this development depend on the following factors:

a. *Extent of the colitis.* Patients with total or near total involvement of the colon are more susceptible than those with partial involvement.
b. *Duration of the colitis.* It is unusual for carcinoma to develop in patients with colitis of less than 10 years duration. The greatest risk of carcinoma developing is in those who have total colitis of long duration. Patients with total involvement of 20 years duration have an annual cancer risk of over 5%.

Carcinoma arising in ulcerative colitis tends to be multifocal, infiltrating, less differentiated and mucus-secreting. It arises mostly from flat mucosa and not from any benign polypoidal lesion which may accompany the colitic process.

In addition to the above it is postulated that there is a carcinogenic potential in some diets. The evidence is

a. The rarity of large bowel cancer in developing countries where high bulk diets are common.
b. The presence of potential carcinogens in bile which can be held in contact with the colonic mucosa or rendered active by bacteria when colonic transit is slow.
c. Possible increase in caecal cancer after cholecystectomy.

Finally, relative selenium deficiency in the diet is thought to be a cofactor.

ASSOCIATED CONDITIONS

Skin changes may occur in association with internal malignant tumours and dermatomyositis and pemphigoid rashes may appear months before the first obvious signs of colonic carcinoma.

SURGICAL PATHOLOGY

Carcinoma of the large bowel has its maximal incidence in the sixth decade and the ratio of females to males is 3:2. About 50% of tumours occur in the sigmoid colon.

Macroscopic features

1. Ulcerative
2. Protuberant
3. Annular or stenosing
4. Polypoidal

Microscopic features

All are adenocarcinomata of the columnar-cell type but features vary according to the degree of cell differentiation and stromal constituents. Mucoid degeneration is not uncommon.

Spread

Direct. Submucous spread is unusual in large bowel cancer which usually invades by direct spread through the layers of the bowel and later erupts on to the surface with infiltration of adjacent structures or dissemination through the peritoneal cavity. 2–3 cm of distal spread may occur in rectal tumours. Those tumours that are below the peritoneal reflexion spread into the perirectal tissue and ultimately the pelvic wall.

Lymphatic. Lymphatic spread occurs along lymph channels which accompany the blood vessels. In 10% of patients where lymph nodes are involved, the primary tumour is confined to the muscle of the bowel wall. In the remaining 90% the tumour has breached the confines of the muscle.

Once lymph node involvement is apparent the prognosis is considerably worsened.

Blood. Invasion of small blood vessels may be quite early and has the same prognostic significance as lymph node involvement. Blood-borne metastases are common in advanced cases when the liver becomes the most frequent site involved as the result of invasion of the portal venous system by tumour cells.

Dukes's classification is a convenient method of describing large bowel cancers.

Dukes's classification
Stage A: Confined to the rectal wall
Stage B: Penetrating the rectal wall
Stage C: Lymph node involvement
       C1—pericolic lymph nodes involved
       C2—mesenteric lymph nodes involved
'Stage D': Distant metastases

Complications

Obstruction. This accounts for 25% of all types of presentation to hospital and occurs with annular or stenosing tumours. Obstruction usually develops insidiously and complete obstruction may be precipitated by impaction of faeces above the tumour. Obstruction is least likely where the bowel is widest—caecum and rectum.

Perforation (5–10% of patients). This may occur at three sites:

1. The malignancy itself
2. A stercoral ulcer just above the malignancy
3. The caecum in the presence of large bowel obstruction

Fistula formation. Rare, and may be either:

1. Internal—when proliferation of the tumour involves the bladder (vesico-colic fistula), the vagina (recto-vaginal fistula) or small bowel (ileo-colic fistula)
2. External—when spontaneous discharge or formal drainage of a pericolic abscess leads to discharge of faecal material on to the skin

Haemorrhage. Severe haemorrhage from a large bowel carcinoma is uncommon. Occult bleeding always occurs. In distal lesions blood may be visible in the stool.

MODES OF PRESENTATION

One third of patients with large bowel cancer present within 3 months of onset of symptoms, one third between 6 and 9 months and one third have had symptoms for over 12 months. Though symptoms vary considerably, they can be collected into two groups:

Carcinoma of the right half of the colon

Abdominal pain or discomfort is the commonest symptom. It may be described as a colicky pain, flatulence,

or a vague dyspepsia but the outstanding feature is that it is commonly related to food and it may be central abdominal or in the right iliac fossa.

Weight loss and anaemia. Weight loss occurs in about half of the patients while lassitude, weakness, anorexia and nausea associated with anaemia and blood loss from the malignancy, may be outstanding features. Unexplained anaemia in a middle-aged individual, particularly a male, should always arouse suspicion.

Acute bowel obstruction. Most often it is only in the later stages of the disease that the features of an acute bowel obstruction occur. When the tumour is close to the ileocaecal valve the features of a low small bowel obstruction will become evident, with severe colicky central abdominal pain, vomiting and central abdominal distension. When the tumour is situated more distally in the right colon (hepatic flexure) distension is late and confined to the right iliac fossa. Caecal distension may be gross, particularly if the ileo-caecal valve remains competent. In these cases vomiting is usually delayed. When the caecum distends its blood supply becomes imperilled and gangrene may develop. Tenderness in the right iliac fossa in the presence of large bowel obstruction is an ominous sign.

Mass in the right iliac fossa. In the presence of a right sided tumour the mass may be due to a distended caecum, a palpable tumour or a peri-colic or peri-caecal abscess following a localized perforation.

A mass in the right iliac fossa must be differentiated from other conditions such as an appendiceal mass or abscess and from caecal distension resulting from obstruction in the left half of the colon.

Miscellaneous modes of presentation. These include the following:

1. Generalized peritonitis following perforation of the caecum, tumour or stercoral ulcer
2. Faecal fistula or peri-caecal abscess after an appendicectomy in which caecal carcinoma has escaped detection
3. Ascites
4. Metastatic disease

Carcinoma of the left half of the colon and rectum

Alteration of bowel habit. This occurs in about two thirds of patients and symptoms include:

1. Alteration in stools which may become watery, small in volume, stained or admixed with flecks or clots of dark blood
2. Increasing constipation

3. Spurious or false diarrhoea, caused by faecal impaction above the tumour, with blood and mucus
4. Diarrhoea alternating with constipation

Large bowel obstruction. Colicky lower abdominal pains, abdominal distension and absolute constipation may occur over a few days with complete obstruction. When obstruction is incomplete there may be repeated attacks of lower abdominal colicky pain with distension.

Miscellaneous modes of presentation. These include the following:

1. Generalized peritonitis due to perforation of the caecum, of the tumour itself or of a stercoral ulcer above the tumour
2. A mass in the left iliac fossa due to peri-colic abscess formation in association with a localized perforation of the colon at or near the tumour site
3. Vesico-colic fistula with frequency and 'burning' or 'scalding' with micturition, haematuria, pneumaturia or faecaluria
4. Severe haemorrhage due to ulceration of the bowel wall by the tumour
5. Distant metastases, e.g. liver and lung

SIGNS

1. Right-sided carcinoma

a. *Tenderness in the right iliac fossa* due to the presence of the malignancy, a peri-colic abscess or a distended caecum
b. *A palpable mass in the right iliac fossa*—which is deeply situated, hard and irregular. It may be fixed by tumour growth or peri-caecal inflammation. Alternatively, a distended caecum may be palpable in the presence of obstruction more distally in the colon.
c. *Abdominal distension* which may be centrally or peripherally situated depending on whether obstruction is predominantly of the small or large bowel. Occasionally, peristaltic waves are visible.
d. *Pallor and weight loss*

2. Left-sided carcinoma

a. *A palpable tumour* in the left iliac fossa is unusual.
b. *A palpable distended caecum* in the right iliac fossa may be apparent in the presence of an acute obstruction to the left side of the colon.
c. *Abdominal distension* and occasionally visible peristaltic waves will be seen in the presence of an acute large bowel obstruction.
d. *Rectal examination* must always be performed as part of the examination of all patients complaining

of rectal haemorrhage or an alteration in bowel habit. A rectal carcinoma can be felt as a mass or an ulcer with a hard raised edge. Occasionally, when the tumour itself is beyond finger reach, a hard and irregular mass can be palpated through the wall of the rectum.
e. *Proctoscopy and sigmoidoscopy* are also essential parts of the examination of such patients. They may reveal blood stained motions, blood descending from a higher level, mucus, or a protuberant, ulcerating or stenosing malignancy. Any lesion seen through the sigmoidoscope requires immediate biopsy. Flexible sigmoidoscopy extends the range to 50 cm.

SPECIAL TESTS

Barium enema. A constant filling defect or a complete obstruction may be outlined by a barium enema. Occasionally, this examination is normal despite the presence of a tumour. This is most likely to occur with caecal or flexural tumours. Clinical features are strongly suggestive of colonic cancer and reasonable doubt still exists in the presence of inconclusive or negative investigations, colonoscopy is indicated.

In the presence of an acute large bowel obstruction an emergency barium enema, using a thin mixture of barium, will demonstrate the level of obstruction when this has not been established on sigmoidoscopy.

Barium meal and follow-through. This may be helpful in outlining lesions close to the ileo-caecal region. However, the procedure may precipitate an obstruction if marked narrowing of the colon is already present.

Plain X-ray of the abdomen. In the presence of obstruction, fluid filled and distended coils of small bowel may be visualized if the obstruction is proximally placed and associated with incompetence of the ileo-caecal valve. Gas-filled and distended large bowel shadows are outstanding features with an obstructing lesion in the lower part of the left colon.

Full blood examination. This is an essential requirement to assess the type and extent of anaemia when pallor, weight loss or blood loss are outstanding features.

Occult blood in stools. False positives are frequent but nevertheless this is a useful test to raise the index of suspicion that an ulcerative lesion exists.

SPECIAL INVESTIGATIONS

Imaging. Though it will not necessarily influence the treatment of the primary tumour, it is of value in overall management for the surgeon to be aware of liver metastases. Ultrasound, Scintiscan and CT scan can all be used, though the last is the most sensitive.

CEA. Carcino-embryonic antigen was first found in the blood in relation to large bowel cancer. It is however not specific so cannot be used for diagnosis. A raised level will usually return to normal after removal of the tumour, so that a subsequent rise means recurrence. Thus baseline and post-excisional values are useful in follow-up.

IVU. It used to be said that an intravenous urogram should be routinely done, particularly in rectal cancer. This is not now generally thought to be the case.

DIFFERENTIAL DIAGNOSIS

Right-sided carcinoma

When only vague abdominal pains or discomfort are present
Particular consideration may have to be given to:

1. Peptic ulceration
2. Cholelithiasis
3. Gastric carcinoma

When weight loss and anaemia are present
Any abdominal malignancy must always be considered. When dyspepsia is associated, gastric carcinoma must be excluded.

When a mass in the right iliac fossa is present
Consideration must be given to:

1. Appendiceal abscess
2. Empyema or mucocele of the gall bladder
3. Renal mass
4. Distended caecum due to obstruction of the left colon
5. Ovarian cyst
6. Miscellaneous causes: fibroid uterus, psoas abscess, Crohn's disease, ileo-caecal tuberculosis

Left-sided carcinoma

When alteration of bowel habit or rectal haemorrhage is present
All patients who present with a recent change of bowel habit or rectal bleeding must have a complete ano-rectal examination to exclude carcinoma.

Other causes of such symptoms include:

1. Benign lesions at the anorectal verge
2. Diverticular disease
3. Inflammatory bowel disease
4. Non-specific colonic symptoms—so-called 'irritable bowel syndrome'

When acute large bowel obstruction is present
Carcinoma is a common cause of acute large bowel obstruction. However, other causes may have to be considered and these include the following:

1. Sigmoid volvulus
2. Stricture of the colon due to diverticulitis, Crohn's disease or ischaemic colitis
3. Impacted faeces
4. Pseudo obstruction (see p. 188)

When other modes of presentation occur

Mass in the left iliac fossa. Diverticulitis of the colon with a peri-colic abscess may be difficult or impossible to distinguish from an abscess caused by carcinoma and it may not be until the affected bowel has been excised and subjected to microscopic examination that the diagnosis becomes certain. On occasions, sigmoidoscopic discovery of the tumour or the presence of blood, either in the rectum or admixed with faeces, together with X-ray demonstration of an irregular filling defect, will indicate the cause as being carcinoma. Amoeboma (p. 198) is another diagnostic pitfall.

Vesico-colic fistula. This is almost always due to carciroma or diverticulitis.

TREATMENT OF CARCINOMA OF THE COLON AND RECTUM

Principles

1. If the tumour is mobile and there is no evidence of secondary spread, an *en bloc* radical resection of the tumour and its vascular supply should be carried out. For tumours of the colon and rectum, gastrointestinal continuity is re-established with an end-to-end anastomosis. For low rectal lesions an abdomino-perineal excision with permanent left iliac fossa colostomy is required. The advent of circular intra-luminal staplers has extended the limits of end-to-end anastomosis for these low rectal tumours.

2. If the tumour is removable but the patient is judged incurable because of the presence of liver or peritoneal metastases, the surgeon is faced with a difficult problem. The points which need to be considered in coming to a decision about the best treatment for an individual patient are as follows:

a. What symptoms require treatment? If there are no serious symptoms perhaps nothing further should be contemplated; but a limited resection (palliative resection) of the primary lesion is usually preferable. Rectal lesions may sometimes be fulgurated with success and radiotherapy is also used in some centres.

If the patient is obstructed an internal bypass procedure should be considered; a de-functioning stoma is poor palliative treatment for a dying patient.

If the patient has a perforation of the bowel, the segment should be excised or at least exteriorized and then vigorous peritoneal toilet carried out.

b. What is the likely survival of the patient? General consideration of the principal systems (heart, lungs, kidneys) and extent of metastatic disease (occasionally hepatic lobectomy for apparently localized and painful metastases can be considered).

3. If the patient is incurable because of widespread secondary deposits, nothing more than sympathetic nursing and the liberal use of analgesics is required.

Management of obstruction

1. Rapid resuscitation of the patient
2. At laparotomy, if the tumour is potentially curable, it should be excised by a radical *en bloc* resection. For obstructing lesions of the right colon a right hemicolectomy with ileo-colonic anastomosis is the treatment of choice. Lesions of the transverse colon, splenic flexure and even left colon, can be treated similarly by an extended right hemicolectomy. For obstructing lesions of the recto-sigmoid area, the resection should probably be followed by an end colostomy and mucus fistula (or oversew of the distal rectum), rather than fashioning an anastomosis. Reconstruction is done later.

Two important conditions must be met before this policy for the treatment of obstruction can be adopted:

a. An experienced surgeon (and anaesthetist) must be available
b. The patient must be reasonably fit

If these conditions are not met, a simple de-functioning stoma (colostomy or caecostomy) should be fashioned and the patient prepared for tumour resection under better conditions.

Chemotherapy in large bowel cancer

The intravenous or oral administration of the chemotherapeutic agent 5-fluorouracil has been shown to be effective against tumour tissue of colonic origin, but in clinical trials the increased survival for the patients in the treated group is little better than for the placebo group. Furthermore, the side effects of therapy and the time spent at hospital for treatment, make a decision about the management of individual patients who have widespread metastatic large bowel cancer extremely difficult.

Operative

PRE-OPERATIVE PREPARATION
Apart from the usual attention to hydration, anaemia and inter-current cardiorespiratory disorders which may be present in elderly patients, the chief special preparation is to make sure the bowel is empty. In unobstructed cases this is achieved either by

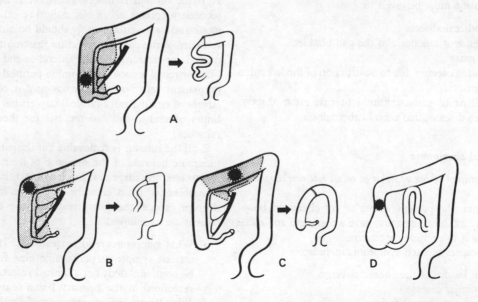

Fig. 29.1 Operations for carcinoma of the right colon **A**. Right hemicolectomy and ileo-transverse anastomosis for carcinoma of the ascending colon **B**. Extended right hemicolectomy for carcinoma of the hepatic flexure **C**. Transverse colectomy and colo-colonic anastomosis for carcinoma of the transverse colon **D**. Palliative ileo-transverse colostomy bypass for obstruction.

a. repeated lavage from below, or

b. whole gut irrigation using large volumes of Hartmann's solution via a nasogastric tube

Antibiotics to 'sterilise the bowel' are no longer widely used, but preventative chemotherapy is given over the operative period (12–24 hours).

When there is obstruction operation becomes more urgent. The bowel cannot be prepared preoperatively but in some instances may be emptied by lavage on the table, so permitting a primary anastomosis. Otherwise the patient is managed as for intestinal obstruction.

The available operations for colon cancer are illustrated in Figs. 29.1 and 29.2. The choice is determined by the position of the growth, whether the resection is curative or palliative, and whether or not obstruction is present.

For cancer of the rectum it used to be felt that an abdomino-perineal excision with permanent colostomy was required for any growth closer to the anus than 7–8 cm in order to remove the lymph nodes in the perirectal area and any distant extension. However the fear of local recurrence seems to have been exaggerated and it is currently customary to carry out an excision of the growth and the proximal lymph node field, provided a cuff of rectum sufficient to make an anastomosis can be obtained. Thus growths down to 3–4 cm from the dentate line can be managed without a colostomy. Continuity is restored either by an anastomosis made from above or endo-anally.

The extensive perineal dissection required for either restorative resection or abdomino-perineal excision interferes with the sacral parasympathetic outflow and may cause

a. urinary retention (worse if in the male there is prostatism)

b. male impotence

Is the same as for any other major operation. A water-soluble contrast enema about the tenth day will identify any anastomotic leakage and will help maintain the highest technical standards which are necessary if the morbidity of this type of surgery is to be reduced.

RESULT OF TREATMENT OF LARGE BOWEL CANCER

This will depend on the site, extent and grade of malignancy but in general it can be said that for Dukes A cases there is a 90% 5-year survival, for Dukes B cases there is a 60% 5-year survival and for Dukes C cases there is a 30% 5-year survival. However, the overall prognosis of patients with rectal cancer is that only 25% survive 5 years.

CARCINOMA OF ANAL CANAL AND ANAL MARGIN

These are rare sites for tumours and account for no more than 3% of ano-rectal tumours. Females are more often affected with anal canal tumours (4:3) and males are more often affected with carcinoma of the anal margin (4:1). There is an association with homosexuality in the male.

Macroscopic and microscopic features

The anal canal extends from the anal verge to the ano-rectal ring and anal canal carcinomata arise most often in the unstable transitional zone of mucosa, which is a narrow area immediately above the anal valves. Here the mucosa is a compromise between large bowel glandular mucosa and squamous mucosa or modified skin below (Fig. 29.3). The zone contains different varieties of

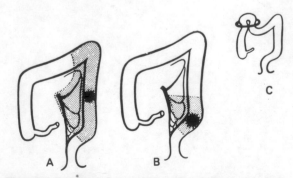

Fig. 29.2 Operations for carcinoma of the left colon A. Left hemicolectomy for carcinoma of the descending or sigmoid colon B. Palliative segmental sigmoid resection C. Loop transverse colostomy for obstruction

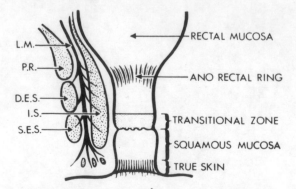

Fig. 29.3 Anal canal L.M. = logitudinal muscle; P.R. = puborectalis; D.E.S. = deep part of external sphincter; I.S. = internal sphincter; S.E.S. = subcutaneous external sphincter

epithelium (transitional, stratified columnar, squamous or combinations).

Anal canal carcinomata are predominantly of the squamous cell type and may be differentiated and keratinizing, or undifferentiated and non-keratinizing.

Anal margin carcinomata are mainly differentiated keratinizing squamous cell tumours but are less common than anal canal tumours.

Spread

DIRECT

Anal canal carcinoma extend mainly upwards by permeation along the submucous plane to the lower third of the rectum. Downward spread appears to be prevented by the anal musculature and the mucosal suspensory ligaments. Spread beyond the wall of the anal canal can lead to involvement of the vagina.

Anal margin carcinoma spread upwards into the anal canal or circumferentially around the anal verge and the peri-anal tissues.

LYMPHATIC

Anal canal carcinoma. Spread to the inguinal lymph nodes follows in about one-third of cases and spread to the superior haemorrhoidal lymph nodes results in about the same proportion. Lateral lymphatic spread along the middle haemorrhoidal vessels may also occur.

Anal margin carcinoma. Spread to the superior haemorrhoidal lymph nodes is exceedingly uncommon but inguinal lymph node involvement occurs in about one-third of cases seen.

BLOOD

Blood spread from either site is most uncommon.

Treatment

The conventional treatment is surgical removal, which nearly always means an abdomino-perineal excision of the rectum. Rarely, in an elderly patient, a local excision may suffice. Because the tumours are squamous in type they are radio-sensitive and thus can be managed by irradiation. This treatment is increasingly used with success but a temporary colostomy is needed while treatment is in progress.

INGUINAL LYMPH NODES

Most surgeons agree that these should not be removed unless they become clinically involved; an ilio-inguinal dissection would then be indicated.

Results

Adequate treatment produces about a 40% 5-year survival rate for carcinoma of the anal canal and about a 50% 5-year survival rate for carcinoma of the anal margin.

30

Perianal conditions

Surgical conditions which affect the perianal region are common, most often present with pain, pruritis or bleeding and are usually due to benign lesions that are easily recognizable.

CLASSIFICATION

1. Anal fissure
2. Haemorrhoids
3. Perianal haematoma
4. Ano-rectal suppuration
5. Pruritis ani
6. Anal papilloma (warts)
7. Proctalgia fugax
8. Pilonidal sinus
9. Anal carcinoma (see Chapter 29)

SURGICAL PATHOLOGY

Anal fissure (fissure-in-ano)

A triangular tear or ulcer at the anal verge which extends into the anal canal and almost always follows the passage of constipated stools.

Most anal fissures occur in the midline posteriorly (90% in males, 60% in females), probably because of the angulation of the anal canal and the relatively unprotected segment of the internal sphincter at this site.

There are two types of fissure:

1. Acute and superficial. In the early stages the tear is superficially situated and its floor contains the longitudinal muscle fibres of the muscularis mucosae. Spasm of the anal sphincter is an outstanding feature and is responsible for marked local pain and tenderness.

2. Chronic and deep. In the later stages the longitudinal muscle fibres in the base of the ulcer become ulcerated and the underlying transverse fibres of the lower part of the internal sphincter are exposed. The ulcer then becomes undermined and indurated and oedema and

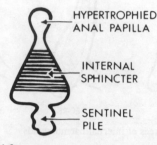

Fig. 30.1 Anal fissure

inflammation of the mucosa at the apex results in a pseudo-polyp or hypertrophied anal papilla. At the opposite end, the skin of the anal verge may hypertrophy to form a skin tag or sentinel pile (Fig. 30.1).

Haemorrhoids (syn. piles)

These form from the prolapse of the cuboidal or columnar mucosa of the anal canal above the anal groove. The mucosal prolapse is associated with congestion of the superior haemorrhoidal venous plexus and some regard piles as being in fact varicosities of this plexus.

The cause of internal haemorrhoids is not exactly known. However, there is increasing evidence that piles are but an exaggeration of the normal anal cushions which, together with the sphincters, maintain continence. When there is much straining at stool, which can occur with constipation or when sphincter tone is high (as often seems to be the case in haemorrhoids) these cushions become engorged and may descend through the sphincters.

Whatever the cause, repeated episodes of prolapse with venous congestion leads to the appearance of primary haemorrhoids at three sites which correspond to the distribution of the superior haemorrhoidal venous plexus (Fig. 30.2). These positions are the left lateral, right anterior, and right posterior. Between these positions secondary haemorrhoids may develop.

There are three degrees of internal haemorrhoid (Fig. 30.3).

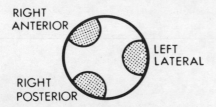

Fig. 30.2 Position of primary haemorrhoids

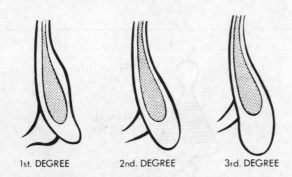

1st. DEGREE   2nd. DEGREE   3rd. DEGREE

Fig. 30.3 Degrees of internal haemorrhoids

1. First degree. Haemorrhoids which bleed but do not prolapse.

2. Second degree. Haemorrhoids which prolapse with defaecation and then reduce spontaneously or can be reduced digitally.

Occasionally the anal sphincter may prevent the return of prolapsing piles and cause oedema and later haemorrhoidal vein thrombosis. Still later the arterial circulation may be jeopardized so that strangulation, sloughing and infection will supervene.

3. Third degree. Haemorrhoids which are persistently prolapsed. The exposed mucosa of the anal canal chronically discharges mucus, which results in peri-anal irritation.

Peri-anal haematoma ('thrombosed' external pile)

An external haemorrhoid, covered by true skin into which there has been an acute submucosal rupture of a tributary of the inferior haemorrhoidal venous plexus.

Spontaneous resolution may occur with resorption of the blood clot leaving a redundant piece of peri-anal skin; alternatively rupture of the skin may occur and be associated with the loss of a small amount of blood, and the formation of an ulcer which slowly heals.

Ano-rectal suppuration

Infection of the peri-anal and peri-rectal spaces with staphylococcal, streptococcal, *E. Coli*, and *Proteus* organisms, may occur.

SOURCE OF INFECTION

Local
1. An anal fissure
2. A peri-anal haematoma
3. A haemorrhoid injection site
4. A hair follicle, sebaceous or apocrine gland
5. Anal glands, situated at the dentate line and ramifying in the wall of the anal canal between the internal and external sphincters—probably the commonest route

Proximal
1. Ulcerative colitis
2. Crohn's disease
3. Carcinoma
4. Actinomycosis
5. Diverticular disease

Proximally situated causes must always be considered if abscesses recur or become chronic.

SITES OF ABSCESS FORMATION

Whatever the source of infection may be, abscess formation can occur at the following sites (Fig. 30.4):

1. Peri-anal abscess. This is commonest, and pus collects just beneath the peri-anal skin close to the anal margin. It usually follows infection of a hair follicle, sebaceous or apocrine gland, or an anal gland.

2. Ischio-rectal abscess. Infection deep within the fat of the ischio-rectal fossa, from the anal glands, a fissure, or spread from a peri-anal abscess, may result in an abscess between the anus, anal canal and sphincters medially and the pelvic wall and obturator internus muscle laterally. Pus may track posteriorly behind the deep

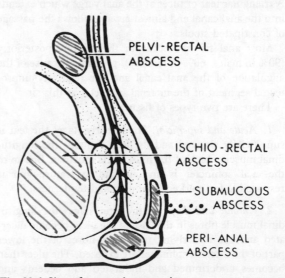

PELVI-RECTAL ABSCESS

ISCHIO-RECTAL ABSCESS

SUBMUCOUS ABSCESS

PERI-ANAL ABSCESS

Fig. 30.4 Sites of anorectal suppuration

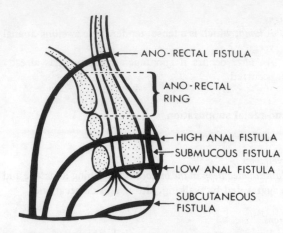

ANO-RECTAL FISTULA

ANO-RECTAL RING

HIGH ANAL FISTULA
SUBMUCOUS FISTULA
LOW ANAL FISTULA

SUBCUTANEOUS FISTULA

Fig. 30.5 Anal fistulae

portion of the external sphincter to involve the opposite ischio-rectal fossa by a horse-shoe shaped track.

3. *Submucous abscess*. Infection of the submucosa of the anal canal may occur from the anal glands, a fissure, or follow the injection of haemorrhoids.

4. *Pelvi-rectal abscess*. This is a rare type of abscess which is situated above the levator ani but deep to the pelvic peritoneum. It most often follows pelvic cellulitis but it may sometimes arise as a complication of ulcerative colitis, Crohn's disease, diverticular disease or rectal carcinoma.

SEQUELAE TO ABSCESS FORMATION

When untreated, an abscess may point and discharge spontaneously into the anal canal, rectum, or peri-anal skin with the development of a complete or incomplete fistula.

The fistulae may be subcutaneous, submucous, low anal, high anal, or ano-rectal (Fig. 30.5).

Pruritus ani

Constant irritation with discomfort or pain in the peri-anal region causes the patient to scratch incessantly. This results in excoriation and infection of the skin with the production of cracks and skin thickening.

The causes for the irritation may be:

1. *Ano-rectal disorders*: prolapsing haemorrhoids, fissure, fistula, carcinoma, proctitis, colitis, threadworms, imperfect cleanliness
2. *Peri-anal skin disorders*: scabies, monilia and other fungal infection; excessive sweating
3. *General disorders*: diabetes, jaundice, drugs, anxiety neurosis
4. *Idiopathic*: most often no cause can be found

Anal papilloma (anal warts, condylomata accuminata)

Anal warts are often multiple, surrounding the anal verge and involving the anal skin up to the dentate line. Individual warts may be sessile or pedunculated and in each patient there is usually a mixture of the two types. A viral aetiology is likely and their high incidence in young male homosexuals infers a venereal route of spread. Cases of malignant change have been reported.

Proctalgia fugax (nocturnal proctalgia)

There is no known pathological basis for this condition but it is included here for completeness.

The term is applied to a recurring paroxysm of intense rectal pain of a stabbing or constricting type, usually occurring in the night. Supposedly it is commonest in highly strung and anxious male adults and often the attacks immediately follow an anxious, frustrating or erotic dream.

Pilonidal sinus

This occurs in the upper natal cleft as a discharging sinus running upwards with lateral, secondarily-infected tracks. Hairy individuals are often affected and 60% of sinuses contain hairs. Pilonoidal sinuses may also occur in the web spaces between the fingers and toes, especially in hairdressers. The lesion is probably acquired and infection with subsequent abscess formation is the commonest complication.

CLINICAL FEATURES

Most often the cause of a perianal condition is easily determined by inspection and gentle palpation of the perineum and anal verge, whereas proctoscopy and sigmoidoscopy may be too painful. However if operation under general anaesthesia is intended then the opportunity is taken to complete the ano-rectal examination particularly if bleeding is the major symptom.

Anal fissure

Symptoms
1. *Pain* is sharp and severe and experienced during and especially after defaecation
2. *Bleeding* is slight and seen as bright blood on the paper
3. *Constipation* is a common accompaniment

Signs
1. *Acute and superficial crack*, which is visible at the anal verge and usually midline posteriorly

2. *Anal sphincter spasm*, usually makes a rectal examination impossible
3. *Chronic and deep ulcer*, which is visible as a triangular ulcer and sometimes associated with a sentinel pile; in the base of the ulcer the circular fibres of the lowest portion of the internal sphincter are visible

Haemorrhoids

Symptoms
1. *Bleeding* which characteristically occurs on defaecation and is usually bright red
2. *Prolapse*—either on straining or all the time
3. *Mucous discharge* when rectal mucosa is exposed.
    Pain, itch, rectal discomfort are often thought by patients (and doctors) to be attributable to piles. Such symptoms and piles may co-exist but there is always another cause.

Signs
The anal verge is normal in 1st degree piles. In second degree there may be hypertrophy of the anal skin verge and, sometimes, a skin 'tag'. Third degree piles are visible as muco-cutaneous bulges.

    1. Digital examination: In first degree piles all that is felt is an increased sphincter tone. Second and third degree piles are usually thickened ano thus distinguishable from the surrounding mucosa.

    2. Proctoscopy. The piles bulge into the instrument at the sites mentioned above. Bleeding and superficial ulceration may be seen. The rectal mucosa is normal.

Diagnosis
To attribute bleeding to piles is dangerous unless the appropriate measures have been taken to exclude other causes, particularly polyps and malignant disease of the left colon and rectum. A careful history—particularly of bowel habit—is helpful but all patients with piles should have at least a rigid sigmoidoscopy and preferably a flexible sigmoidoscopic examination of the left colon. If there is continuing doubt, colonoscopy and barium enema are indicated.

Peri-anal haematoma

Symptoms
1. *Pain* is of acute onset and often experienced after straining at defaecation
2. *A lump*, which appears at the anal verge
3. *Haemorrhage* is in the form of a small amount of clotted blood when spontaneous rupture occurs and which is followed by dramatic relief of pain

Signs
1. *A lump*, which is a tense, tender, blue swelling at anal verge
2. *An ulcer* occurs if spontaneous rupture has already occurred

Ano-rectal suppuration

1. PERI-ANAL ABSCESS

Symptoms
Pain situated deep in the buttock is throbbing in nature and is aggravated by walking, sitting and defaecation.

Signs
1. *Pyrexia and toxaemia* are usually absent
2. *A lump*, which is red, hot and tender to touch and appearing superficial; overlying cellulitis is common
3. *Digital examination*. A tender lump is felt outside the wall of the anal canal and just beneath the peri-anal skin

2. ISCHIO-RECTAL ABSCESS

Symptoms
Pain situated deep in the buttock is throbbing in nature and is aggravated by walking, sitting and defaecation.

Signs
1. *Pyrexia and toxaemia* may be present
2. *Absence of superficial signs of inflammation*
3. *Digital examination*. There is a tender lump outside the wall of the anal canal but extending above the ano-rectal ring; occasionally it may be bilateral when the posterior communication between the two fossae may be felt as a tender swelling.

3. SUBMUCOUS ABSCESS

Symptoms
Pain, which is usually mild but aggravated by walking, sitting and defaecation.

Signs
1. *Pyrexia and toxaemia* may be present
2. *Absence of external signs of inflammation*
3. *Digital examination*. Extreme tenderness is found over a superficial lump which is usually situated in the mild line posteriorly.

Pilonidal sinus

Pain in the posterior anus with a discharge or, when infected, a hot tender lump felt laterally, are the usual clinical findings, and needs to be differentiated from a perianal abscess.

TREATMENT

Anal fissure

1. ACUTE AND SUPERFICIAL FISSURE
Treatment is conservative, particularly if the patient is of the co-operative type when measures taken include the following:

1. Sedation or tranquillization when required
2. Regulation of bowel habit
3. Local analgesic ointments or suppositories
4. Digital dilatation under local anaesthetic

2. CHRONIC AND DEEP FISSURE
When the fissure becomes chronic and indurated conservative treatment is unlikely to be of value. Then the following procedures can be performed:

a. *Anal stretch*. This has not become a standard treatment though it has its advocates. It may be associated with a higher incidence of unhealed or recurrent fissures and then the following methods should be used.

b. *Lateral sphincterotomy*. Through a left lateral incision at the anal margin a small flap of mucosa is elevated and the lower portion of the internal sphincter is divided. It is considered by those who use this method that both anal wound and fissure healing occur more rapidly.

c. *Posterior sphincterotomy*. The lower portion of the internal sphincter is divided through the base of the fissure.

d. *Posterior sphincterotomy and fissurectomy*. In addition to the sphincterotomy the fibrotic tissue around the fissure together with any hypertrophied anal papilla and sentinel pile, is excised.

Haemorrhoids

There are three methods of treatment:

1. REASSURANCE AND CORRECTION OF CONSTIPATION
Once a complete ano-rectal examination has been performed and the patient reassured that no malignancy is present, nothing more than regulation of bowel habit may be necessary, particularly if the haemorrhoids are of a minor degree and associated with minimal symptoms. As with diverticular disease, fibre in the form of bran may be helpful.

2. INJECTION

Indications
a. First degree haemorrhoids
b. Second degree haemorrhoids if haemorrhage is the major problem

Aim
This is to create submucous perivenous fibrosis at the base of the pile with a sclerosant solution which will obliterate the superior haemorrhoidal venous plexus. Injections have no effect on prolapse. The injection is made into the base of the pile and may have to be repeated once or twice.

The probability of haemorrhage from the haemorrhoidal area being controlled by injection is very high. Consequently if blood loss is unaffected by this treatment a more sinister cause should always be suspected and a barium enema becomes essential.

3. OPERATIVE

Indications
a. Third degree haemorrhoids
b. Second degree haemorrhoids when prolapse is the major problem, or when injections have failed to control haemorrhage in a patient in whom more serious causes for haemorrhage have been eliminated

Methods
Many techniques of dealing with haemorrhoids have been devised, but those which have gained popularity are as follows:

a. *Anal stretch*. This method is based on the premise that haemorrhoids are due to a high anal sphincter pressure and that stretching the anal canal and lower rectum with four fingers of both hands and keeping it stretched by the frequent use of a special anal dilator will cure the disease. Though the procedure is still on trial it is rapidly achieving a place in the treatment of haemorrhoids. It is certainly a minor procedure which can be done on a short stay or outpatient basis. Its success rate is about 75–80% and thus the number of patients requiring a more radical approach is reduced   Lord's procedure

b. *Excision and low ligation*. This is the most popular method. Each pile and its related peri-anal skin or skin tag is pulled down and a V-shaped cut is made through the peri-anal skin and carried up on each side of the pile so that the pile is freed from the underlying tissues to expose the inner border of the lower end of the internal sphincter. The base of the pile is then transfixed and excised. When the operation is completed the patient is left with three raw areas in the peri-anal skin which take anything from 3–6 weeks to heal. The end results are usually excellent.

c. *Submucous excision*. This is accomplished by raising mucocutaneous flaps on either side of the pile and dissecting the tissue contained within between the mucosa and the internal sphincter. It is designed to preserve mucosa to cover the raw areas so that the post-operative pain is minimized in order that healing will occur more rapidly.

d. *Rubber band ligation*. This relatively simple procedure of ligation the pile base as an outpatient has been shown recently to be as effective as more radical procedures.

Recurrent haemorrhoids

The recurrence rate after surgical treatment is difficult to estimate. Mucosal prolapse between the primary haemorrhoid sites is probably caused by secondary haemorrhoids and not a true recurrence. It does appear however that preservation of the mucosa at operation (sub-mucous excision) may pre-dispose to later recurrence.

Peri-anal haematoma

There are two methods of treatment.

1. Conservative

Most peri-anal haematomata subside spontaneously within a week and during this time analgesics can be prescribed.

2. Operative

In the acute stage when pain is severe and incapacitating immediate relief is gained by evacuation of the blood clot through a small incision made in the peri-anal skin over the haematoma. Then simple daily dressings are required until healing occurs.

Ano-rectal suppuration

There is no place for conservative treatment; early operation is essential to prevent rupture of the abscess and possible anal fistula formation.

Operative treatment entails the following:

1. Incision

Incisions are made radially to the anal canal at the anterior and posterior margins of the abscess. Fat lobules and necrotic debris are removed from the abscess cavity. Pus swabs are taken and sent for culture under aerobic and anaerobic conditions. With large abscesses an extra incision may be required between the other incisions. If an ischio-rectal abscess affects both sides then the procedure is repeated on the other side of the anal canal.

2. Establishment of free drainage

Once the pus and debris have been removed and haemostosis achieved, thin latex tubing (Paul's tubing 1.5 cm in diameter) is passed through adjacent incisions; the ends are overlapped and sutured to each other. This leaves a snug loop of tubing around the skin bridge which can be left in place until all induration and pus discharge has stopped. The loops are then simply cut and removed.

The purpose of this technique is to preserve peri-anal skin which is not diseased.

3. Search for anal fistulae

It is probably wise, especially for the inexperienced surgeon, *not* to look for a fistula at the first operation. If the bacteriological swab grows *Staph. aureus* then a fistula is very unlikely to be present. However, if gut organisms are present then a second examination under anaesthetic should be carried out about one week after the first, the fistulous tract looked for and, if found, laid open. On the rare occasion that a 'high' fistula is identified, the patient should be referred to a surgeon who has a special interest in these problems, because the chance of making the patient incontinent is significantly large.

Pruritus ani

Treatment includes the following measures:

1. Correction of general causative factors (diabetes, jaundice, psychiatric disorders)
2. Correction of local causative factors (fissure, haemorrhoids, rectal prolapse, proctitis) and personal hygiene
3. The use of soothing lotions or ointments containing calamine and zine oxide and phenol, or hydrocortisone

Anal papilloma

1. Conservative

Local application of a 25% podophyllin solution suspended in Tinc. Benz. Co. and painted on to the warts, but not intervening skin, may be effective. Two or more applications are usually necessary and excoriation of the normal perianal skin is a problem. Early results with anti-viral vaccination are encouraging.

2. Operative

Excision of anal warts under general anaesthesia is indicated for residual warts after podophyllin treatment or in extensive lesions. The skin is infiltrated with a weak adrenaline solution, individual warts are excised preserving intervening normal skin and bleeding is controlled by diathermy. Diathermy of large areas of normal skin will cause anal stenosis. A meticulous search for lesions in the anal canal is necessary to avoid recurrence.

Pilonidal sinus

Conservative treatment with antibiotics is of little value whether discharging or with abscess formation. The aims of treatment are to excise all the tracks and prevent recurrence.

The surgical options include:

1. Radical excision with primary suture closure, with or without a Z-plasty or similar refashioning of the natal cleft
2. Wide excision, laying open the wound and allow healing by secondary intention

3. Excision of the skin pits and aggressive local toilet, with brushings of the lateral tracks

For pilonidal abscess simple incision and drainage is preferable, in the first instance, followed by definitive treatment at a later date.

31

Gastro-intestinal haemorrhage

Gastro-intestinal haemorrhage is essentially a management problem needing the right decision at the right time and close co-operation between gastroenterologist and surgeon. Only by defining accurately the source of bleeding, defining the high risk group of patients and acting quickly will a successful outcome be achieved.

Though theoretically an artificial separation, from a management point of view it is useful to divide gastro-intestinal haemorrhage into two groups:

1. Upper gastro-intestinal bleeding
2. Bleeding per rectum

UPPER GASTRO-INTESTINAL BLEEDING

The vomiting of blood, often associated with melaena, may be a serious and alarming event, necessitating rapid judgement and technical skill for successful management. However, haemorrhage may be less severe, so that diagnosis and definitive management can be performed more at leisure.

Haematemesis must be distinguished from haemoptysis. With the latter, the blood is bright red, frothy and alkaline in reaction and it may be associated with symptoms of respiratory disease. Occasionally, the vomiting of port or claret may be confused with upper gastro-intestinal haemorrhage!

Melaena is the inevitable consequence of a significant haemorrhage into the upper gastro-intestinal tract. A varying degree of digestive alteration in the spilt blood makes the bowel content dark. Melaena may follow haematemesis or, particularly in bleeding beyond the pylorus (as, for example, a posterior duodenal ulcer), be the only symptom and sign. It is dangerous to assume that melaena is less serious than haematemesis or that the occurrence of one or the other identifies the source of the bleeding.

CLASSIFICATION OF CAUSES

1. Oesophageal

a. Varices
b. Peptic oesophagitis

c. Carcinoma (rarely)
d. Foreign body

2. Stomach

a. Peptic ulcer
b. Gastric erosions and gastritis
c. Carcinoma
d. Hiatus hernia
e. Mallory-Weiss syndrome (oesophago-gastric tear)
f. Benign tumours (polyps with superficial ulcer)
g. Foreign body, e.g. naso-gastric tube

3. Duodenum

a. Peptic ulcer
b. Diverticulum

4. Miscellaneous

a. Disorders of gastro-intestinal blood vessels, e.g. pseudoxanthoma elasticum, Ehlers–Danlos syndrome
b. Aneurysm of the splenic artery
c. Generalized disorders such as uraemia

The commoner causes of haematemesis are
1. Peptic ulcer—70–90% of instances
2. Mallory–Weiss syndrome
3. Acute gastric erosions or multiple ulcers
4. Portal hypertension—perhaps 5% of cases but this varies from place to place

Less common causes are
1. Carcinoma of the stomach
2. Hiatus hernia and peptic oesophagitis

SURGICAL PATHOLOGY

Chronic peptic ulcer

80% of all bleeding ulcers are duodenal. Haemorrhage may come from hyperaemic mucosa at the margin, from granulation tissue in the base, or from eroded blood vessels which may be either in the wall of the stomach or duodenum, or outside these organs. Haemorrhage in the latter situation is always caused by a large penetrating ulcer and torrential haemorrhage is likely to occur from the left gastric, splenic or gastro-duodenal arteries. The magnitude of the haemorrhage bears no relationship to the presence or absence of atherosclerosis but is dependent upon the degree to which the vessel is held open or encased by fibrous tissue.

Acute lesions

Acute gastric and duodenal lesions, variously labelled acute peptic ulcer, acute gastritis, acute gastric erosions and haemorrhagic duodenitis, are known to occur. Ulcers may follow burns (Curling's ulcer), head injuries and intracranial operations (Cushing's ulcer), administration of steroids, aspirin, indomethacin or phenylbutazone. Acute ulceration has also been noted after myocardial infarction, severe temperature changes, severe infections and physical or emotional stress. The causation of these lesions is discussed in more detail on p. 148.

Portal hypertension

Obstruction of the portal venous system causes the development of a collateral circulation to transport portal blood into the systemic system. A most important and potentially dangerous collateral circulation is that in the submucosa of the oesophagus and stomach, formed by anastomoses of tributaries of the left gastric and short gastric veins with oesophageal veins. These anastomotic channels become varicose in the presence of an elevated portal venous pressure and may rupture, causing severe haemorrhage.

Carcinoma of the stomach

A slow ooze of blood from an ulcerated malignancy is not uncommon. However, more invasive tumours may be associated with erosion of larger gastric or extra gastric vessels, leading to profuse haemorrhage.

Hiatus hernia

Peptic oesophagitis associated with a sliding hiatus hernia can lead to ulceration and haemorrhage of the lower oesophagus.

Mallory–Weiss syndrome

When vomiting occurs there is usually a relatively orderly sequence of events in which paroxysmal contraction of the abdominal wall is associated with diaphragmatic relaxation and reverse peristalsis in the stomach. The oesophagus usually offers no bar to the ejection of stomach contents. Occasionally however, the oesophagus may not relax, either because co-ordination is lost (as in a very drunk individual) or when social pressures lead to inhibition. In such circumstances many of the prodromata of vomiting takes place: there is a dramatic rise in intragastric tension so that a pressure cone is driven up into the lower oesophagus. The consequence is either full thickness rupture into the pleural cavity or a mucosal tear. The latter gives rise to bleeding, which constitutes the Mallory–Weiss syndrome.

CLINICAL FEATURES

Chronic peptic ulceration will be suspected when there is a long history of dyspepsia with pain related to meals. There may be a history of previous haemorrhages, requiring admission to hospital, and a past barium meal may have shown a duodenal or gastric ulcer. Though suggestive, this evidence should not automatically lead to the assumption that the bleeding is from an ulcer.

Alternatively, the patient may be a known cirrhotic and/or alcoholic, when portal hypertension should be suspected. The presence of hepatomegaly, splenomegaly, palmar erythema, spider naevi, gynaecomastia, testicular atrophy, ascites, jaundice and a tremor indicate liver insufficiency. Again, bleeding may be coming from another source.

On other occasions, a history of aspirin ingestion, in the absence of other features, may suggest an acute erosion.

In Mallory–Weiss syndrome, characteristically there has been a drinking bout and either frank vomiting or retching. The latter may have been forgotten. If vomiting occurs it does *not* initially contain blood. After a varying period of minutes or hours there is haematemesis which may be single or multiple. Clinical examination is, as in most circumstances of bleeding, often negative. Stigmata of alcoholic liver disease may divert attention away from an oesophageal tear and suggest varices.

SPECIAL INVESTIGATIONS

The introduction of fiberoptic endoscopes makes it possible to ascertain the source of upper gastro-intestinal bleeding with some ease. Though as yet there is little evidence to suggest that mortality and morbidity is much altered by early and precise anatomical diagnosis, it is rational to find a cause as soon as possible. In the individual patient this may be of great importance. Thus, where facilities are available, endoscopy should be carried out:

1. At once when bleeding continues. It may be necessary to wash the stomach out vigorously to see a lesion.
2. As early as is convenient if the bleeding has stopped

Fiberoptic oesophago-gastro-duodenoscopy establishes the diagnosis in upwards of 90% of instances. Barium meal is less reliable (60%) and has the slight disadvantage that it may demonstrate a lesion (such as a duodenal ulcer) which is *not* the source of the bleeding. However, it is sufficiently valuable that it should be used urgently if either endoscopy is unavailable or has failed to demonstrate the lesion.

MANAGEMENT

Early consultation between physician and surgeon is the basis upon which proper management of haematemesis should be conducted. The surgeon's role may be to act immediately when life is threatened but more commonly the haemorrhage is less catastrophic and operation is not urgently required. He may later be asked to operate to control repeated haemorrhages or to undertake a curative procedure.

There are three common groups of patients with haematemesis: those with a history indicative of chronic peptic ulceration, those with portal hypertension and those with no ulcer history. The latter usually have an acute erosion, Mallory–Weiss syndrome or a silent chronic peptic ulcer.

All patients with haematemesis should be admitted to hospital. When blood loss is minimal, time may be taken for a detailed history and examination but in the presence of a seriously depleted circulating blood volume, no time should be lost in resuscitating the patient.

The management of haematemesis may be considered under the following headings:

1. Resuscitation
2. Establishment of a diagnosis
3. Specific management to secure haemostasis and treat the cause

Resuscitation

An initial assessment must be made to determine whether blood transfusion is necessary or not. The patient's account of the amount of blood lost is often misleading and the decision to transfuse may need to be made from other considerations.

Thus, if the patient is in shock with pallor, sweating, a lowered blood pressure and an elevated pulse rate, or if he is not, but has a haemoglobin below 10 g/dl and an elevated blood urea concentration, or is showing signs of continuing haemorrhage, transfusion is certainly required. The indications may need to be modified for patients known to be previously hypertensive or anaemic.

If transfusion and treatment of shock is necessary, the following routine is used:

1. Strict rest in bed
2. Establish an intravenous line for volume replacement. It is desirable to have a central line to measure central venous pressure which may provide a more sensitive way of assessing changes in blood volume.
3. Draw blood for grouping and cross matching, for haemoglobin estimation and base line values of electrolyte and urea concentrations.
4. Administer an opiate (morphine, pethidine) in small doses and preferably intravenously.
5. Pass a naso-gastric tube to empty the stomach and to provide early warning of further bleeding. Opinion varies about the advisability of this.
6. Arrange for repeated observations of pulse, blood pressure and respiration and for the recording of any blood lost.
7. Nil by mouth

The further signs of continued or repeated bleeding are:

1. Rising pulse and respiration rate and falling arterial blood pressure and central venous pressure
2. Increased restlessness, sweating and pallor
3. Failure of blood pressure to improve despite transfusion thought adequate
4. Fall of blood pressure during transfusion
5. Fall of blood pressure after an initial response to transfusion
6. Repeated or persistent aspiration of fresh blood from nasogastric tube

Establishment of a diagnosis

Once shock and hypovolaemia have been corrected, time can be taken to elicit a detailed history and make a thorough physical examination.

Management of specific conditions

SURGERY IN BLEEDING PEPTIC ULCER
Operation is indicated:

1. When bleeding is massive and continuous
2. When a patient who has bled has a further haemodynamically significant bleed (i.e. fall in CVP or arterial pressure, rise in pulse rate)
3. When there is a co-existent systemic condition—incipient heart failure, poor respiratory function—which

will make survival less likely if the patient bleeds again
4. Usually when there is pyloric stenosis
5. When at endoscopy there is a visible vessel—bleeding or not—in the ulcer base

Age is closely related to the majority of these.

Endoscopic laser photo-coagulation offers an alternative to surgery in the elderly and patients with co-existent cardio-respiratory disease. Early results with the laser are encouraging.

Choice of operation
Unlike perforation, where a simple operation on the ulcer is all that is necessary, control of bleeding requires reduction in acid secretion.

The alternatives are:

1. For duodenal ulcer
   a. Polya gastrectomy—effective, but a large operation for a patient often not in a good condition
   b. Vagotomy, underunning of the bleeding point and drainage, either by pyloroplasty (using the incision made to get at the ulcer) or gastroenterostomy
   c. Highly selective vagotomy and underunning of the bleeding point
2. For gastric ulcer
   Billroth I gastrectomy—usually technically easy

SURGERY IN ACUTE EROSIVE BLEEDING, STRESS ULCER AND MALLORY–WEISS SYNDROME

1. Erosive bleeding. Obviously surgery should be avoided. However, if cimetidine does not work, a subtotal gastrectomy with Billroth I reconstruction is the best procedure. Very occasionally, the patient bleeds from the gastric remnant and a total gastrectomy has to be done.

2. Stress ulcer. Again, operation should be avoided in these often seriously ill and septic patients. If required, vagotomy, underrun and a drainage operation is the treatment of choice but the mortality is high.

3. Mallory–Weiss syndrome. Only rarely do these patients need surgery. However, procrastination can be fatal. It is a relatively simple matter to underrun the tear after opening the stomach.

BLEEDING OESOPHAGEAL VARICES
On occasions, it may be difficult to be sure that the haemorrhage is in fact from varices, when associated peptic ulceration and alcoholic gastritis may be possible causes.

Mallory–Weiss syndrome is, for obvious reasons, common in alcoholics. Full endoscopy is highly desirable and is quite safe with the flexible instrument.

The emergency management of bleeding oesophageal varices should include the following:

1. Resuscitation
2. Prevention of intraluminal protein breakdown
3. Securing haemostasis

Resuscitation
As haemorrhage from oesophageal varices tends to be repeated, the patient should be admitted to hospital and placed under continuous observation regardless of the size of the initial haemorrhage. Also, as patients with gastro-intestinal haemorrhage may need operation, perhaps urgently, they should be assessed jointly by a physician and surgeon at the earliest possible time.

Blood transfusions are given when shock is present and if possible fresh blood is used to alleviate temporarily deficiencies in clotting factors and platelets which are frequently present in patients with parenchymal liver disease. Sedation in patients with liver disease should be cautious.

Prevention of protein breakdown
In liver disease and when there are porto-systemic communications, products of bacterial digestion (one of which is ammonia) can escape more readily across the liver 'barrier' into the general circulation. When there is a large amount of blood in the gut, the production of these substances increases and 'porto-systemic encephalopathy' or 'hepatic coma' may develop. To prevent this, the number of organisms in the bowel and their division should both be decreased.

1. The bowel is washed out from below and a cathartic such as magnesium sulphate administered by mouth.
2. Neomycin is given by mouth, 1 g every 4 hours. This agent is not absorbed and does significantly reduce the number of organisms in the colon. In addition, the patient is kept on a low protein intake.

Securing haemostasis
There are four methods available:

1. Vasopressin or octapressin (synthetic vasopressin). This drug lowers the portal venous pressure as the result of constriction of the splanchnic arterioles. 20 units are given intravenously over 20 minutes in 200 ml of 5% dextrose. Its effect lasts up to 1 hour and during this time abdominal colic, pallor and bowel actions may occur. 20 units can be repeated 4 hourly, but the effectiveness decreases with successive doses.

Disadvantages:

a. Short-lived unpleasant side-effects
b. Should not be given in the presence of myocardial ischaemia, as it is a coronary vasoconstrictor

2. Sengstaken–Blakemore tube. A double balloon tube: the lower balloon in the stomach locates the upper balloon over the varices.

The balloons must be deflated after 24 hours and if haemorrhage recurs they may be inflated for a further 24 hours. If haemorrhage begins again after the second inflation, direct control of the bleeding is indicated.

The disadvantages of oesophageal tamponade include:

a. Discomfort of the procedure
b. Oesophageal ulceration
c. Too much traction may lead to pharyngeal obstruction and asphyxia
d. Aspiration of pharyngeal secretions may lead to pulmonary complications
e. Traction on the tube may cause necrosis of the nares
f. Vomiting of inflated bag into the pharynx may cause airway obstruction

3. Direct surgery on the bleeding point. There have been a number of methods advocated but none is uniformly successful.

a. Transaction of the stomach or oesophagus—portoazygos disconnection, now usually done with the circular stapler
b. Direct ligature of varices either through the stomach or through the oesophagus
c. Sclerosant injection of the varices via the oesophagoscope. At the moment this seems the most promising technique.

4. Subsequent management. The outcome in portal hypertension, if bleeding is controlled, rests entirely on the state of the liver. In extrahepatic block (which usually follows thrombosis of the portal vein in the neonate) the liver is normal and survival should be indefinite. Intrahepatic block is most often caused by alcoholic cirrhosis, chronic active hepatitis or more rarely primary biliary cirrhosis. The first is usually steadily progressive unless drinking ceases and less than 20% of those who bleed from oesophageal varices are likely to survive 5 years. The second and third are less predictable and long survival may be possible. The liver disease of schistosomiasis though it produces portal hypertension is also moderately benign.

Until recently it has been usual to offer a portosystemic shunt to a fit patient who has bled from oesophageal varices, with the exception of young children with extrahepatic block, who are better managed conservatively. Fitness is broadly assessed under Child's criteria (Table 31.1).

Only patients in Grade A are suitable for shunting. The current favoured shunt joins the distal cut end of the splenic vein to the left renal vein (Fig. 31.1) but many other shunts have been used—portocaval, mesentericocaval.

Table 31.1 Child's grading of severity of liver disease in portal hypertension.

	Serum bilirubin	Serum albumin	Clinical stigmata (ascites, encephalopathy)
Grade A	Normal	35 g/l	None
Grade B	20–50 mmol/l	30–35 g/l	Mild, easily controlled
Grade C	> 50 mmol/l	< 30 g/l	Severe and uncontrolled

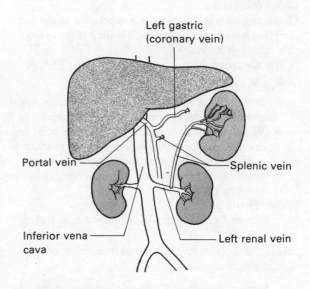

Fig. 31.1 Distal spleno-renal (Warren) shunt for portal hypertension

The alternative to a decompression procedure is repeated sclerotherapy. Though still under trial, the results are encouraging and, of course, the procedure can be used in Grade B and C patients.

BLEEDING PER RECTUM

The passage of blood per rectum is a common symptom, most often due to haemorrhoids, but any lesion of the small or large bowel may be implicated.

Blood which enters the gastro-intestinal tract proximal to the ileo-caecal valve mixes with liquid intestinal content and also undergoes some degree of digestive alteration. Therefore unless the bleeding is massive, it is unusual in proximal lesions for the patient to present with passage of bright blood per rectum but rather with anaemia, change in bowel habit or the passage of melaena or maroon-coloured stool.

CLASSIFICATION OF CAUSES

Small bowel

1. Meckel's diverticulum
2. Intussusception
3. Mesenteric infarction
4. Aorto-enteric fistula
5. Arterio-venous malformations
6. Tumours

Large bowel

1. Carcinoma
2. Neoplastic polyps
3. Diverticular disease
4. Ulcerative procto-colitis
5. Crohn's colitis
6. Ischaemic colitis
7. Vascular ectasia (arterio-venous malformations)
8. Endometriosis

Perianal

1. Internal haemorrhoids
2. Anal fissure
3. Perianal haematoma
4. Anal carcinoma

The common causes of bleeding per rectum are:

1. Internal haemorrhoids
2. Anal fissure
3. Large bowel cancer

The common causes of massive bleeding per rectum are:

1. Diverticular disease
2. Vascular ectasia
3. Upper gastro-intestinal bleeding
4. Aorto-enteric fistula

DIAGNOSIS OF THE CAUSE OF BLEEDING PER RECTUM

This is established from a consideration of the usual triad of history, general examination and special investigations.

History

NATURE OF HAEMORRHAGE

1. Colour. The loss of bright blood per rectum indicates that the source is situated in the anal canal or rec-tum. The passage of darker blood indicates that the source is situated at a higher level, in the small or large bowel.

2. Clots. The loss of clotted blood almost always indicates a source above the haemorrhoidal-bearing area.

3. Squirt or drip with defaecation. The loss of bright blood with defaecation as a squirt or drip is characteristic of internal haemorrhoids.

4. Smear on paper. A smear of bright blood on the paper at the end of defaecation occurs with internal hae-morrhoids and anal fissure.

5. Profuse loss. This is uncommon but usually occurs in the absence of prodromal symptoms, and the com-moner causes are listed above.

6. Mixed with stool. Blood mixed with or adherent to the surface of the stool indicates a colonic or upper rectal lesion.

PERINEAL PAIN

Associated perineal pain occurs with anal fissure, stran-gulated haemorrhoids, carcinoma of the anal canal or carcinoma of the rectum involving the anal canal.

ABDOMINAL PAIN

Abdominal pain or discomfort is a common symptom of carcinoma of the colon in the presence of incomplete obstruction.

Recurrent pain in the left iliac fossa in association with an irregular bowel habit frequently occurs in diverticu-lar disease.

Severe left-sided abdominal pain with bloody diar-rhoea occurs with acute ischaemic colitis and acute and severe ulcerative colitis.

Colicky central abdominal pains may occur when bouts of small bowel intussusception are due to gastro-intestinal polyposis (hereditary polyposis, juvenile poly-posis, Peutz–Jeghers syndrome i.e., hamartomatous polyps).

PROLAPSE

This occurs typically with second and third degree hae-morrhoids. In children, juvenile polyps may prolapse beyond the anal verge on defaecation.

DIARRHOEA

Bloody diarrhoea or the passage of mucus occurs with ulcerative colitis, villous adenoma, or mucus-secreting and ulcerated tumours.

ALTERATION IN BOWEL HABIT

All patients complaining of the passage of blood per rec-tum must be questioned carefully about bowel habit.

Alternating constipation and diarrhoea, spurious diarrhoea, increasing need for the taking of purgatives or a feeling of incomplete evacuation, make it imperative that a complete investigation should be performed in order to establish the presence or absence of a colonic or rectal malignancy.

ABDOMINAL DISTENSION

Abdominal distension and rectal haemorrhage are strongly indicative of a colonic malignancy.

SYMPTOMS OF ANAEMIA

Although rectal haemorrhage is usually an obvious symptom causing the patient to seek medical advice at once, chronic and unrecognized blood loss may have been present for some time, due to haemorrhoids or a 'silent' colonic tumour. Then tiredness, loss of energy, breathlessness on exertion and increasing pallor, result from an iron deficiency anaemia. Angina may develop in an individual with pre-existing asymptomatic cardiac disease.

MISCELLANEOUS SYMPTOMS

Weight loss. This may be a feature of advanced colonic malignancy or chronic ulcerative colitis.

Disturbance of micturition. Frequency, scalding, and haematuria may suggest bladder involvement by carcinoma of the colon or rectum, diverticulitis, ulcerative colitis or Crohn's disease.

Rectal haemorrhage with menses. Blood loss per rectum during menstruation is characteristic of the rare condition of colonic endometriosis.

Family history

This is obtained with hereditary polyposis and sometimes with haemorrhoids.

Examination

General

A particular search is made for:

1. Anaemia, which indicates chronic blood loss
2. Weight loss, which suggests a malignant cause
3. Lymph node enlargement, which suggests a malignant cause

Abdominal

1. An abdominal mass, when situated in the left iliac fossa, usually indicates diverticulitis or carcinoma of the colon, and when situated in the right iliac fossa suggests carcinoma.
2. Abdominal distension, in association with hyperre-sonance, indicates some degree of obstruction which is usually due to carcinoma of the colon.

Ano-rectal examination

This is an essential requirement for any patient complaining of blood loss per rectum.

1. Position of patient: the left lateral position with the hips and knee flexed and the buttocks protruding over the edge of the examination couch.

2. Inspection. With the buttocks separated an anal fissure can always be seen as a crack or triangular ulcer at the anal verge in the midline posteriorly or anteriorly with or without a 'sentinel pile'. Fissures situated in unusual positions should arouse suspicion of some other pathological process (ulcerative colitis or Crohn's disease of the colon) particularly when associated with diarrhoea.

Anal sphincter spasm and pain associated with a fissure make it undesirable to perform proctoscopy and sigmoidoscopy. Then one should wait until the fissure has been treated before proceeding with the assessment, except when symptoms and signs suggest a more sinister and proximally situated lesion, when these further examinations will be indicated under general anaesthesia.

Carcinoma of the anal verge will be seen as an ulcer with heaped-up margins.

3. Patient straining. Prolapsing second degree haemorrhoids which are not visible on inspection will become obvious when the patient strains, when a squirt or a drip of bright blood may be seen. Third degree haemorrhoids, which are chronically prolapsed, will also be made more apparent on straining. Occasionally a pedunculated polyp may appear at the anal verge on straining.

4. Palpation. Digital examination will reveal tumours which are situated within 10 cm of the anal verge. Typically, a carcinoma of the rectum is felt as a hard ulcer crater with heaped-up margins; a benign villous adenoma is so soft and slippery that it is difficult to delineate and may even be overlooked; while a sessile benign polyp is usually felt as a firm smooth nodule.

5. Proctoscopy enables lesions felt digitally to be seen and biopsied and is particularly useful in the assessment of internal haemorrhoids (see p. 215).

6. Sigmoidoscopy must always form part of the routine examination.

It is important that no bowel washout or enema be given before sigmoidoscopy as clots or blood-stained faeces which indicate a pathological process situated beyond the reach of the sigmoidoscope may be removed. If faeces prevent a satisfactory view from being obtained, there should be no hesitation in repeating the examination at a later date. The observation of normal formed faeces is an important negative finding.

As with proctoscopy, any suspicious area visualized should be biopsied and subjected to histological scrutiny.

Whenever a sigmoidoscopy is performed, the length of bowel visualized must be recorded, together with the level of any abnormality seen. In about 20% of cases it is impossible to manipulate the sigmoidoscope beyond the recto-sigmoid area.

7. Fiberoptic flexible sigmoidoscope. This instrument allows for easier passage along the bowel and the distance visualized can often be considerably increased.

Special tests

1. Barium enema. This is not an essential requirement for all patients complaining of blood loss per rectum. Most often the cause will have been established by the examinations already described but when the extent of disease has not been determined (ulcerative colitis or diverticulitis) or if the history leaves doubt as to whether the cause is trivial or more serious, then a barium enema is advisable.

A double contrast barium study is preferable as greater definition of the mucosal lining can be demonstrated which is of particular relevance for demonstrating polyps.

2. Colonoscopy. The development of flexible endoscopes is now such that the whole colon can be visualized. Though a little tedious to perform, and requiring X-ray control, the method is finding increasing application in:

a. Diagnosis and treatment of colonic polyps
b. Differential diagnosis of causes of bleeding
c. Surveillance in inflammatory bowel disease

3. Selective angiography. In unusual situations when the source of gastro-intestinal haemorrhage cannot be ascertained, selective coeliac axis, superior mesenteric or inferior mesenteric angiography may be performed. By this method haemangiomatous or possibly arteriovenous malformations may be demonstrated.

4. Scintillation scan. ⁹⁹ᵐTechnetium-sulphur colloid, when injected intravenously, is rapidly cleared by the liver so that blood extravasated into the bowel lumen results in pooling of the technetium with a local area of increased activity. The technique is simple and accurate and useful in selecting patients for angiography.

5. Isotope studies. In cases of chronic anaemia when intestinal blood loss is suspected but conventional tests have not demonstrated a lesion, the patient's red cells can be labelled with ⁵¹Cr, re-injected and the faeces collected and the radioactivity assessed. Blood loss of 5 ml per day or greater can be determined by this technique.

6. Laparotomy. Occasionally all investigations prove negative and if rectal haemorrhage continues, or if symptoms suggest a malignant cause, then investigations should be repeated after an interval of 6–8 weeks. If no further information is thus gained, or if doubt still exists, laparotomy is indicated. Seldom will this step be proved to have been unnecessary.

SPECIFIC CLINICAL SYNDROMES

Meckel's diverticulum

Ectopic gastric mucosa in the neck or base of a Meckel's diverticulum may cause ulceration and bleeding. In children, abdominal pain usually precedes the passage of blood per rectum, whereas adults present with anaemia. Contrast radiology is of little benefit but scintillation scan may be diagnostic. Exploratory laparotomy is most rewarding and provides long lasting benefit.

Intussusception

Children in their first decade present with sudden onset of abdominal pain, vomiting and the passage of a 'red-currant-jelly' stool. A mass in the right iliac fossa may be palpable and barium enema is both diagnostic and sometimes therapeutic. In adults the presentation is that of acute intestinal obstruction and the intussusceptum is usually a polyp or a carcinoma; laparotomy is necessary.

Ischaemic bowel disease

Ischaemic bowel disease presents in two patterns:

1. Acute infarction
This is usually the result of an arterial embolism or thrombosis, but may also occur with mesenteric venous obstruction. The superior or inferior mesenteric arteries may be occluded with either small or large bowel infarction. Predisposing causes include atrial fibrillation, recent myocardial infarction with sluggish perfusion and atherosclerosis. Patients present with acute abdominal pain, shock, profuse diarrhoea and the passage of blood per rectum. Treatment is urgent laparotomy and a combination of embolectomy and bowel resection.

2. Ischaemic colitis
This refers to small-vessel occlusion of the colon, which results in infarction, stricture-formation or resolution (see p. 197).

Aorto-enteric fistula

Erosion of an aortic prosthesis into the third part of the duodenum and subsequent fistula formation may follow aortic reconstructive surgery, particularly aneurysm repair. The diagnosis should always be kept in mind in patients presenting with bleeding per rectum or haematemesis who have had previous aortic surgery. Urgent laparotomy, removal of the prosthesis and axillo-bifemoral graft is the treatment of choice.

Arteriovenous malformations (vascular ectasia)

These hamartomata occur in the small and large bowel, and in particular are commonly localized to the caecum and right colon and are being increasingly recognized as the source of bleeding in massive colonic haemorrhage.

Diverticular haemorrhage

The source of bleeding is usually a small ulcer overlying an intramural vessel and coexistent pericolic inflammation or abscess is unusual. The patient is characteristically elderly, hypertensive with no recent bowel symptoms and presents with acute explosive fresh rectal bleeding. The bleeding usually completely resolves in all but 10% of cases. Selective arteriography is useful in the small group of patients with persistent bleeding.

MANAGEMENT OF MASSIVE BLEEDING PER RECTUM

The principles of surgical management or similar as for acute upper gastrointestinal bleeding, namely:

1. Resuscitation
2. Diagnosis of the cause
3. Definitive surgical treatment

   To these must be added

4. Exclude an upper gastro-intestinal source of bleeding
5. Test for any bleeding diathesis.

As endoscopy is the cornerstone of diagnosis in upper gastro-intestinal bleeding, so selective arteriography is mandatory in massive bleeding per rectum.

Surgery in small bowel bleeding

If the small bowel is the source of bleeding, then the site may sometimes be localized by isolating the small bowel into a number of segments with clamps; the segment containing the bleeder will distend. Segmental resection is then performed. When bleeding is not rapid nor the site obvious then a colonoscope may be inserted into the small bowel via an enterotomy.

Surgery in large bowel bleeding

Pre-operative selective arteriography will in the majority of cases identify the site of bleeding, and segmental colectomy or hemi-colectomy can be performed. If arteriography is not available or localization is not precise then sub-total colectomy and ileo-rectal anastomosis is the operation of choice.

32

External herniae

A hernia is a protrusion of the whole or part of a viscus from its normal position through an opening in the wall of its containing cavity.

An external hernia is a protrusion of a viscus from the peritoneal cavity into an abnormal position, the commonest site being inguinal.

CLASSIFICATION

1. Inguinal
2. Femoral
3. Umbilical and para umbilical
4. Epigastric
5. Incisional
6. Obturator
7. Spigelian
8. Lumbar
9. Gluteal
10. Sciatic
11. Perineal

The commoner herniae are: inguinal, femoral, umbilical and para-umbilical.

PREDISPOSING FACTORS

All herniae occur at the sites of weakness or potential weakness of the abdominal wall which are acted on by a continued or repeated increase in abdominal pressure. Frequently such sites are where blood vessels and other structures enter or leave the abdominal or thoracic cavity.

1. Congenital defect. A congenital peritoneal sac predisposes to hernia formation in early life and can result in:

a. Persistence of processus vaginalis allowing indirect inguinal hernia formation
b. Incomplete obliteration of umbilicus allowing umbilical hernia formation
c. Patent canal of Nück allowing indirect inguinal hernia formation in females

d. Persistent communication between abdominal and thoracic cavity

2. Acquired defect. Weakness of the anterior abdominal wall can result from.

a. Surgical incisions causing incisional herniae
b. Muscle weakness due to obesity with fatty infiltration, pregnancy, wasting diseases, normal ageing processes, poliomyelitis and nerve division, e.g. a higher incidence of inguinal hernia following appendicectomy due to ilio-inguinal nerve injury

PRECIPITATING FACTORS

Herniation occurs when the intra-abdominal pressure is rapidly raised by such factors as:

1. Chronic cough
2. Straining at defaecation
3. Bladder-neck or urethral obstruction
4. Parturition
5. Vomiting
6. Severe muscular effort
7. Ascitic fluid may fill an existing sac and so render it obvious

SURGICAL PATHOLOGY

The sac

An external abdominal hernia usually has a peritoneal sac with a neck, body and fundus which completely contains any extruded contents. However, a sliding hernia incompletely contains its contents when sigmoid colon, caecum or bladder is involved; in this variety the sac is deficient posteriorly or, put another way, the sac is formed by the viscus.

The contents

The contents may comprise:

1. Omentum
2. Bowel

3. Portion of circumference of bowel (Richter's hernia)
4. Meckel's diverticulum (Littré's hernia)
5. Two loops of bowel (Maydl's hernia)
6. Bladder

The contents may be:

1. *Reducible* when they can be completely emptied from the sac by external pressure
2. *Irreducible* when they cannot be completely emptied from the sac because of adhesions formed between the contents and the peritoneal sac, or because of retention of faeces in large bowel in the sac (incarceration), or because of fibrosis and constriction of the neck of the sac. The term *incarcerated*, which may also be used to describe either irreducible or obstructed hernia, is probably best avoided.

PRINCIPLES OF TREATMENT OF HERNIAE

These principles apply to the treatment of uncomplicated (reducible) herniae.

No treatment

This will be indicated in symptomless and easily reducible herniae (except femoral) in patients with severe general ill health.

Truss

In infants up to 1 year of age reducible indirect inguinal and umbilical herniae may occasionally be treated with a truss in the hope that by keeping contents out of the sac the normal obliterative processes will proceed. However, natural closure of a sac is no longer possible after 1 year or if the hernia reappears during the trial with the truss. The method is not strongly recommended.

In adults with easily reducible inguinal herniae, a truss is indicated only if operation is refused or contraindicated because of general debility; a truss used in healthy young adults has disadvantages in being an encumbrance and in being associated with pressure atrophy of the inguinal muscles and of causing the development of adhesions between the sac and its contents.

Operation

PRINCIPLES OF OPERATIVE MANAGEMENT

1. Pre-operative. Precipitating factors should, whenever possible, be controlled; in particular obesity, constipation, bladder-neck obstruction, chronic cough and smoking. Instruction in breathing exercises is a valuable measure aimed at improving the patient's general health and reducing the risk of recurrent hernia postoperatively.

2. Operative. The following manoeuvres are used alone or in combination:

a. Herniotomy. This is simply excision of the sac at its neck. For indirect inguinal hernia in infants or children this is all that is necessary. For direct hernia in adults, with a diffuse bulge of the posterior wall, herniotomy is undesirable and may lead to bladder injury.
b. Herniorrhaphy. This is closure of the defect with local tissues. The defect may be: the deep inguinal ring; the posterior wall of the inguinal canal (transversalis fascia); or the femoral ring.
c. Hernioplasty. This strictly means the strengthening of a defect with a patch or inlay of living material such as fascia lata or skin, but it has come to include the replacement of a defect by an inlay or darn with some absorbable or non-absorbable foreign material.

3. Post-operative. The continued avoidance of pre-operative factors which might precipitate hernial recurrence.

PRINCIPLES OF OPERATIVE REPAIR

The strength of a hernia repair depends in particular on four factors:

1. Reconstitution of anatomy. Herniae disturb the normal anatomy which should be reconstructed to as near as normal as possible, e.g. reconstitution of tranversalis fascia in inguinal hernia

2. Apposition of fascial, aponeurotic or tendonous structures. Scar tissue formation is promoted when fibrous structures are apposed by sutures. Suturing muscle to fascia neither promotes sound healing nor reconstitutes anatomy.

3. The absence of tension. The function of any suture material, whether absorbable or non-absorbable, is one of approximation only. When sutures are inserted under tension they cut out and the tissues separate and return to their original positions.

4. Suture material and fibroblastic reaction. Suture material must retain its strength until the formation of healthy scar tissue, as the ultimate strength of the repair is dependent not on the suture but on the laying down of collagen by fibroblasts. Absorbable sutures stimulate a brisk inflammatory response which subsides when they fragment and are absorbed after 3–4 weeks. This is insufficient time for consolidation of strength. Non-absorbable monofilament material, on the other hand, is walled off by fibroblasts and multifilament material is walled off and invaded by fibroblasts, while an open mesh becomes part of the permanent fibrous tissue reparative process.

Monofilament materials have an additional advantage in that they do not cause local trauma, an acute inflammatory response or have crevices in which bacteria can lodge. Thus they are the materials of choice.

CAUSES OF RECURRENT HERNIAE

1. Pre-operative. Any factor that predisposes to faulty or delayed healing

2. Operative. Any factor involving faulty technique, with *failure to*:

a. Follow the principles of operative repair
b. Identify an indirect sac and ligate it at its neck
c. Perform a herniorrhaphy in the presence of a defect
d. Adequately repair a defect, particularly transversalis fascia
e. Achieve adequate haemostasis, predisposing to wound haematoma and infection
f. Close the medial corner of the posterior wall of the inguinal canal between the conjoint tendon, pubic tubercle and inguinal ligament. This predisposes to direct hernia recurrence.

3. Post-operative

a. Persistence of pre-operative factors
b. Wound haematoma
c. Wound infection

INGUINAL HERNIA

This is the commonest type of hernia in both males and females.

Surgical anatomy

The inguinal canal is an oblique passage or intermuscular split about 4 cm long in the lower part of the abdominal wall, passing downwards and medially from the internal inguinal ring to the external inguinal ring. Through the canal passes the spermatic cord in the male and the round ligament in the female.

The external ring is formed by a V slit in the external oblique aponeurosis and is situated 1 cm above and lateral to the pubic tubercle (Fig. 32.1). It transmits the vas deferens, the testicular artery (branch of the aorta), the artery of the vas (branch of the inferior vesical), the cremasteric artery (branch of the inferior epigastric), the pampiniform plexus of veins, the ilio-inguinal nerve, the genital branch of the genito-femoral nerve and the processus vaginalis when present.

The anterior wall of the inguinal canal is made up of the arching fibres of the internal oblique muscle laterally

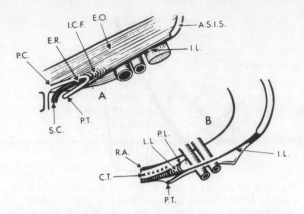

Fig. 32.1 External oblique and external ring **A.** Anterior view: A.S.I.S. anterior superior iliac spine; I.L. inguinal ligament; E.O. external oblique aponeurosis; I.C.F. intercrural fibres; E.R. external ring; P.C. pubic crest; P.T. pubic tubercle; S.C. spermatic cord. **B.** Superior view: C.T. conjoint tendon insertion; R.A. rectus abdominis insertion; L.L. lacunar ligament (Gimbernat's ligament), P.L. pectineal ligament (Astley Cooper's ligament); P.T. pubic tubercle I.L. inguinal ligament.

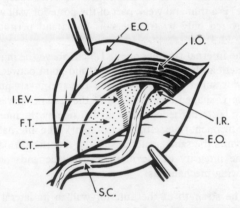

Fig. 32.2 Internal oblique and inguinal canal (external oblique aponeurosis reflected): E.O. = reflected external oblique aponeurosis; I.O. = arching muscle of internal oblique; C.T. = conjoint tendon; F.T. = fascia transversalis; I.E.V. = inferior epigastric vessel; I.R. = internal inguinal ring; S.C. = spermatic cord.

and the aponeurosis of the external oblique medially. Both structures are covered by superficial fascia, subcutaneous fat and skin.

The floor of the inguinal canal is formed by the gutter of the inguinal ligament laterally and the lacunar ligament (Gimbernat's ligament) medially.

The roof of the inguinal canal is formed by the lower borders of the internal oblique and transversus abdominis muscles (Fig. 32.2)

The posterior wall of the canal consists of the conjoint tendon medially (the fused common insertion of the

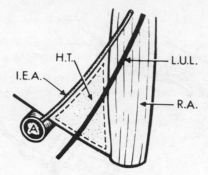

Fig. 32.3 Hesselbach's triangle: H.T. = Hesselbach's triangle; I.E.A. inferior epigastric artery; L.U.L. = lateral umbilical ligament (obliterated umbilical artery); R.A. = rectus abdominis; A. = femoral artery.

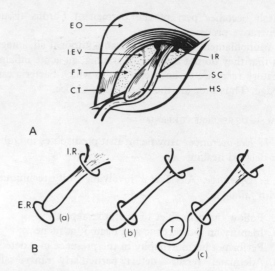

Fig. 32.4 Indirect inguinal hernia **A.** External oblique reflected: E.O. = external oblique; I.E.V. = inferior epigastric vessels; F.T. = fascia transversalis; C.T. = conjoint tendon; H.S. = hernial sac; S.C. = spermatic cord; I R. = internal ring. **B.** Hernial sacs (**a**) bubonocele (**b**) funicular (**c**) complete (scrotal): I.R. = internal ring; E.R. = external ring; T. = testis.

internal oblique and transversus abdominis muscles into the pubic crest) and the lateral umbilical ligament, the inferior epigastric artery and the fascia transversalis, laterally. The triangular area bounded by the inferior epigastric artery, the inguinal ligament and the lateral border of the rectus abdominis muscle (Hesselbach's triangle) is a thin and weak part of the posterior wall which is covered only by transversalis fascia and peritoneum (Fig. 32.3)

The internal ring lies about 1.5 cm above the inguinal ligament at the *mid-inguinal point* (mid-point between the anterior superior iliac spine and the symphysis pubis). It is a U-shaped condensation of the fascia transversalis which is strengthened on its medial side by the interfoveolar ligament (Hesselbach's ligament). The internal ring transmits the same structures as the superficial ring.

The integrity of the inguinal canal depends on the following mechanisms:

1. The strength of the anterior wall in its lateral part when contraction of the external oblique narrows the external ring
2. The strength of the posterior wall in its medial part when contraction of the internal oblique and the transversus abdominis muscles straightens the conjoint tendon
3. The upward and lateral movement of the U-shaped internal ring.

Types of inguinal herniae

1. INDIRECT
This enters the inguinal canal through the internal inguinal ring lateral to the inferior epigastric vessels and traverses the full length of the canal in front of the cord (Fig. 32.4A).

Indirect inguinal herniae are usually congenital in origin and they may be subdivided into:

a. Bubonocele
b. Funicular
c. Complete or scrotal (Fig. 32.4B)

The coverings of an indirect inguinal hernia are:

a. *Peritoneum*
b. *Extraperitoneal fat*
c. *Internal spermatic fascia* (derived from the fascia transversalis at the internal ring)
d. *Cremaster muscle and fascia* (derived from the muscle of internal oblique and transversus abdominis and the areolar tissue between these muscles)
e. *External spermatic fascia* (derived from the crura of the external ring—external oblique aponeurosis)
f. *Superficial fascia and skin*

2. DIRECT
Usually a diffuse bulge of the medial portion of the posterior wall of the inguinal canal medial to the inferior epigastric vessels and which is behind, above, or below the cord (Fig. 32.5A). Direct inguinal herniae are acquired, with the exception of a rare type in which there is a rigid circular defect in the conjoint tendon (Ogilvie's hernia, Fig. 32.5B).

The coverings of a direct inguinal hernia are:

a. *Peritoneum*
b. *Fascia transversalis*
c. *Conjoint tendon* (if the hernia passes medial to the lateral umbilical ligament)

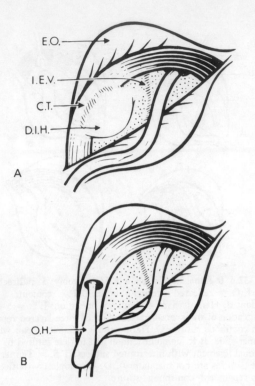

Fig. 32.5 Direct inguinal hernia **A**: E.O. = external oblique reflected; I.E.V. = inferior epigastric vessels; C.T. attenuated conjoint tendon; D.I.H. = direct hernial sac; **B**: O.H. = congenital direct hernia (Ogilvie hernia).

d. *External oblique aponeurosis*
e. *Superficial fascia and skin*

3. INDIRECT AND DIRECT
(Dual hernia, pantaloon hernia or saddle bag hernia.) This presents with dual sacs straddling the inferior epigastric vessels.

Clinical features

Indirect inguinal herniae occur at all ages and when caused by a persistence of the processus vaginalis they present soon after birth or in adolescence.

Direct inguinal herniae occur most often in the middle-aged or elderly as an acquired condition.

SYMPTOMS
1. *A lump.* This appears in the groin, sometimes after a bout of strenuous exercise and disappears on lying down unless irreducible.
2. *Discomfort or pain.* Discomfort in the groin is common and is probably the result of stretching of the neck of the sac but severe pain in the lump or in the abdomen usually indicates obstruction or strangulation.
3. *Vomiting.* This suggests obstruction or strangulation.

SIGNS
General
Special attention must be paid to the following:

1. *Precipitating factors*, especially chronic lung disease, urinary obstruction, colonic disorders and previous appendicectomy
2. *Signs of obstruction or strangulation*, particularly dehydration, shock and peritonitis

Local
1. *Inspection* with the patient standing and coughing
   a. An indirect inguinal hernia passes downwards and medially towards the scrotum.
   b. A direct inguinal hernia protrudes directly forwards in the inner part of the inguinal canal.
2. *Palpation*
   a. An indirect inguinal hernia, when reducible, returns in an upward and lateral direction and it is prevented from returning by pressure over the internal ring at the mid inguinal point.
      A small inguinal hernia (bubonocele) may not be detectable unless the little finger invaginates the scrotum and is passed into the external ring when an impulse will be felt when the patient coughs. This is an uncomfortable examination and should be done only if there is doubt.
   b. A direct inguinal hernia is seldom large enough to enter the scrotum and, when it is reducible, it returns directly backwards. Since it lies medial to the internal ring it cannot be controlled by pressure over this site and with a finger in the external ring the cough impulse is directed forwards.

Whether the hernia is indirect or direct it is important to assess the nature of the contents of the sac; intestine gurgles on reduction of the hernia but omentum does not.

When making a local assessment of an inguinal hernia it is important to remember the following three points:

1. It is sometimes impossible to decide clinically whether an inguinal hernia is direct or indirect.
2. A tense, tender, irreducible hernia (most often an indirect hernia), in the absence of abdominal pain is simply irreducible. However when persistent pain, loss of cough impulse and perhaps oedema and reddening of the skin over the hernia are present, together with other signs of intestinal obstruction, strangulation of bowel must be suspected. An obstructed hernia cannot be distinguished clinically from a strangulated one; the distinction can only be made at operation which, in the presence of symptoms and signs of bowel obstruction, is an urgent requirement.

3. An absent cough impulse alone does not indicate strangulation of bowel as the hernia sac may be plugged with omentum. Omental strangulation is likely when a tense, tender, irreducible hernia is present in the absence of features of bowel obstruction.

DIFFERENTIAL DIAGNOSIS OF A GROIN LUMP

1. Femoral hernia. A femoral hernia appears in the groin below the medial end of the inguinal ligament, lateral to the pubic tubercle and enlarges upward over the inguinal ligament, whereas an inguinal hernia appears above the inguinal ligament, medial to the pubic tubercle and enlarges downwards and medially.

2. Inguinal lymph nodes. When inguinal lymph nodes are palpable they may be confused with an irreducible femoral hernia but they are usually multiple and below the inguinal ligament.

3. Saphena varix. This is associated with long saphenous varicosities. The varix lies below the inguinal ligament and disappears when the limb is elevated; it imparts a thrill and bruit when the patient coughs (Cruveilhier's sign).

4. Femoral aneurysm. This is usually due to atherosclerosis but it may follow trauma. The aneurysm lies below the inguinal ligament and is associated with expansile pulsation.

5. Encysted hydrocele of the cord. This appears as a tense irreducible swelling anywhere along the cord. It moves downwards when traction is exerted on the testis.

6. Hydrocele of the canal of Nuck. This appears as an irreducible, tense, cystic swelling in the superficial ring of a young female, and is a cyst replacing the distal round ligament.

7. Lipoma of the cord. This may produce features similar to those of an encysted hydrocele, or it may be indistinguishable from an irreducible hernia.

8. An incompletely descended testis emerging from the external ring. A hernia is usually also present.

9. Ectopic testis. A testis situated in the superficial inguinal pouch or at the root of the penis may cause confusion but again the absence of a testis from the scrotum indicates maldescent of the testis.

10. Very large scrotal herniae in the elderly.
In these the integrity of the inguinal canal has been completely disrupted and removal of the cord and testis enables the inguinal canal to be obliterated

COMPLICATED INGUINAL HERNIAE
Obstructed or strangulated inguinal herniae require urgent operation. A short period of pre-operative resuscitation with intravenous fluids is indicated when dehydration is present.

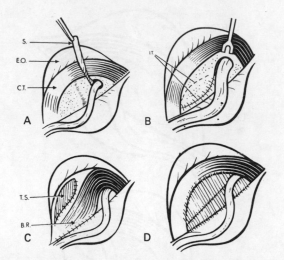

Fig. 32.6 Inguinal hernia repair **A.**Herniotomy: S. indirect sac; E.O. = reflected external oblique; C.T. = conjoint tendon; **B.** Herniorrhapy—Shouldice operation: I.T. = imbrication of transversalis fascia (first of three-layered repair) with continous suture. **C.** Herniorrhapy—Bassini repair with Tanner slide: B.R. conjoint tendon and muscle sutured to inguinal ligament with interrupted sutures; T.S. = Tanner slide (sutures are not mandatory). **D.** Hernioplasty—lattice darn repair with continuous suture.

At operation one of the three following situations will be encountered:

1. The hernia reduces on opening the external oblique and dividing the external ring. This is the commonest occurrence. After the sac is opened, the involved loop of bowel is found and assessed for viability. When it is not viable, resection is performed; the hernia is then repaired in the usual manner.

2. The hernia reduces spontaneously under general anaesthetic.

a. The operation is continued and on opening the hernial sac the loop of bowel or portion of omentum which has been involved in the hernia is most often located just deep to the internal ring through which it can be delivered and its viability assessed.
b. When the involved bowel loop cannot be located, provided there were no pre-operative signs of peritonitis and there is no haemorrhage, brown or faeculent effusion present, the hernia is simply repaired in the usual manner.
c. When the viscus cannot be located, but when there are pre-operative signs of peritonitis or there is 'tell tale' peritoneal fluid present in the sac, then a formal laparotomy must be performed to locate the involved bowel.

3. *The hernia is not reduced after dividing the external ring*. This is usually due to a tight neck of the sac or adhesions, and the constriction ring causing the tightness plus the adhesions must be divided, the contents of the sac dealt with as necessary and repair of the defect performed.

Operations on complicated hernia are best covered with a broad spectrum antibiotic, to reduce the incidence of wound infection, should a bowel resection be necessary.

Treatment

UNCOMPLICATED INGUINAL HERNIAE

The general principles outlined on p. 232 apply to inguinal herniae.

Operation is the most satisfactory treatment and should be advised whenever possible.

There are many operations available and an equally impressive variety of suture materials may be used; the following plan is regarded as an acceptable one for routine use.

There are four groups of patients:

1. Indirect inguinal herniae in children and adolescents. In these there is a normal posterior wall to the inguinal canal and, if there has been no stretching of the internal ring, herniotomy alone is sufficient.

2. Indirect inguinal herniae in healthy adults. These patients have good inguinal musculature and an intact posterior wall of the inguinal canal but when the internal ring is stretched and widened then the following steps are required:

a. *Herniotomy* (Fig. 32.6A)

b. *Herniorrhaphy*. The Shouldice operation incorporates all the principles of operative repair (p. 232), closing the hernial defect with local tissues. All three layers of the abdominal wall are strengthened using monofilament non-absorbable sutures. The transversalis fascia is divided and reconstituted by imbrication (double-breasting, Fig. 32.6B), the fascia of the conjoined transversalis and internal oblique is approximated to the inguinal ligament by imbrication and the divided external oblique is similarly closed by double-breasting. Recurrence rates of less than 1% at 5 years illustrate the effectiveness if this repair. The Bassini operation, as practised, involves tightening the internal ring, plication of the posterior wall and suturing the conjoined muscle to the inguinal ligament, starting at the medial end. Tension is relieved by an oblique relaxing incision in the anterior rectus sheath allowing easier approximation of muscle to inguinal ligament (Tanner's slide, Fig. 32.6C) The

Bassini operation maintains its popularity despite a high recurrence rate and non-compliance with sound principles.

c. *Hernioplasty*. With healthy tissues and a small defect, repair using fascia lata or plastic mesh is unnecessary; however, routine use of a darn with non-absorbable mono-filament sutures and incorporating posterior wall plication and approximation of conjoined muscle to inguinal ligament has gained in popularity (Fig. 32.6D)

3. Large indirect herniae, direct herniae, and recurrent herniae. In these there is a weakened and often attenuated posterior wall of the inguinal canal and the following are required:

a. *Herniotomy*. This is performed except for direct hernial bulges when the sac is inverted, or sliding herniae when it is impossible to excise the sac completely.

b. *Hernioplasty*. The internal ring is tightened and the fascia transversalis is plicated; then a patch of fascia lata, an inlay of plastic mesh, or a darn with monofilament or multifilament nylon, linen thread or wire is essential to replace the posterior wall of the canal (Fig. 32.6D).

FEMORAL HERNIA

The majority of femoral herniae are acquired and occur more frequently in middle-aged and elderly females in whom increased abdominal pressure during pregnancy was probably an initiating factor. However, in females as a group, inguinal hernia is commoner than femoral hernia.

Surgical anatomy

The femoral sheath is composed of a funnel-shaped prolongation of the fascia transversalis in front and the fascia iliaca behind, and it contains the femoral vessels. The sheath is separated from the medial side of the femoral vein by a space, the femoral canal, which contains fat, lymph channels from the deep inguinal glands, the lymph gland of Cloquet, and, under abnormal conditions, a femoral hernia. The canal is about 2 cm long.

The femoral ring is the abdominal end of the femoral canal and is bounded anteriorly by the inguinal ligament, medially by the crescentic edge of the lacunar ligament (Gimbernat's ligament), posteriorly by the pectineal line of the horizontal ramus of the pubis and the pectineal ligament (ligament of Astley Cooper), and laterally by the femoral vein (Fig. 32.7). All these boundaries are rigid except the femoral vein.

In 30% of cases the pubic branch of the inferior epigastric artery replaces the obturator artery when there is

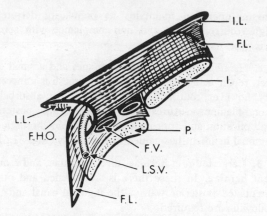

Fig. 32.7 Formation of the femoral hernial orifice: I.L. = inguinal ligament; F.L. = fascia lata; I. iliacus muscle; P. = pectineus muscle; F.V. = femoral vein; L.S.V. = long saphenous vein; L.L. = lacunar ligament; F.H.O. = femoral hernial orifice.

a 10: 1 chance of it passing medial to the neck of a femoral hernia. In this position it is vulnerable if the lacunar ligament is divided to widen the femoral ring.

The femoral hernial orifice is the superficial end of the femoral canal. It is well formed only in the presence of a femoral hernia when condensation of the fascia lata of the thigh at the saphenous opening becomes more apparent (Fig. 32.7)

When a femoral hernia enlarges it passes through the saphenous opening of the fascia lata up over the inguinal ligament in the subcutaneous plane superficial to the superficial fascia (Scarpa's fascia).

The coverings of a femoral hernia are as follows:

1. Peritoneum
2. Extraperitoneal fat
3. Fused transversalis fascia, and fascia lata
4. Cribriform fascia
5. Subcutaneous fat and skin

OTHER TYPES OF FEMORAL HERNIAE

The majority of femoral herniae pass through the femoral canal but rare types occur and these are:

1. Prevascular hernia. This passes in front of the femoral artery and is sometimes associated with congenital dislocation of the hip (Narath's hernia).

2. Pectineal hernia. This passes behind the femoral vessels between the pectineus muscle and its fascia (Cloquet's hernia).

3. External femoral hernia. This passes lateral to the femoral artery (Hesselbach's hernia).

4. Lacunar hernia. This passes through the lacunar ligament of Gimbernat (Langier's hernia).

Clinical features

Patients with femoral herniae present in one of two ways:

1. With a lump. This is usually a small globular swelling situated below and lateral to the pubic tubercle. It is apparent on standing or straining but may disappear on lying down.

2. With obstruction or strangulation. The femoral ring is small and narrow and is surrounded by rigid structures with the exception of the femoral vein. This anatomical arrangement predisposes to irreducibility and strangulation of hernial contents. The obstructing agent is either the neck of the sac, or the femoral ring itself.

The lump becomes tense, tender and irreducible and the overlying skin may be oedematous when strangulation is present.

In addition the features of a small bowel obstruction are apparent with abdominal pain and vomiting.

It should be remembered that an obstructed femoral hernia, particularly with a Richter's type of strangulation, may be extremely difficult to detect in an obese patient and it may be overlooked unless a very careful search is made.

DIFFERENTIAL DIAGNOSIS
See Inguinal Hernia

Treatment

There is no place for conservative treatment of femoral herniae for two reasons: (1) no truss can be fitted to control the femoral ring; (2) there is always a risk of strangulation.

OPERATION
This may be performed by one of three methods:

1. Supra-inguinal. A midline vertical (Henry's incision), a vertical para-rectal (McEvedy's incision) or a transverse incision in the skin crease above the inguinal ligament is used, and an extraperitoneal approach is made behind the inguinal canal to the fundus of the sac which is opened and emptied of its contents. The sac is then reduced from the groin into the abdomen where it is excised.

A herniorrhaphy is performed by suturing the inguinal ligament or the conjoint tendon to the pectineal ligament.

The operation has the advantages of providing optimum conditions for dealing with gangrenous bowel and for repair of the femoral ring; it has however a disadvantage in that there is imperfect access to the fundus of the sac which may make its removal difficult.

2. Inguinal (Lotheissen operation). A transverse inguinal incision is used as for an inguinal hernia operation, the inguinal canal is opened and its posterior wall incised (with or without division of the inferior epigastric vessels). An extraperitoneal approach is then made to the sac and the femoral ring which are then dealt with in the same way as in the supra-inguinal operation.

The operation has the disadvantage that the inguinal canal is transgressed and inguinal herniorrhaphy is also required.

3. Sub-inguinal (Lockwood operation). A transverse-incision is made directly over the swelling in the groin and the sac is separated from its layers of fat and fascia and then opened, emptied and tied off. A herniorrhaphy is performed by suturing the inguinal ligament to the pectineal fascia; alternatively a purse-string suture, starting at the inner end of the inguinal ligament and picking up Gimbernat's ligament, pectineal fascia, and the lateral side of the saphenous opening and its fascia lata, may be used.

The operation has the disadvantage of making it difficult to resect bowel when gangrene is present, or to ligate the sac at its neck. In addition there is largely theoretical disadvantage of possible damage to the abnormal obturator artery if incision of Gimbernat's ligament is performed to facilitate reduction of the contents of the hernial sac.

The operation has the advantages of being speedy, simple and may be performed with ease under local anaesthesia.

For obstructed and strangulated femoral herniae the supra-inguinal and inguinal approaches are recommended as they provide optimal circumstances for dealing with the contents of the sac, access to the peritoneal cavity, better access for herniorraphy and exposure of an aberrant obturatory artery.

UMBILICAL HERNIA

Exomphalos. This is a rare neonatal condition due to an anomaly of the second stage of gut rotation when the midgut loop fails to return into the abdominal cavity during the tenth week of fetal life, and presents at birth as two types:

1. Exomphalus minor. The sac is small and the umbilical cord attached is at its summit. Treatment involves twisting the cord, so facilitating reduction of the sac, and this is maintained by a firm dressing for 2 weeks.

2. Exomphalus major. The sac is large and contains small and large bowel and often part of the liver, whilst the umbilical cord is at the inferior margin of the sac. Surgical repair is urgent as rupture and subsequent peritonitis is liable to occur. Principles of repair involve constructing skin flaps or using synthetic material to cover the defect, and definitive repair performed at a later date but the prognosis is often poor.

Umbilical hernia of infancy. This occurs through a defect in the umbilical cicatrax during the first few days of life. A hernial sac protrudes as a small knob at the umbilicus and it is most apparent when the child cries or strains.

Umbilical herniae are reducible and they rarely strangulate.

Treatment is conservative as most disappear within 12–18 months; in the meantime they may be retained by a simple pad. Occasionally they persist after this period and operation is then recommended. The sac is excised through a transverse sub-umbilical incision and the small fibrous defect is closed with a few interrupted sutures.

Para-umbilical hernia. In the majority of cases this occurs as an acquired condition in middle-aged, obese, multiparous women in whom there is often an initial small defect in the linea alba just above the umbilicus. The peritoneal sac is often preceded by the extrusion of a small knuckle of extraperitoneal fat through the tendinous fibres of the linea alba.

As the hernia enlarges the peritoneal sac cannot enlarge indefinitely because of the fixation of the peritoneum about the umbilicus. It splits and the contents, which are most often omentum and, in very large herniae, transverse colon and small bowel, become loculated and adherent. For these reasons a large para-umbilical hernia is seldom reducible and strangulation is likely to occur.

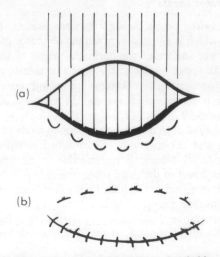

Fig. 32.8 Mayo repair (a) interrupted non-absorbable mattress sutures (b) Completion of overlap

Treatment is operative because of the risk of complications particularly when the hernia is irreducible. The standard practice is to perform a Mayo's operation which entails a transverse elliptical incision with excision of the umbilicus, redundant skin and the fibro-peritoneal sac and then to incise the rectus sheath on each side of the defect. Closure is effected by overlapping the upper and lower flaps with interrupted mattress sutures (Fig. 32.8) Large defects may be closed with plastic mesh.

EPIGASTRIC HERNIA

This is a midline protrusion of extraperitoneal fat, and occasionally a small peritoneal sac, through a defect or defects in the linea alba, usually in fit, muscular males under 40.

It presents as a small irreducible hernia often situated midway between the xiphisternum and the umbilicus and is usually felt more easily than it is seen.

Many epigastric herniae are symptomless but pain, discomfort or digestive disturbances may occur and simulate peptic ulceration or gall bladder disease.

Treatment entails excision of the knuckle of fat and any associated hernial sac and repair of the defect by longitudinal suture or by a transverse overlap operation of the Ma:yo type if the defect is larger than usual.

INCISIONAL HERNIA

This is discussed in Chapter 5.

MISCELLANEOUS HERNIAE

Obturator hernia

An acquired hernia through the fibro-osseous obturator canal which is situated between the obturator groove on the lower surface of the horizontal ramus of the pubis and the upper border of the obturator membrane. The canal transmits the obturator nerve and vessels. The hernia is commoner in women and usually occurs after the age of 50.

Intestinal obstruction is the common mode of persentation and the diagnosis is established at laparotomy. Occasionally a lump is recognizable in the upper and medial aspect of the thigh when pain may be referred to the inner aspect of the knee by the geniculate branch of the obturator nerve.

At operation the sac and its contents are reduced into the abdomen but herniorrhaphy is impossible because of the rigid nature of the canal and the presence of the obturator nerve.

Spigelian hernia

A herniation through the linear semilunaris at the outer border of the rectus abdominis muscle which occurs about halfway between the pubis and umbilicus (at about the level of the semilunar fold of Douglas).

It is probably an acquired condition and may be confused with a direct inguinal hernia, although it is usually situated higher and more medial.

Treatment is operative as the hernia is liable to strangulate.

Lumbar hernia

Either an incisional hernia following a loin incision or a spontaneous occurrence through the inferior lumbar triangle of Petit bounded by the iliac crest, the posterior edge of the external oblique and the anterior edge of the latissimus dorsi, or through the superior lumbar space bounded by the twelfth rib, the lower border of serratus posterior inferior, the anterior border of sacrospinalis and the internal oblique.

Herniae through these anatomically weak places are wide-necked and reducible and usually controlled by a surgical belt.

Gluteal hernia

Occurs through the greater sciatic notch either above or below pyriformis muscle. Most often it is diagnosed at laparotomy for the relief of a bowel obstruction; rarely is a gluteal swelling palpable.

Treatment is operative.

Sciatic hernia

A protrusion through the lesser sciatic notch and is usually discovered at operation for bowel obstruction; very rarely does it present as a gluteal swelling or cause pain in the distribution of the sciatic nerve.

Perineal hernia

Most often occurs as an incisional hernia after an abdominoperineal excision of the rectum. It may also occur in middle-aged or elderly women through an extension or persistence of the recto-vaginal pouch or as a protrusion of a sac between the bladder and the vagina.

33

Testis and epididymis

Disorders of the testis and epididymis are common and, with the exception of imperfect testicular descent, they all give rise to solid or cystic scrotal swellings.

CLASSIFICATION OF DISORDERS

Testis and epididymis

1. Imperfect descent
2. Inflammation
3. Tumours
4. Torsion
5. Cysts

Spermatic cord

Varicocele

Tunica vaginalis

1. Hydrocele
2. Haematocele

TESTIS AND EPIDIDYMIS

IMPERFECT DESCENT

The testis develops from coelomic epithelium and mesoderm of the urogenital ridge in the posterior wall of the coelomic cavity. It joins with the mesonephric duct system which forms the epididymis and the vas deferens and descends to reach the internal inguinal ring at 7 months gestation, then passes along the inguinal canal to reach the external ring at 8 months and enters the scrotum at birth.

During its descent the testis is preceded by a prolongation of peritoneum (processus vaginalis) which projects into the foetal scrotum. The testis slides down behind the processus vaginalis which normally becomes obliterated at birth to form the innermost covering of the testis (tunica vaginalis).

A strand of fibro-muscular mesoblastic tissue (the gubernaculum) attaches itself to the lower pole of the testis during fetal life preceding it into the scrotum and, together with intra-abdominal pressure, probably brings about normal descent of the testis.

Testicular descent may be imperfect and result in:

1. Undescended testis. Descent may be arrested along the *normal pathway* as the result of some local factor such as adhesions or a shortened vas deferens or testicular vessels; and, unless the testis is placed in the scrotum by the age of 5 years, spermatogenesis is likely to be affected. Interstitial cell development will, however, proceed normally and secondary sex characters will be unaffected.

The normally placed testis develops in three stages: the resting stage (0–5 years), the growth stage (5–10 years) and the maturation stage (10 years and throughout adolescence). In the growth stage spermatogonia begin to appear and seminiferous tubules become tortuous and it is in this stage that an abnormally-placed testis undergoes imperfect but reversible spermatogenesis. Permanent and irreversible changes in the maturation stage will occur if the testis is not in the scrotum by the time the boy is 10 years old.

Unilateral undescended testes are about four times as common as bilateral; occasionally bilateral undescended testes are associated with some general endocrine abnormality with hypogenitalism and obesity.

Complications of an undescended testis include all diseases peculiar to a normally-placed testis but in addition there is an increased risk of the following:

a. Defective spermatogenesis and sterility if bilaterally undescended
b. Torsion
c. Trauma
d. Inguinal hernia, which occurs in about 90% of cases
e. Malignancy, which is about 50 times commoner than in a normally placed testis, occurs most often in an abdominally situated testis

2. Ectopic testis. Testicular descent takes place along the inguinal canal and beyond the external ring but the testis is guided to an ectopic position (probably by gubernacular fibres) so that it comes to be superficial to the external oblique muscle, at the root of the penis, in the perineum, or in the upper and medial part of the thigh.

3. Retractile testis. Testicular descent occurs normally and excessive cremasteric muscle activity draws the testis up into the inguinal canal.

History

Always ask the mother if two testicles were present at birth. The newborn's scrotum is lax and both testicles are usually clearly visible. If the parent's answer is 'yes' a provisional diagnosis of retractile testes can be made.

Clinical examination

The proper clinical examination of a child who is said to have an undescended testis is critical. Relaxation of both child and mother must be achieved! The crucial monoeuvre is to get above the testis by putting the hand over the inguinal canal just lateral to the external ring. Firm pressure is exerted downwards and medially so as to trap a testis that lies outside the ring and push it towards the scrotum. In such circumstances the retractile testis will nearly always be displaced into the scrotum. An inguinal ectopic testis will slip under the fingers.

The following suggest an undescended testis rather than a retractile one:

a. A testis cannot be felt in the conscious child
b. The scrotum on the affected side is underdeveloped
c. A hernia is present. Sometimes the bulge of a hernia may be mistaken for a testis.

Treatment

Treatment of undescended and maldescended testes is as follows:

1. *Undescended testis.* Operation is indicated well before puberty and as early as possible if both endocrine and reproductive function is to be preserved. The principle of this operation is wide mobilization of the cord and anatomical replacement in the scrotum. Repair of the associated inguinal hernia may be necessary. Numerous methods have been devised for securing the testis in the scrotum but these are much less important than that it should be freely mobile *to descend.*
2. *Ectopic testis.* An ectopic testis, like the undescended testis, must be placed in the scrotum before it is damaged by defective maturation—i.e. as soon as possible and certainly before puberty. The cord is usually of normal length and the operation easy.
3. *Retractile testis.* Reassure the parents and leave the child alone.
4. *Hormone therapy.* While there was a vogue for gonadotrophin therapy in the management of this condition, this approach has now been virtually abandoned.

INFLAMMATION

Inflammation of the testis may present in the following forms:

Acute epididymo-orchitis

This inflammatory process of the epididymis and testes frequently occurs in young men without the isolation of any organism. If an organism is isolated it is usually of the coliform species or a gonococcus. The mumps virus is well known for its ability to produce orchitis and in some instances it has been postulated that reflux of urine along the vas results in a chemical epididymitis.

Infecting organisms are believed to travel along the vas deferens in a retrograde manner to reach the epididymis before spreading to involve the testis. Alternative routes of infection are the bloodstream and lymphatics of the vas deferens but the exact means by which infection occurs has not been clearly established.

CLINICAL FEATURES

Symptoms
1. Malaise and fever
2. Painful swelling of the testis of gradual onset and increasing in severity over several days
3. Dysuria and frequency, often
4. Urethral discharge, rare

Signs
1. Pyrexia
2. Reddened and oedematous scrotum
3. Thickened cord
4. Painful swollen testis and epididymis which cannot be distinguished separately
5. A small secondary hydrocele is often present

Special tests
1. Microscopy and culture of urine—usually negative
2. Microscopy and culture of any urethral discharge
3. Intravenous urography and cysto-urethroscopy if bladder or bladder-neck disease is suspected.

Differential diagnosis
Torsion of the testicle may be difficult to distinguish from acute epididymo-orchitis but features of the former include:

1. It occurs almost entirely in children and adolescents
2. There is occasionally a history of previous attacks
3. There is a sudden onset of severe lower abdominal and testicular pain, often accompanied by vomiting
4. There is an absence of urinary symptoms
5. The testis is usually situated high in the scrotum

Pyrexia may be present in both conditions but it is usually greater in epididymo-orchitis. *If there is any doubt the testis should be explored.*

TREATMENT

1. Rest in bed, elevation of the scrotum and analgesics
2. Administration of a broad spectrum antibiotic after urine and any urethral discharge has been sampled for microscopy and culture. If the causative organism is isolated the appropriate antibiotic is given
3. Incision and drainage if abscess formation occurs

Chronic epididymo-orchitis

This may follow acute epididymo-orchitis, particularly in elderly patients with recurrent urinary tract infections. It may also be a sequel to urogenital tuberculosis, especially when the kidney is involved. Spread of infection is initially to the globus minor of the epididymis and later, by way of the vasa efferentia, to the testis.

TUBERCULOUS EPIDIDYMO-ORCHITIS

The possible modes of infection of the epididymis by tubercle bacilli are the same as for acute epididymo-orchitis. In some cases, particularly young adults, blood spread from a primary infection in the lung appears most likely, especially when tuberculosis is also present at other sites.

Tuberculous epididymo-orchitis progresses slowly; it may be bilateral and associated with involvement of the prostate and seminal vesicles. The epididymis becomes hard and nodular but as caseation progresses it softens and becomes adherent to the posterior scrotal skin where a sinus may form. The cord becomes thickened and nodular and spread to the testis results in the formation of an irregular mass filling the scrotal compartment. There is sometimes a small hydrocele.

When tuberculosis exists elsewhere in the urogenital tract there may be a 'sterile pyuria' in the sense that the urine is sterile to the usual culture methods but usually tubercle bacilli can be cultured from the urine by an appropriate technique.

Tuberculous epididymo-orchitis may be difficult to distinguish from a testicular tumour or syphilitic orchitis without careful and repeated examinations of the urine for acid-fast bacilli.

Treatment

1. Intensive and prolonged chemotherapy with combinations of streptomycin, para-aminosalicylic acid and isoniazid hydrazine
2. Surgery and epididymectomy or epididymo-orchidectomy will be indicated for a chronic scrotal sinus

TUMOURS OF THE TESTIS

These usually occur in men under the age of 40 years. The majority are malignant but they are rare and represent less than 1% of all male cancers.

The testis has two functions, the production of spermatozoa and hormones and there are three cell types concerned in these processes:

1. Germ cells are spermatogenic cells which line the seminiferous tubules and produce spermatozoa in four stages (spermatogonia, primary spermatocytes, secondary spermatocytes and spermatids).

2. Sertoli cells are the cells in the seminiferous tubules which provide a supporting framework and perhaps nourishment for the developing spermatozoa. They also produce oestrogens and are probably under the control of the follicular stimulating hormone of the pituitary gland.

3. Leydig cells are interstitial cells in the lobules of the testis specialized to produce androgens which stimulate and maintain sex characteristics. They are probably stimulated by the luteinizing hormone of the pituitary gland.

Surgical pathology

Imperfect descent is thought to be an important predisposing factor to malignant change.

CLASSIFICATION OF TESTICULAR TUMOURS

Neoplasms of the testes may be either primary or secondary. The primary tumours are derived principally from the germinal epithelium. It is believed that the germinal tumours arise from a totipotent germ cell. This totipotent cell is thought to be capable of giving rise to either a seminoma or an embryonal carcinoma which in turn can develop either along 'extra-embryonic' lines (yolk sac tumour, choriocarcinoma) or 'intraembryonic' lines (teratoma).

Germinal
These represent more than 96% of all tumours.

1. Seminoma
2. Embryonal carcinoma
3. Teratoma
4. Choriocarcinoma

Non-germinal
These represent less than 4% of all tumours.

1. Sertoli cell tumour (sertolioma, tubular adenoma)
2. Leydig cell tumour (interstitioma)
3. Orchioblastoma (gynandroblastoma)

4. Supporting tissue tumours: fibroma, lipoma, angioma, rhabdomyoma, neurofibroma, sarcoma, carcinoma of the rete testis, lymphoma

GERMINAL TUMOURS

1. Seminoma. This is the commonest tumour. It arises from the germinal epithelium of the seminiferous tubules in a patient usually between 30 and 40 years of age.

Macroscopically it is a hard, smooth, fleshy tumour; its cut surface is homogeneous and creamy and fibrous septa give the appearance of lobulation.

Microscopically there is considerable variation with large clear polyhedral cells resembling spermatogonia and small lymphocyte-like cells with dark nuclei resembling spermatids. The cells are arranged in clumps or sheets.

Spread is usually by the lymphatics accompanying the cord to reach the para-aortic nodes. The inguinal lymph nodes are not involved unless local spread to the tunica vaginalis or scrotum has occurred. Bloodstream spread, particularly to the liver and lung, is generally a late manifestation.

Hormone effects may occur infrequently and cause feminization.

2. Embryonal carcinoma: the name is reserved for a highly malignant tumour in which the cells lack uniformity and come to resemble embryonal fetal germinal epithelium in a syncytium.

3. Teratoma is highly malignant and rapidly growing tumour which appears between 20 and 30 years and contains structures from all three germinal layers—ectoderm, mesoderm and endoderm.

Macroscopically there is great complexity; the tumour may be smooth or irregular, soft or hard; the cut surface may be cystic, haemorrhagic, necrotic or fleshy.

Microscopically a combination of derivatives from the three primary germinal layers is present, with epithelium, hair, glands, bone, cartilage, muscle, fat and fibrous tissue.

4. Choriocarcinoma. This is a rare tumour which is regarded as a variant of an embryonal carcinoma in which elements of chorionic tissue are present. Occasionally it may be extra-genital in position (mediastinum, retroperitoneum, liver or pineal gland).

Macroscopically the chorionic material appears as a blood clot.

Microscopically there is evidence of both elements of chorionic tissue, with an undifferentiated and primitive syncytium which retains its power to erode blood vessels, and polygonal granular cells (Langhans layer).

Hormone effects are often pronounced and high levels of chorionic gonadotrophins may be excreted in the urine.

NON-GERMINAL TUMOURS

These are exceedingly rare benign tumours, but are of interest because of their hormonal effects.

1. Sertoli cell tumour. A common tumour in dogs; when it occurs in man feminization results.

Microscopically sertoli cells occur in compact alveolar masses. They are slender and pyramidal shaped with oval nuclei and cytoplasm extends to the lumen of the seminiferous tubules as slender processes to which may be attached heads of spermatozoa.

2. Leydig cell tumour (interstitial cell tumour) accounts for about 1% of all testicular tumours and is by far the most remarkable.

Microscopically the tumour consists of large, round, slightly acid-staining cells with dark, round nuclei arranged in a pattern strongly suggestive of liver cords.

There is an excess androgen production, and is responsible for the production of precocious puberty when it appears in prepubertal years. However, for some unknown reason, feminization occurs in about 50% of cases when it appears in post-pubertal years.

3. Supporting tissue tumours and orchioblastomas are very rare and not associated with hormone production.

Clinical features

Symptoms

Testicular tumours may present the following features:

1. A painless testicular lump only noted after minor trauma
2. A slightly painful testicular lump growing rapidly over weeks or months
3. A hydrocele, which is associated with 5% of testicular tumours
4. Weight loss, malaise, cough due to metastatic spread to lungs and lymph nodes
5. Feminizing effects, particularly gynaecomastia

Signs

1. Local

    a. A painless, swollen and hard testis
    b. A small secondary hydrocele

2. General
   A search is made for metastases, particularly in the para-aortic chain of lymph nodes, and for evidence of feminization.

Staging
Perhaps the single most important step in the management of a testicular tumour is its staging. To stage a tumour adequately the following investigations are required:

a. Serum alpha fetoprotein (tumour marker)
b. Serum human chorionic gonadotrophin (tumour marker)
c. Chest X-ray

(all prior to orchiectomy)

d. Lung tomography
e. Intravenous urogram
f. Lymphangiography

The last three investigations, which have been used to detect lymph node or lung involvement, may become superceded by CT scanning of the chest and abdomen.

Stage I   No clinical evidence of disease. Tumour markers return to normal after orchiectomy.
Stage II   Demonstrable involvement of the para-aortic nodes
Stage III Involvement of the mediastinal lymph nodes and parenchymal metastases

Treatment of malignant testicular tumours

SEMINOMA
Stage I   Inguinal orchiectomy and radiotherapy to the para-aortic nodes (2500–3000 rad)
Stage II   Inguinal orchiectomy and radiotherapy to the para-aortic and mediastinal nodes
Stage III This stage will require elements of the above and chemotherapy. The agents in common use are cis-platinum, vinblastine and methotrexate.

NON-SEMINOMATOUS TUMOURS
Stage I   Inguinal orchiectomy and para-aortic lymph node dissection. In some centres para-aortic node irradiation is preferred, but it would seem that node dissection has marginally better survival figures.
Stage II   Requires combined therapy, and this may include surgery to remove bulky lymph node metastases and chemotherapy
Stage III Chemotherapy and surgical removal of large metastases if possible

Prognosis

SEMINOMA
For stage one and two disease the 5-year survival is 98% and 75% respectively.

NON-SEMINOMATOUS TUMOURS
For stage one and two disease 5-year survivals of 85% and 75% can be anticipated with the advent of triple agent chemotherapy.

TORSION

This is a surgical emergency which is commonly referred to as torsion of the testis, though the twist is always in the lowest part of the spermatic cord or the mesorchium.

Predisposing factors

Abnormalities, which are often bilateral, said to predispose to torsion include:

1. Long mesorchium
2. Horizontal testis
3. Ectopic testis
4. Capacious tunica vaginalis
5. Well developed spiral cremaster muscle

Surgical pathology

The cord usually twists from without inwards; occasionally the cord may untwist spontaneously but in the majority of cases necrosis of the testis will occur unless operation is performed. Operation must be performed as rapidly as possible if damage is to be minimized.

Clinical features

There is a sudden onset of lower abdominal and testicular pain. The localization of the pain to the T12, L1 segment of the abdomen (the developmental origin of the testes) can cause diagnostic confusion unless the condition is thought of and the testis and scrotum are carefully examined.

The testis is swollen and drawn up and a small hydrocele is often present in an oedematous scrotum.

Differential diagnosis

See epididymo-orchitis

Treatment

This is always operative when the diagnosis is certain or

when epididymo-orchitis cannot be excluded. The steps of the operation are to:

1. Expose the testis and untwist the cord or mesorchium
2. Establish viability—return of colour and free bleeding
3. Fix testis to tunica vaginalis
4. Perform orchidectomy if testis is not viable
5. Fix the opposite testis

CYSTS OF THE EPIDIDYMIS

These are common and may be unilateral or bilateral, single or multilocular cysts. They lie above and behind the testis and contain crystal clear fluid or opalescent fluid and spermatozoa.

Most probably they arise from vestigal remnants in the epididymis or vasa efferentia; the pedunculated hydatid of Morgagni; the appendix of the epididymis; and the paradidymis or organ of Giraldes (all being remnants of the mesonephric or Wolffian duct system); or the sessile hydatid of Morgagni or appendix testis (remnants of the paramesonephric or Mullerian duct system). Alternatively they may be acquired as retention cysts of the vasa efferentia.

Cysts which communicate with the seminiferous tubules and contain spermatozoa are sometimes referred to as spermatoceles, but the differentiation is of no practical value.

Treatment by excision is indicated if cysts are large enough to cause persistent pain or discomfort but most do not require any treatment.

May undergo torsion ∴ Testicular pain.

SPERMATIC CORD

VARICOCELE

It is commonly held that a varicocele is a dilatation and elongation of the pampiniform plexus of veins. The plexus is a mass of intercommunicating veins accompanying the testicular artery in the spermatic cord which joins to form 2 or 3 testicular veins in the inguinal canal and one testicular vein at the level of the internal inguinal ring. Almost invariably the left side is involved. While the angle of entry of the left spermatic vein into the renal vein has been invoked to explain this left sided preponderance, this seems to be a too simple explanation.

Clinical features

A 'worm-like' collection in the scrotum which is visible and palpable on standing.

Pain of a dull dragging nature which may extend into the groin.

Depression of spermatogenesis may occur and is presumably due to impaired heat loss in the scrotum. It is said that unless the testes are kept at a temperature of 2.5°C below rectal temperature normal spermatogenesis will not occur.

Treatment

Conservative. Reassurance and a suspensory bandage usually suffices and tight Y-front underpants may relieve ache and discomfort.

Operative. This is indicated rarely for infertility or continuing pain and discomfort.

The standard operation entails ligature of testicular veins in the inguinal canal. An alternative method is to explore the scrotum and divide the cremasteric veins, but damage to the testicular artery is a hazard of this approach.

TUNICA VAGINALIS

HYDROCELE

A collection of fluid within the tunica vaginalis.

Primary hydrocele

There is no associated disease of the underlying testis or epididymis and the hydrocele may be:

1. Congenital
2. Infantile
3. Vaginal
4. An encysted hydrocele of the cord (Fig. 33.1)

Secondary hydrocele

There is underlying inflammation or a neoplasm of the testis or epididymis.

SURGICAL PATHOLOGY
In a primary hydrocele of the congenital type there is

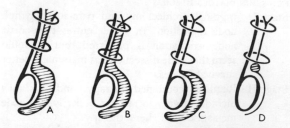

Fig. 33.1 Types of hydrocele **A.** Congenital **B.** Infantile **C.** Vaginal (commonest) **D.** Encysted hydrocele of cord

incomplete obliteration of the processus vaginalis and the tunica vaginalis is distended with peritoneal fluid. In the infantile and the encysted types there is partial obliteration of the processus vaginalis. In the common vaginal type of hydrocele the tunica vaginalis is distended with varying amounts of straw-coloured fluid the origin of which is unknown. In long standing cases the tunica vaginalis becomes thickened and the underlying testis and epididymis flattened.

In secondary hydroceles the fluid collection in the tunica vaginalis may be rapid as in acute epididymo-orchitis or torsion of the testis, or slow as with chronic inflammation or testicular tumours. The fluid is usually an exudate which in the presence of a tumour is often blood-stained.

CLINICAL FEATURES

A hydrocele presents as a tense or lax unilocular translucent scrotal swelling which may be emptied on lying down if it is congenital in type.

The testis cannot be clearly separated from the hydrocele which lies anterior to it.

TREATMENT

Aspiration

This is essential when the hydrocele appears in adults so that the underlying testis can be accurately palpated for any underlying disorder. The site for aspiration in the scrotum is usually anterior but it must be carefully determined by transillumination so that the testis can be avoided. Aspiration may be repeated for recurring tense hydroceles associated with discomfort and techniques have been described for the installation of sclerosing agents into the hydrocele which will prevent the reaccumulation of fluid.

Operation

This is the method of choice when repeated aspirations fail to control the hydrocele.

The tunica vaginalis can be partially excised and everted behind the epididymis if it is thin-walled (Jaboulay's operation); alternatively it can be completely excised if it is thick-walled and chronic. Meticulous haemostasis is particularly important.

HAEMATOCELE

This may follow trauma to the scrotum, or after an inguinal or scrotal operation or aspiration of a hydrocele.

A tense painful swelling occurs which is treated by scrotal elevation, bed rest and analgesics.

Its major importance is often in the differential diagnosis of an enlarged testis.

34

Urinary tract disorders

SYMPTOMS

Many symptoms may be associated with urinary tract disease. However, there are three that between them cover most urological presentations: pain, haematuria and disordered micturition.

Pain

Pain results from:

1. Obstruction of the flow of urine with muscular contraction and distension proximal to the site. Thus a stone in the pelvic-ureteric junction or ureter produces:

   a. Colic
   b. Distension pain—dragging, continuous—in the loin

2. Inflammation of any level of the urinary tract—continuous pain associated also with 'burning' on micturition
3. Expansion by a tumour causing capsular distension. This produces a dragging aching pain which may become more severe if haemorrhage occurs into the tumour substance.

Haematuria

Haematuria occurs as a result of:

1. Parenchymal renal bleeding
   a. Anticoagulants
   b. Micro infarcts, e.g. in subacute bacterial endocarditis
   c. Nephritis
2. Any renal tract disorder from renal pelvis to urethra which can cause a breached or ulcerated surface

   a. External trauma
   b. Calculus and foreign bodies—internal trauma
   c. Inflammation—acute or chronic (tuberculosis)

Difficulty with micturition

Difficulty with micturition includes:

1. Obstructive symptoms which range from hesitancy and poor stream to complete obstruction
2. Disorders of control—chiefly continence

By far the commonest cause of *obstructive symptoms* in the male is benign prostatic hypertrophy. Other causes are:

1. Lesions of the bladder—malignant tumour and calculus
2. Carcinoma of the prostate
3. Urethral stricture from previous injury or inflammation (usually gonorrhoea)

Disorders of control may occur in prostatic disease in men because of mechanical interference with the internal sphincter. In both sexes they may be the consequence of interference with the nervous mechanism of the bladder:

1. Spinal cord trauma or compression (e.g. by tuberculosis or tumour)
2. Degenerative diseases—subacute combined degeneration, disseminated sclerosis
3. Damage to pelvic nerves—e.g. at surgery

In females, incontinence follows pelvic floor trauma in childbirth where it is usually, but not uniformly, associated with prolapse.

SURGICAL PATHOLOGY

Urinary calculi

The mode of formation of urinary calculi remains uncertain.

There are two types of urinary calculi:

1. Primary calculi are those which develop in an apparently normal urinary tract in the presence of acid urine and when there is usually some metabolic disturbance. There is usually no nidus upon which crystallization occurs. It is possible that these calculi develop in renal papillae as subepithelial plaques which later cause erosion of the papillae and allow subsequent precipitation of urinary crystalloids.

2. Secondary calculi develop in an infected and alkaline urine where bacteria, debris and products of inflammation act as a nidus for the precipitation of urinary crystalloids.

The various types of urinary calculi are:

1. Calcium oxalate calculi which are radio-opaque, solitary, hard and whitish, with sharp projections, and occur in an alkaline urine (*mulberry calculi*). These account for about 80% of urinary tract calculi.
2. Phosphate calculi which occur in strongly alkaline urine infected with urea-splitting organisms such as *B.proteus* and *E.coli*. These are dirty white, chalky, radio-opaque calculi which may reach considerable size and fill calyceal systems (staghorn calculi). They are composed of calcium, magnesium and ammonium phosphate (triple phosphate) and account for about 10% of all urinary tract calculi.
3. Uric acid calculi which are radiolucent, multiple and faceted. They form in acid urine and account for about 10% of urinary calculi.
4. Cystine calculi are marginally radio-opaque due to the high sulphur content. They result from an inborn error of tubular function which is manifest by increased excretion of a number of amino-acids, of which cystine is the least soluble.
5. Xanthine and phenyl pyruvate stones are very rare and result from metabolic abnormalities.

PREDISPOSING FACTORS TO CALCULUS FORMATION
1. Dehydration
2. Metabolic disorders—hyperparathyroidism
3. Stasis
4. Infection
5. Diet
6. Lack of urinary inhibitors of crystalization

COMPLICATIONS OF URINARY CALCULI

1. Obstruction. Most urinary calculi form in the kidney or the bladder and small calculi can be passed from the kidney along the full length of the urinary tract. Impaction and obstruction is most likely to occur at the pelvi-ureteric junction or in the ureter, either at the level where it crosses the common iliac vessels or where it is about to enter the bladder.

In the case of a solitary kidney or if the stones are bilateral, this may lead to anuria.

2. Infection. Obstruction of the urinary tract predisposes to hydronephrosis, hydro-ureter and infection, which may then lead to pyonephrosis with rapid destruction of the kidney.

3. Stricture formation and malignancy are rare sequelae of stones.

Urinary tuberculosis

Tuberculous infection of the kidneys usually represents haematogenous spread from a distant site such as the lung, cervical lymph nodes, gut or bone; occasionally it is part of a generalized miliary tuberculosis.

The earliest lesions are multiple foci in the renal cortex close to the medulla, which may either heal without symptoms or radiological changes, or aggregate, caseate and ulcerate into a calyx. In the latter case, spread of tubercle bacilli is likely to occur by means of the urine or the lymphatics to other parts of the renal tract and the bladder, prostate, seminal vesicles and epididymis are particularly likely to be involved.

If the disease is untreated, extensive destruction of the renal parenchyma, with pyonephrosis or perinephric abscess may occur; occasionally the kidney is completely destroyed and replaced by a caseous or calcified mass (autonephrectomy).

Ureteric involvement may lead to obstruction with consequent hydronephrosis while bladder involvement is associated with haematuria in the early stages and later intractable frequency as fibrosis and contraction occur.

Renal tumours

These arise from the kidney or the renal pelvis and account for about 2% of all malignancies of the body.

KIDNEY TUMOURS
1. *Benign*. Angioma, adenoma or haemangioma are rare but occasionally responsible for haematuria.
2. *Malignant*. There are two types:

a. Adenocarcinoma (hypernephroma, Grawitz tumour, clear cell carcinoma). This accounts for about 75% of all renal tumours and occurs more frequently in males over 40 years of age. It arises from renal tubules and not, as was once supposed, from adrenal rests. 'Hypernephroma' is therefore an undesirable term.

Macroscopically it appears as a well-encapsulated tumour usually near one or other poles of the kidney; the cut surface is characteristically golden yellow and honey-combed with radiating septa and areas of haemorrhage and necrosis.

Microscopically there are sheets, columns or clumps of large cuboidal or columnar cells with clear cytoplasm and small darkly staining nuclei. The cytoplasm contains glycogen, cholesterol and fat which account for the yellow colour of the tumour.

The stroma is rich in thin-walled delicate blood vessels.

Spread of the tumour may occur by the following routes:

(i) *Direct*. Expansion of the tumour may slowly encroach upon the calyceal system which it finally invades to cause haematuria.

(ii) *Bloodstream*. The renal vein and inferior vena cava are involved in about 40% of cases. Thus metastases in bones, particularly the spine, pelvis, ribs, humerus and the lungs are likely to occur.

(iii) *Lymphatic*. To the para-aortic and renal lymph nodes.

b. Nephroblastoma (embryoma, adenosarcoma, Wilms's tumour). This is an anaplastic mixed connective tissue tumour which accounts for about 10% of renal tumours, 20% of all malignancies in children and over 50% of malignancies in infants. It occurs mainly between the ages of 0–3 years, but never after 7 years.

The origin of the tumour is disputed, but it is generally believed to be derived from a mesodermal malformation which may represent misplaced nephrogenic mesenchyme or remnants of the mesonephros.

Macroscopically it appears as a pale grey or 'brain-like' tumour which grows rapidly to compress the surrounding kidney; its cut surface shows areas of necrosis, haemorrhage, softening and cyst formation.

Microscopically there is considerable variation of connective tissue elements (spindle cells, cartilage, muscle, bone) and epithelial elements (primitive renal tubules, irregular acini, clumps or columns of cells). Connective tissue or sarcomatous elements usually predominate.

Spread directly to adjacent structures is common, while blood-stream and lymphatic spread occurs later than with adenocarcinoma.

RENAL PELVIS TUMOURS
Account for about 10% of all renal tumours.

a. Transitional cell carcinomas arise as solitary or multiple tumours from the transitional epithelium of the renal pelvis. Recently, a significant association has been established between analgesic abuse and this type of tumour. It would appear that a 'field change' occurs in the epithelium and other tumours may appear in the urinary tract.

b. Squamous cell carcinoma. This is a rare tumour of the urinary tract and may arise from epithelium which shows metaplastic or leukoplakic changes due to chronic irritation from a renal calculus.

Bladder tumours

Epithelial tumours account for at least 95% of all primary bladder tumours. Connective tissue tumours (myoma, fibroma, angioma and sarcoma) are rare.

PREDISPOSING FACTORS

1. Aniline dyes. Workers in chemical and dye industries, in the clothing trade, and those concerned with the production of coloured magazines and comics, may be exposed to alpha or beta naphthylamine, benzidine, auramine or magenta dyes, which are carcinogenic substances. It is known that persons exposed to beta naphthylamine have a 60 times greater chance of developing carcinoma of the bladder than the general population and those exposed to benzidine a 19 times greater chance.

2. Tryptophane metabolism. Abnormal tryptophane metabolism in otherwise normal people and in some leukaemic patients, when there is difficulty in metabolizing pyridoxine, may predispose to the development of carcinoma of the bladder.

3. Bladder irritation. Infestation of the perivesical veins by the trematode *Schistosoma haematobium* and subsequent ulceration and chronic infection of the bladder wall may predispose to squamous cell carcinoma.

4. Miscellaneous. Adenocarcinomas may develop in urachal remnants.

Macroscopically epithelial tumours of the bladder may be papillary, solid, or partly papillary and partly solid.

These tumours are often multiple and, although any part of the bladder may be involved, they are particularly common at the base and trigone and around the ureteric orifices.

Microscopically. A number of histological appearances have been described.

a. Benign papilloma. This has a central core of connective tissue supporting a thin layer of regular transitional cells identical with those of normal bladder mucosa.

b. Malignant tumours
Carcinoma in situ: this is characterised by a thin abnormal epithelium with moderate to marked variation in nuclear size.

Grade I: in these tumours there is invasion of the lamina propria and the cells are uniform without significant pleomorphism.

Grade II: has moderate nuclear variability and a loss of the basement membrane.

Grade III: characterized by highly pleomorphic cells with loss of maturation.

To these types may be added two rarer tumours: squamous cell carcinoma, which grows slowly and metastasizes late, and adenocarcinoma, which usually arises in the base of the bladder or occasionally from the dome (when it probably arises from a urachal remnant).

Spread of epithelial tumours may be:

1. *Direct*, to infiltrate the bladder wall, prostate, urethra, vagina, colon and rectum. When situated close to the ureteric orifices obstruction with hydro-ureter and hydronephrosis can occur.
2. *Lymphatic*, to the perivesical, iliac and para-aortic nodes, particularly with solid tumours
3. *Blood-stream*, to the liver, lungs and bones, particularly in the case of solid tumours
4. *Implantation*, to involve other parts of the bladder or an abdominal operation wound

Staging of epithelial tumours is determined after a complete urological examination:

T1S The tumour is confined to the epithelium

T1 The tumour involves the epithelium and extends through the lamina propria

T2 The tumour has invaded the superficial layers of the detrusor muscle

T3 The tumour has infiltrated deeply into the detrusor muscle and may extend into the perivesical fat but is still mobile

T4 The tumour involves contiguous structures and is fixed

The prognosis of epithelial tumours depends on the following factors:

1. Histological grade
2. Clinical stage

Of the two, the stage is probably the most important determinant of outcome. However, the two are often difficult to separate as the high grade tumours tend to have a high stage at the time of diagnosis.

Thus once a tumour has a solid component, an anaplastic epithelium and is at stage T2 or beyond, the outlook is poor.

Carcinoma of the prostate

This is the commonest malignancy of the genito-urinary tract and it accounts for about 10% of all male malignancies. It occurs most commonly after the age of 60 and it is rare below the age of 50 years.

Macroscopically it starts in the outer zones of the prostate, particularly in the posterior lobe, and grows as a hard, pale, nodular tumour.

Microscopically it is usually a differentiated adenocarcinoma in a well-developed fibrous stroma; occasionally it is anaplastic.

Spread of carcinoma of the prostate may be:

1. *Direct*, upwards and laterally to the peri-prostatic tissues, bladder, urethra and seminal vesicles, is usually slow. Posterior spread to the rectal wall is unusual and it appears to be limited by the fascia of Denonvillier; however perirectal spread occasionally leads to a rectal stricture.
2. *Lymphatic*, to the internal iliac, para-aortic and mediastinal nodes is common and early. Retrograde spread to the inguinal nodes may also occur as a late manifestation.
3. *Blood-stream*, to bone is characteristic of prostatic carcinoma and osteosclerotic lesions are particularly likely to affect the pelvis, lumbar spine and upper femora. The mode of involvement of bone is disputed but it may be by way of the systemic circulation or by way of a communication between the prostatic venous plexus and the pelvic and vertebral veins. Spread may also occur to the liver, lungs, skin, skull and other sites.

Benign prostatomegaly

The prostate, which is a fibro-muscular organ permeated by glandular elements, commonly enlarges by the formation of an adenomatous mass in men over the age of 45.

Glandular and fibro-muscular hyperplasia predominantly affects the lateral and middle lobes with the formation of nodules which enlarge and compress the peripheral parts of the prostate to form a false capsule.

However, the extent of the enlargement does not correlate with the severity of the urinary symptoms.

The cause for benign hypertrophy of the prostate is not known but may be related to changes in the oestrogen-androgen ratio in aging men.

Effects of prostatomegaly with outflow obstruction

1. *Bladder*. This undergoes hypertrophy with increased vascularity, trabeculation and diverticula formation. Stagnation of urine may lead to infection and the development of vesical calculi.
2. *Ureters*. Dilatation and reflux of urine occur.
3. *Kidneys*. Calyceal dilatation, pyelonephritis and later impaired renal function will occur.

Haematuria in association with prostatomegaly may be

due to varicose vesical or prostatic veins, or to an associated cystitis or vesical calculus.

INVESTIGATION OF A PATIENT WITH HAEMATURIA

The presence of blood in the urine always demands full urological evaluation.

HISTORY

The history is of considerable importance in the management of patients with haematuria.

Age. Special attention should be paid to age. Often the age of the patient will provide a valuable guide to the likely cause of haematuria. Haematuria in young children suggests a congenital cause, whereas in an elderly person it suggests a malignant one.

Confirmation of haematuria. It is important by means of the history to try to confirm that the patient has had haematuria. In some instances patients may confuse dark or coloured urine with haematuria, and so it is important to try to determine whether the patient noticed whether the urine was cloudy as well as discoloured. Red cells will make the urine opalescent. In women it is also important to establish that blood has come from the urinary tract and not from the vagina. This is particularly important in postmenopausal women who may sometimes mistake postmenopausal bleeding for haematuria. In those circumstances the two can readily be distinguished by asking the patient whether there was spotting or staining of her underwear.

Pain. The presence of pain suggests either an inflammatory or an obstructive process. If there is no pain, then one is more likely to be dealing with a neoplastic process or a renal parenchymal problem such as glomerulonephritis.

Trauma. It is necessary, particularly in young people, to exclude trauma as a possible cause for haematuria, and in young children minor trauma may produce haematuria and thereby unmask a congenital abnormality.

Drugs. It is important to determine whether patients are on anticoagulant therapy. Haematuria should not be ignored in these circumstances unless there has been gross bleeding from other sites. Often the anti-coagulants will cause bleeding from an unsuspected bladder malignancy, or because the patient is on anticoagulants more diligent examination of urine will show up previously unnoticed haematuria.

Past history. It is important to obtain information about previous problems as many disease processes that cause haematuria, such as calculi and urothelial tumours, are recurrent.

SIGNS

General. A careful search is made for evidence of a medical cause for the haematuria, for features of widespread metastases from a urinary tract malignancy and for renal failure.

Local. A renal swelling is occasionally palpable with renal carcinoma or hydronephrosis.

A bladder tumour is occasionally palpable on bimanual examination at which time its degree of fixation must be noted.

A distended bladder may be palpable suprapubically in the presence of bladder-neck obstruction due to prostatomegaly or prostatic carcinoma.

When benign hypertrophy of the lateral lobes is present rectal examination reveals an enlarged firm elastic prostate with well-demarcated median and lateral grooves; alternatively ar irregular, nodular, hard prostate in association with obliteration of the grooves, fixation of the rectal mucosa and lateral and upward spread indicates carcinoma.

INVESTIGATION

1. *Examination of the urine.* Culture of a mid stream specimen of urine should be performed before any treatment is undertaken. A sterile pyuria is due to tumour, analgesic nephropathy or tuberculosis until proven otherwise. Depending on the age of the patient it is also very important to examine a recently voided specimen of urine for casts. Failure to examine urine samples carefully for casts may lead to an inappropriate pattern of investigation.

2. *Exfoliative cytology.* In patients over the age of 50 or if a urothelial malignancy is suspected, urine should be sent for cytologic examination.

3. If casts have not been detected, then the patient should have an *intravenous urogram.* The only common exception would be young female patients in whom the degree of haematuria has been minimal and has almost certainly been the result of a lower urinary tract infection.

4. *Cytoscopy.* This should be performed unless some specific abnormality has been detected either in the urine or after the intravenous urogram. If all previous investigations are normal cystoscopy is required, as the intravenous urogram does not define bladder lesions sufficiently well to avoid this step.

It is important to point out that many conditions that cause haematuria do so episodically, and so, if on the basis of the history a clinician is convinced that there has been significant haematuria, all the above investigations need to be performed even though the urine is now clear of blood on microscopy. Thus the importance of taking a careful history in the management of this problem. If after these investigations no abnormality is found and the urine is clear of blood, then the most prudent course is to wait and cystoscope the patient, if possible during the next episode of haematuria. This will provide the best chance of establishing the diagnosis and if there is no bladder lesion, it is usually possible to determine which ureter the bleeding is coming from, thus allowing selective renal arteriography to be performed.

MANAGEMENT OF COMMON DISORDERS

Urinary calculi

PROPHYLAXIS
1. Encourage a high fluid intake to achieve an output of 1.5l per day.
2. Provide dietary advice, depending upon the nature of the stone.
3. Correct metabolic abnormalities, such as hyperparathyroidism due to a parathyroid tumour.
4. Correct any urinary tract obstruction and prevent infection.
5. In patients with recurrent calcium-containing stones, the use of thiazide diuretics or cellulose phosphate may be beneficial. In the case of patients with uric acid stones, alkalization of the urine and allopurinol are valuable in preventing recurrence.

Renal calculi

INDICATIONS FOR OPERATION
1. Obstruction
2. Size of stone. In most instances small stones are best left alone. However, once the stone becomes greater than 1 cm in diameter and is causing obstruction, then it is unlikely to pass spontaneously and it is preferably removed electively. Sometimes the stones can be very large and form a calculus (staghorn) which is moulded to the shape of the calyceal system. Whilst these stones may produce few symptoms, they are best removed when first diagnosed.
3. Infection. A combination of obstruction and infection can have disastrous consequences, and whenever these two co-exist the obstruction must be relieved.

TYPE OF OPERATION

1. Nephrolithotomy. The renal substance is incised over the stone and the stone removed. This approach is usually used if a stone is imprisoned in a calyx or where there is an intrarenal pelvis which is unsatisfactory for an extended pyelolithotomy.

2. Pyelolithotomy. In this operation the stone is removed from the renal pelvis after the posterior surface of the renal pelvis has been cleared and opened. Greater exposure can be obtained by dissecting into the renal sinus.

3. Partial nephrectomy. This approach is occasionally used if there is a large number of calculi in a lower calyx and there is considerable distortion and damage of the calyceal system.

4. Nephrectomy. It is unusual to need to undertake nephrectomy for a stone and as renal calculus disease is frequently a bilateral problem, functioning renal tissue should be preserved wherever possible.

Ureteric calculi

The hallmarks of treatment are:
1. Pain relief
2. Maintenance of an adequate fluid intake
2. Mobilization of the patient

INDICATIONS FOR OPERATION
1. Stone too large to pass, usually greater than 1 cm
2. Failure of a moderate sized stone 0.5–1 cm in size to progress over a 4–6 week interval
3. Severe or continuous pain
4. Infection
5. Anuria

The operations available for ureteric calculi include the following:

1. Endoscopic manipulation. It is sometimes possible to remove stones from the lower end of the ureter using a special basket extractor. It is also possible to remove stones from the upper ureter by passing a nylon loop attached to a ureteric catheter above the stone and allowing the catheter to fall out drawing the stone down with it. By this means quite large ureteric stones can be removed.

2. Ureterolithotomy. Stones can be removed by an extraperitoneal route if it is thought that they will not pass spontaneously and are causing obstruction.

Urinary tuberculosis

There is now little place for surgery in the management of urinary tuberculosis. The treatment of choice is rest, diet and the prolonged administration of antituberculosis drugs. The treatment needs to be administered until the urine is sterile. The principal indication for surgical treatment is ureteric stricturing. This will often occur after therapy and so patients need to be carefully followed. In many instances the stricturing can be overcome by periodic endoscopic dilatation using ureteric catheters. In rare instances severe contraction of the bladder may occur after treatment and ileocystoplasty or some other bladder enlarging procedure may need to be undertaken to overcome disabling frequency.

Renal tumours

a. ADENOCARCINOMA

Presentation. The most common reasons for presentation are:

1. Haematuria
2. Loin pain
3. A renal mass

Others reasons for presentation may be as a result of:

1. Systemic effects of the tumour, such as fever, malaise or weight loss
2. Metastatic spread, either to lungs, skin or bone (pathological fracture)
3. Endocrine effects on either haemopoietic, hepatic or skeletal systems

Investigations. 1. To diagnose the tumour the following investigations are usually required:

a. An intravenous urogram — to indicate a space-occupying lesion
b. Ultrasound—to confirm its solid nature
c. Arteriography or CT scan—for final confirmation

2. To stage the tumour a bone scan and a chest X-ray are usually performed. However, recent studies would suggest that if the serum alkaline phosphatase is elevated, this is invariably associated with bony metastases and so an elevated alkaline phosphatase may preclude the need to undertake a bone scan.

Treatment. The treatment of choice is nephrectomy with removal of the kidney and its perinephric fat. While radiotherapy and chemotherapy have been used in the treatment of this condition, to date their addition has appeared to contribute little to improving patient survival.

b. NEPHROBLASTOMA

The treatment of choice is excision of the tumour followed by chemotherapy.

Renal pelvis tumours

Presentation. Haematuria is the most common reason for presentation.

Diagnosis. An intravenous urogram will usually indicate some distortion of the calyceal system, however this may need to be confirmed by a retrograde ureterogram.

Also the presence of abnormal cells in the urine will assist in the confirmation of a filling defect seen on either the intravenous urogram or retrograde ureterogram.

Treatment. Wherever possible, nephro-ureterectomy is indicated. The ureter, plus a cuff of bladder mucosa, needs to be removed because there appears to be a field change, and hence the entire urothelium on that side needs to be ablated. These tumours usually have a poor prognosis and do not respond to either radiotherapy or single-agent chemotherapy. After nephrectomy patients will require repeat urograms and cystoscopies because of the possibility of recurrence in the remaining urothelium.

Bladder tumours

Presentation. Most patients present with haematuria.

Diagnosis. Whilst the intravenous urogram may be diagnostic, cystoscopy is necessary to confirm the diagnosis and stage the tumour.

Treatment. The treatment options for this condition are:

1. Endoscopic. This approach is usually satisfactory for TI tumours and for some T2 tumours. However, this approach may be inadequate for some high grade T2 tumours, and these patients will need to be followed carefully with repeated endoscopic examinations.

An adjunct to endoscopic treatment of T1 tumours is the intravesical installation of agents such as thiotepa and adriamycin. These agents may have some effect on developed tumours, however their most valuable role is in reducing the recurrence of these tumours.

2. Total cystectomy and urinary diversion. This approach is usually restricted to T2 tumours and some T3 tumours where it is believed the tumour has not spread to the draining lymph nodes. It is usually preceded with radiotherapy to the bladder and lymph nodes in an attempt to sterilise the nodes prior to surgery. This is a major procedure and the general fitness of the patient needs to be carefully assessed before subjecting them to this form of surgery. It is also important that the tumour has been very carefully staged to minimise the likelihood that there are metastases at the time of operation.

3. Radiotherapy. If the tumour is extensive or the patient unsuitable for radical surgery, the treatment of choice is radiotherapy. This is usually given to the tumour and to the iliac lymph nodes. The dose of radiotherapy used is usually between 5500 and 6000 rad.

4. Chemotherapy. A wide range of agents have been tried in carcinoma of the bladder, but to-date results have been disappointing.

Carcinoma of the prostate

On the basis of the history it is often impossible to separate patients with obstructive symptoms due to benign prostatic hyperplasia from those with carcinoma. The key to the diagnosis is rectal examination. If on rectal examination the prostate feels hard, is irregular or has a well defined nodule, a carcinoma should be suspected. The diagnosis can then be confirmed by biopsy which may be achieved by

a. Aspiration biopsy
b. Needle biopsy
c. Transurethral resection

The aspiration technique appears superior as it has minimal complications and can be performed as an outpatient investigation.

Staging. The important steps in staging a prostatic carcinoma are:

1. Rectal examination with determination of tumour size.
2. Serum acid phosphatase measurement
3. Bone scan
4. Radiological studies, including an intravenous urogram

Stage A: These are tumours that are confined to the prostate but are not detectable on clinical examination. The diagnosis is made on histological criteria from tissue obtained at operation.

Stage B: These tumours are evident on rectal examination. This can be subdivided into:

B1 N a palpable nodule surrounded by normal prostatic tissue
B1 palpable involvement of entire lobe, and
B2 palpable involvement of both lobes.

Stage C: Palpable extra-prostatic tumour, in other words spread beyond the capsule, but no evidence of metastases.

Stage D: where there are lymph nodes or other metastatic involvement.

Treatment. At present the treatment of carcinoma of the prostate is strongly linked to the stage of the disease at the time of diagnosis.

Stages A and B1 are the only stages that are now thought suitable for radical surgery. North American studies have shown very good long-term results for radical prostatectomy and inguinal lymphadenectomy for Stage B1 disease. The alternative approach is to treat all localized disease, Stages A, B and C, with radiotherapy to the prostate. If the disease has spread beyond the prostate, anti-androgen therapy is the treatment of choice.

Suppression of androgens can be achieved either by orchidectomy or by the administration of stilboestrol. The problems associated with orchidectomy are:

1. That an operation is required
2. Patient acceptance cannot always be obtained, and
3. Hot flushes post-orchidectomy can be difficult to control

These problems however appear to be preferable to:

Gynaecomastia
Testicular atrophy
Loss of pubic and facial hair
Fluid retention
Cardiovascular complications

that are associated with oestrogen administration. It would seem that as far as survival and control of the malignancy is concerned, there is little to choose between orchidectomy and oestrogens.

Benign prostatomegaly

Indications for operation:

1. Acute urinary retention
2. Chronic retention with overflow
3. Significant symptoms

Whilst the first two are clear indications for surgery in an appropriately aged patient, the last indication is by no means as clear cut. Thus it is important to take a careful history and to cover the following points.

1. Nature of the stream
2. Hesitancy
3. Frequency of micturition by day and by night
4. Urgency or urge incontinence
5. Ability to completely empty the bladder
6. Infection

Examination. The examination may not be contributory and the most important observation is to determine whether the gland feels benign or malignant. The size of the gland may dictate the surgical approach that is used to overcome the obstruction but as previously indicated, size does not help in determining whether a patient requires prostatectomy. Small glands can be associated with disabling urinary symptoms and conversely, large glands may be associated with minimal symptoms and require no intervention.

Investigations.

1. A midstream specimen of urine is required to exclude infection
2. Serum creatinine to assess renal function
3. An intravenous urogram

4. Measurement of urine flow rates and urodynamic studies if diagnostic uncertainty exists

However, the value of routine intravenous urography in the management of patients with outflow obstruction has been questioned and needs further scrutiny.

Type of operation. In most instances the obstruction due to the prostate can be overcome by transurethral resection.

The relative indications for open operation are:

1. Size. Very large glands may be best treated by an open operation and the size of gland that can be dealt with endoscopically is often dependent upon the experience of the surgeon.
2. Large bladder stones that cannot be crushed
3. A history of previous urethral strictures
4. Diverticula that are narrow-necked, fail to empty and thus require excision

COMPLICATIONS OF PROSTATIC SURGERY

1. Infection and septicaemia. The most dangerous complication of prostatic surgery is still septicaemia. Every attempt needs to be made to prevent this from occurring and no patients should undergo prostatic surgery if the urine is infected.

2. Haemorrhage. Bleeding, both primary and secondary, can complicate prostatic surgery. The important principles are to wash out the clot and ensure that the bladder can drain freely. Providing this is done and adequate transfusion is maintained, it is unusual that bleeding presents a major problem. If, however, frequent bladder washouts are required, then the risk of infection increases and antibiotic prophylaxis is advisable.

3. Incontinence. Sphincteric damage post-prostatectomy still occurs. However, with improved endoscopic equipment this is now much less frequent.

4. Stricture. Any urethral instrumentation can lead to stricture formation, and deterioration in the urinary stream post-prostatectomy should make the clinician consider this possibility.

5. Bladder neck stenosis. This complication which is due to severe fibrosis of the bladder neck is much less frequent than urethral stricture formation, but also needs to be considered if a patient experiences voiding difficulties after prostatectomy.

Other uncommon perioperative complications of transurethral surgery are bladder perforation and hyponatremia as a result of excessive fluid absorption during the procedure. This latter complication can be minimised by limiting resecting time and ensuring that the reservoir is always less than 60 cm above the symphysis pubis.

MANAGEMENT OF RETENTION

The management of acute retention of urine may be considered under the following headings:

1. Establishing diagnosis
2. Relief of the retention
3. Treatment of the cause

(2. and 3. are sometimes combined as a single stage)

Diagnosis

IS IT RETENTION AND NOT ANURIA?
A palpable bladder rising out of the pelvis will settle the issue. Occasionally a catheter must be passed if the bladder is impalpable or to prove that a mass which is felt is or is not bladder.

WHAT IS THE CAUSE?

Age of patient
If the patient is 60 years or over the most likely cause is benign prostatomegaly or prostatic carcinoma.

PAST HISTORY

1. Symptoms of bladder neck obstruction. These usually indicate the presence of a benign or malignant prostatic enlargement and include hesitancy, urgency, dribbling, nocturia, bed wetting, poor stream flow and calibre, scalding (present only in infection) and haematuria.

   There may have been previous attacks of acute retention of urine precipitated by a heavy intake of alcohol.
2. Urethral trauma. Instrumentation, or venereal disease may suggest urethral stricture formation.
3. Recent surgery—hernia repair, haemorrhoidectomy
4. Haematuria may accompany carcinoma of the bladder or vesical calculus.
5. The use of autonomic depressant drugs for hypertension may be the cause of a 'nervous' retention.
6. Neurological disorders or recent symptoms suggesting a neurological problem

EXAMINATION

1. General. Look particularly for evidence of dehydration and uraemia which are more likely to occur with acute-on-chronic retention.

2. Local.

a. The renal areas are palpated for swellings which may indicate hydronephrosis and for tenderness which may suggest the presence of stones or infection in the kidney.

b. The lines of the ureters are palpated for tenderness which may suggest the presence of an associated stone.

c. The bladder is palpated.

d. The testis and epididymis and the cord are palpated on each side for evidence of swellings which may indicate a recent epididymo-orchitis. Their atrophy on the other hand will suggest previous inflammation.

e. The bulbous and penile urethra are palpated for evidence of scars from previous sinuses or thickenings around strictured sites.

f. A rectal examination is essential, remembering that it is impossible to assess accurately the size of the prostate in the presence of a full bladder. However, it should be possible to judge whether the gland is obviously benign or malignant from its contour and consistency. If it is smooth, elastic and uniformly enlarged and the lateral sulci are present and the rectal mucosa moves over it readily, then it is almost certainly benign.

From a consideration of the above it is nearly always possible to establish the likely cause.

Relief of retention

Ideally all patients with *acute* retention of urine should be admitted to hospital without any attempt having been made at catheterization beforehand.

There are two groups of patients: (1) those who pass urine spontaneously after simple measures; (2) those who require preliminary drainage.

THOSE WHO PASS URINE SPONTANEOUSLY AFTER SIMPLE MEASURES

An injection of morphine for pain together with a hot bath and the sound of a running tap, or correction of constipation, may be enough to enable the patient to void spontaneously.

Once the retention is overcome the patient is assessed for elective prostatectomy—which is often still required.

THOSE WHO REQUIRE PRELIMINARY DRAINAGE

When simple measures fail to relieve retention then one of the following methods will be required:

Urethral catheterization

Catheterization should be performed under strict aseptic conditions. Care must be taken to ensure that an adequate amount of a lubricating agent, preferably one containing a local anaesthetic, is introduced into the urethra. A 16 Ch. Foley catheter should then be passed slowly into the bladder and the bladder should be decom-

pressed. Patients with chronic retention and an elevated serum creatinine may have a significant diuresis and will require careful supervision if severe disturbances in fluid and electrolyte balance are to be avoided.

Suprapubic drainage

This is indicated when urethral catheterization has failed to overcome the obstruction. Percutaneous puncture of the full bladder is the treatment of choice.

URINARY INCONTINENCE

Urinary incontinence may be defined as the involuntary loss of urine. In clinical practice there are four main groups:

1. Stress incontinence
2. Urge incontinence
3. Overflow incontinence
4. Total incontinence

STRESS INCONTINENCE

This most commonly occurs in women, but may occur in men after prostatectomy.

History

The patient normally complains of a loss of small to moderate amounts of urine during any activity that increases intra-abdominal pressure, such as sneezing or coughing. The patient is not incontinent at night. In order to assess the extent of patients' incontinence it is important to determine the amount and nature of the protective clothing needed to keep them dry.

Examination

The presence of stress incontinence should be confirmed by getting the patient to cough and strain, both lying and standing. In women it is also important to determine whether there is an associated uterine prolapse, as this may need to be corrected as well as the stress incontinence.

Investigation

If stress incontinence cannot be readily demonstrated, a cystogram and a cystometrogram may need to be performed. In some instances patients have symptoms of both stress and urge incontinence, and in this situation a cystometrogram can be very valuable in demonstrating detrusor instability which is discussed more fully later.

Treatment

Unless the degree of incontinence is minor, the only effective treatment available is surgery. While many approaches are available, both vaginal and suprapubic, their principal aims are to support the bladder neck, bring the urethra closer to the symphysis pubis and elevate the bladder neck so that it is 'intra-abdominal'.

URGE INCONTINENCE

Occurs in both men and women, and may co-exist with stress incontinence. In men it is usually due to detrusor instability secondary to obstruction, whereas in women instability can occur frequently without any evidence of obstruction.

History

The patient complains of frequency, severe urgency and urge incontinence by day and nocturia. In men it is neccessary to determine whether they also have obstructive symptoms.

Examination

It is important to exclude stress incontinence and also to exclude neurological disorders, as the first manifestation of demyelinating diseases such as multiple sclerosis, may be urinary symptoms.

Investigation

In men it is usually clear that the incontinence is due to prostatic obstruction, and the routine evaluations outlined previously in this chapter should be undertaken.

In women the cause of the urgency is not always evident and to establish the diagnosis it may be necessary to undertake cystometry. The value of cystometry is that if the urgency is due to inappropriate contractions of the detrusor, i.e. an unstable bladder, abnormal contractions will be provoked during the filling phase of the cystometrogram.

Treatment

1. Urgency—unstable bladder (motor)
If it is established that the urgency is due to detrusor instability, then bladder training, bio-feedback and anticholingergic drugs, such as propantheline bromide, have all been found to be useful.

2. Urgency—sensory
This group of patients have no detectable abnormality on the filling cystometrogram apart from feeling an urgent desire to void after 100–200 ml of filling. These individuals may be helped by bladder training or bio-feedback, and in some cases symptoms can be improved by trigonal diathermy or urethrotomy.

OVERFLOW INCONTINENCE

Occurs mainly in men, and is due to decompensation of the detrusor as a result of prolonged obstruction.

History

A history of obstructive symptoms needs to be sought for and also diseases, such as diabetes, that may cause autonomic degeneration and an atonic bladder which will lead to poor emptying and dribbling.

Examination

The diagnostic finding is a grossly distended, readily palpable, non-tender bladder.

Investigations

These should be aimed at determining renal function, as in many cases there will be gross renal impairment due to back pressure that follows the chronic obstruction, as well as establishing the cause for the decompensated bladder.

If an atonic bladder is suspected on history, then a cystometrogram can be performed but in most cases the history clearly establishes the cause of the incontinence.

TOTAL INCONTINENCE

In this situation the patient is continuously wet with the bladder acting more as a conduit than a reservoir.

History

The patient complains of permanent wetness and in many instances there will be a history of either a urological operation or symptoms consistent with a neurological problem.

Examination

There may be evidence of a neurological deficit and it is important to determine anal sphincter tone and peri-anal sensation as part of the routine clinical assessment.

Treatment

In some cases, provided bladder function is normal, reconstructive surgery or artificial sphincters can restore urinary control. If reconstructive surgery is inappropriate, some form of appliance is necessary to collect the urine in men or a permanent indwelling catheter can be used in both sexes. A permanent catheter should be used as a last resort. Occasionally urinary diversion is applicable in the management of urinary incontinence.

Venous and related conditions of the lower limb

Four conditions need to be considered

a. Varicose veins
b. Ulceration of the leg
c. Venous thrombosis and pulmonary embolism
d. Swelling of the lower limb

VARICOSE VEINS

Varicose veins are dilated, lengthened and tortuous veins of the superficial venous system of the lower limb. Varicosities of the lower oesophageal and superior haemorrhoidal venous plexuses are excluded here.

SURGICAL ANATOMY

1. Superficial venous system—the system of veins in the subcutaneous tissues

a. Long saphenous vein. This vein arises from the dorsal venous arch on the medial aspect of the foot and courses in front of the medial malleolus up the leg and thigh superficial to the deep fascia before it empties into the femoral vein after passing through the fossa ovalis. It contains more than 12 valves. Just before its junction with the femoral vein, the proximal end of the long saphenous vein usually receives four tributaries: the superficial circumflex iliac, the superficial epigastric and the superficial and deep external pudendal veins. However, considerable variations may occur and any of these tributaries may empty directly into the femoral vein. The long saphenous vein may be duplicated. It may even course up the leg deep to the deep fascia (Fig. 35.1).

b. Short saphenous vein. This vein arises from the dorsal venous arch on the lateral border of the foot behind the lateral malleolus and courses upwards superficial to the deep fascia in the midline of the calf to pierce the deep fascia over the popliteal fossa and enter the popliteal vein. It receives tributaries which pierce the deep fascia from the calf muscles. There are however many

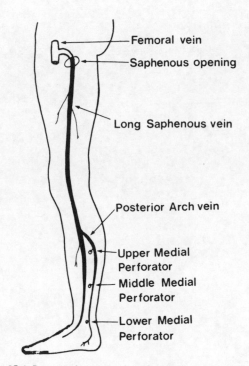

Fig. 35.1 Long saphenous and perforating veins. Medial side of the leg.

variations in its length and depth of course and in its communications with the long saphenous system (Fig. 35.2).

2. Perforator system

The perforating or communicating veins are valved structures passing through the deep fascia and connecting the superficial venous system to the deep system. Under normal conditions they allow blood to flow only from the superficial to the deep system. Incompetence of valves guarding the perforators allows transmission of pressure from deep to superficial systems and reverse flow during exercise.

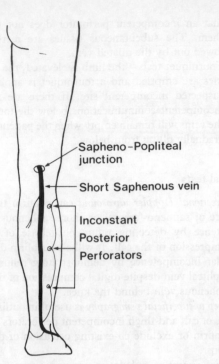

Fig. 35.2 Short saphenous and perforating veins. Posterior aspect of the leg.

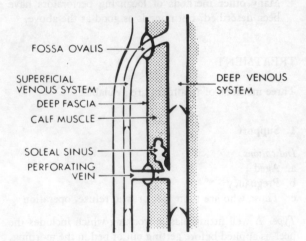

Fig. 35.3 Superficial and deep venous system of lower limb

3. Deep venous system

This is a well supported system comprising the femoral and popliteal veins, veins or venae comitantes accompanying the anterior tibial, posterior tibial and peroneal arteries as well as the valveless blood lakes in the calf muscles (Fig. 35.3). The system communicates with the superficial system at the following sites:

a. Sapheno-femoral junction constantly
b. Subsartorial canal by inconstant perforators
c. Short sapheno-popliteal junction constantly
d. Medial aspect of the leg by perforators
e. Posterior aspect of the leg by inconstant perforators

4. Internal iliac vein and veins of round ligament

Gluteal veins run back from the labia and perineum and upper and inner aspect of the thigh and pass beneath the lower fold of gluteus maximus to enter the pelvis and internal iliac venous system. Veins accompanying the round ligament drain the labia majora and converge into the inguinal canal to enter the ovarian veins.

In pregnancy vulval varicosities are a common occurrence; they are a combination of gluteal veins round ligament veins and superficial and deep external pudendal tributaries of the long saphenous system.

SURGICAL PATHOLOGY

At rest there is little difference between the pressure in the superficial and deep systems. However, on exercise in the normal limb, the muscle pump propels blood centrally, pressure falls in the deep system and blood is 'aspirated' from the superficial system so that pressure also falls in that system. In contrast, if the superficial to deep valves are incompetent, the muscle pump forces blood into the superficial system, preventing the normal fall in pressure. Thus, superficial venous hypertension on exercise because of incompetent deep to superficial valves is the hallmark of varices and the cause of the problem.

The cause of incompetent valves are:

1. Absence at specific sites such as sapheno-femoral in the groin and sapheno-popliteal behind the knee, which seems to have a hereditary element.
2. Thrombosis in either the superficial or the deep system. The valves at the perforator sites are destroyed. In addition, those in recanalized deep veins may be damaged so increasing deep venous hypertension or, if recanalization does not take place, high pressure persists behind the block.

Other contributing factors are:

1. Hormones of pregnancy (progesterone and relaxin), which dilate not only uterine veins but also lower limb veins causing valvular mechanisms to become incompetent. This hormonal effect is maximal in the first three months, a time when the uterus is incapable of producing mechanical obstruction to the iliac veins.
2. Over-active muscle pump in which it is postulated that continuous calf muscle activity of an excessive nature may actually force blood through the perforating system in a reverse direction causing perforator

valve disruption. There is no real evidence to sub-stantiate this concept; there are however many patients with varicose veins in whom no predisposing factor is apparent.

CLINICAL FEATURES

Symptoms

1. The vast majority of superficial varices do not have a demonstrable causative background. However symptoms may be present in relation to:

a. Pregnancy
b. Deep vein thrombosis
c. Pelvic obstruction

2. Symptoms
a. Disfigurement
b. Ache or pain, which may occasionally be 'bursting' and severe in nature, when perforator incompetence is likely to be apparent
c. Pigmentation
d. Swelling
e. Eczema, which may be dry and scaly, or moist, itchy and infected

Signs

1. Of the cause
Pregnancy, pelvic tumours, or previous deep vein thrombosis may be apparent.

2. Of the effect
Two questions must be answered:

   a. Which system is varicose? Inspection of the front and back of the limb with the patient standing will establish whether the long or short saphenous system, or both sys-tems, are varicose.

   b. Which perforator or perforators are incompetent? Sapheno-femoral incompetence is evident from a palpa-ble thrill and a bruit on auscultation, when the patient coughs. Leg perforator incompetence is evident from the following:

   (i) An ankle flare—caused by venular dilatation and most apparent over a triangle centred at the medial malleolus (varicular triangle)
   (ii) A 'blow-out'—a visible varix often situated over the site of a constant medial leg perforator
   (iii) A palpable pit—caused by enlargement of the defect in the deep fascia which transmits the perforators. Both the blowout and the pit may be spurious in

that an incompetent perforator does not underlie them. The subcutaneous tissues are merely hol-lowed out by the dilated vein.
   (iv) Tourniquet tests—the limb is elevated, the varicos-ities are emptied and a tourniquet is applied to a suspected incompetent site. If there are not any incompetent communications below the tourniquet the veins will remain empty when the patient stands, gradually filling from below.

Special tests

1. *Directional Doppler ultrasound* can confirm the pres-ence of sapheno-femoral or short saphenous incom-petence by detecting reflux on release of manual compression of the calf. It will also confirm deep val-vular incompetence by demonstrating reflux in the popliteal vein despite digital compression of the short saphenous vein behind the knee.
2. *Deep to superficial venography* is useful in outlining the site of calf and thigh incompetent perforators and can confirm or exclude co-existing occlusion of the deep veins
3. *Measurement of ambulatory venous pressures* (in a vein on the foot), while a tourniquet controls the super-ficial veins, will confirm deep venous incompetence.
4. Many other methods of localizing perforators have been described, but none is as good as the above.

TREATMENT

Three methods of treatment are available:

1. Support

Indications
a. Aged
b. Pregnancy
c. Those who are unfit for, or who refuse, operation

Type. A well fitting elastic stocking which includes the heel, is applied before getting out of bed in the morning.

2. Injections

Indications
a. Post-operative recurrences
b. Troublesome vulval varicosities
c. As an alternative to surgery

   The usual method has been to inject a sclerosant sol-ution such as 5% ethanolamine oleate (Ethamolin) or 3% sodium tetradecyl sulphate into the varicosities so that intravascular clotting will occur and cause obliteration of the veins. However recanalization is always likely to occur and allow subsequent reformation of varicosities.

The principle can, however, be modified by injecting the sclerosant solution into an empty varicose tributary and maintaining compression over the site for a few weeks in the hope that clotting can be avoided and intravascular granulation tissue will form which will later become fibrous and obliterate the vein lumen permanently (compression sclerotherapy). The injections can be repeated at various sites in the leg but the total amount of sclerosant should not exceed 10–12 ml otherwise haemolytic effects may occur. Also the injections must always be intravascular or skin ulceration may occur.

When compression sclerotherapy is used the compression is maintained by sorbo-rubber pads over the injection sites which are maintained in position by crepe bandage and a full length two-way stretch elastic yarn stocking; it is important to maintain day and night compression for about two weeks after which time the situation is reassessed and further injections and bandages are applied for another two weeks or until the sclerosed veins are no longer tender. Even well done injection sclerotherapy does not work if there is significant deep to superficial incompetence. Thus preliminary surgery is usually a prerequisite to sclerotherapy.

3. Surgery

The principles of the operation are to:

a. Secure incompetent perforator sites
b. Remove the varicosities

The operation entails a dissection of the saphenofemoral junction with division of its tributaries and ligation of the saphenous vein flush with the femoral vein; other incompetent perforator sites (including the saphenopopliteal) are isolated subfascially and then ligated, and varicose systems may be removed with the aid of wire strippers. Smaller varicose tributaries may be avulsed, ligated, punctured, or injected. The wide variety of methods used testifies to the difficulty of ridding some patients of their varices. However, though a cosmetic cure may be difficult, effective interruption of sites of incompetence does relieve symptoms.

ULCERATION OF THE LEG

Ulceration of the leg is a common problem and while those ulcers due to disorders of the venous system account for about 75% of cases there are a number of other possible causes to be considered.

CLASSIFICATION OF CAUSES

1. Venous (by far the commonest)
2. Arterial
3. Traumatic
4. Infective
5. Neuropathic
6. Neoplastic
7. Cryopathic
8. Idiopathic
9. Self-inflicted
10. Miscellaneous

The commoner causes are
1. Venous
2. Arterial
3. Traumatic

VENOUS ULCERATION

Surgical pathology

Leakage of blood under high pressure from the deep veins into the superficial system, particularly in the region of a constantly placed perforator over the medial side of the leg results in venular dilatation (ankle flare) and leathery induration and pigmentation of the skin as the result of stagnation of the circulation, The final cause of poor oxygenation is deposition of fibrin outside the capillary wall. These are pre-ulceration changes and, if the high pressure leakage is allowed to continue, skin ischaemia can occur and ulceration results. Still later, the superficial veins may attract to themselves an increased arterial circulation with the formation of arteriovenous fistulae and arterial blood by-passes the capillary circulation causing the ischaemic process to be prepetuated. This is particularly likely to occur with long-standing ulceration. Trauma and infection may be associated factors.

Clinical features

Patients may or may not have a definite past history of deep vein thrombophlebitis and they may or may not have visible varicosities of the superficial system.

However, there is little doubt that (a) most patients have had a previous deep vein thrombosis and (b) in those who have not (usually men) there is massive sapheno-femoral incompetence.

SIGNS
1. Varicose veins
2. Perforator incompetence

3. The ulcer itself. In over 90% of cases the ulcer will be situated in the distal third of the medial side of the leg.

Treatment

There are two methods available:

1. CONSERVATIVE

Indications
a. Severe ulceration of long duration associated with wide areas of skin involvement with dense fibrosis and brawny swelling
b. Eczema, which may be dry and coarse, scaly, moist or infected
c. Pre-operative preparation for surgery
d. As an alternative to surgery

Those ulcers associated with considerable degrees of peripheral arterial occlusive disease and/or arteriovenous fistulae are extremely difficult to treat and in only a few cases are cures possible.

Method
This depends on whether the ulcer is clean or infected. The latter includes those patients with moist or septic eczema.

a. Clean ulcer
(i) Correct any general disorder, in particular obesity, cardiac failure, anaemia or any debilitating illness.
(ii) Rest the patient in bed with the foot of the bed elevated about 9 inches (22 cm). This will heal the majority of ulcers not complicated by peripheral arterial disease. However, such treatment is not always practicable.
(iii) Apply dressings and compression bandages. A satisfactory regimen was to apply zinc cream to the ulcer, olive oil to the dry surrounding skin and calamine lotion to eczematous areas that itch. Dry gauze is then placed over the ulcer and a felt pad or sponge rubber piece, cut to a size approximating that of the ulcer, is held over the site by a crepe bandage. Over this is applied a one-way stretch elastic bandage from the base of the toes including the heel, up to the knees using a good one half overlap with firm and even pressure, particularly around the foot and ankle.

The patient must be instructed in the efficient application of the bandages so that oedema can be relieved, the pumping and massaging effects of the leg muscles can be assisted and dilated veins and incompetent perforators can be compressed.

Dressings and bandaging are performed as frequently as is necessary; this may be at least twice a week. Once the ulcer has healed the patient may be instructed to wear an efficiently fitted rubberized cotton or nylon stocking. The heel should be included and it must extend from the bases of the toes to at least just below the knee. For maximum benefit the stocking should be applied before rising each morning. It may be discarded at night, provided the foot end of the bed is elevated, or during the day for short periods when calf muscle massage is carried out.

b. Infected ulcer
The aim is to convert an infected ulcer into a clean one and then treat as above.

(i) Swab for culture and sensitivity.
(ii) Apply Eusol soaked gauze to the ulcer frequently to remove slough and pus. Other methods of removing slough have become available but are expensive.
(iii) Omit the use of zinc cream to the ulcer; otherwise all the principles of clean ulcer treatment are carried out.
(iv) Avoid the use of local antibiotics; these are unnecessary and may be dangerous if a sensitivity reaction or a resistant organism develops. Systemic antibiotics are however required in the presence of cellulitis, lymphangitis and lymphadenitis.
(v) Rest the patient in bed if the infective process shows signs of spreading or if the ulcer is requiring frequent toilets.

Once the infection has been controlled the ulcer is treated along the lines indicated for a clean ulcer.

c. Injection sclerotherapy (see p. 262)
Injections of sclerosant are used to obliterate incompetent perforating veins

2. OPERATIVE

Indications
a. Small ulcers with localized changes in the surrounding tissues
b. More extensive ulcers over 2.5 cm in diameter, with a surrounding area of induration over 5 cm in diameter where healing is difficult to achieve or to maintain by conservative means
c. Ulcers in patients with a normal deep venous system

Contraindications
a. Severe ulceration with wide areas of skin deterioration and diffuse brawny oedema. In these cases skin necrosis may occur after a perforator dissection.
b. Presence of infected ulcers or moist or infected eczema
c. An obstructed deep venous system

The operation

This may include:

a. A subfascial perforator dissection
b. Excision of the ulcer, which includes excision of nearby unhealthy skin down to healthy fascia or muscle, and the application of a split skin graft to the defect
c. Treatment of associated varicose veins

OTHER LEG ULCERS

Surgical pathology

ARTERIAL ULCER

Such ulcers are caused by skin ischaemia usually in association with atherosclerotic peripheral vascular disease. Ulceration occurs commonly on the toes, dorsum of the foot anterior tibial area or the heel and appears as patches of dry gangrene.

Buerger's disease (thrombo-angiitis obliterans), a disease of men aged between 20 and 40, may also be associated with skin gangrene.

TRAUMATIC ULCER

This is most likely to occur where skin is closely applied to bony prominences, e.g., shin, malleoli and the back of the heel. Plaster sores and bedsores may be included in this group. A common lesion particularly in the elderly is where a flap of skin is raised by trauma, with its base distally. Though it is replaced it often undergoes necrosis.

INFECTIVE ULCER

a. Pyogenic ulcer. Inoculation with staphylococcal organisms may be so potent as to result in abscess formation and skin necrosis.

b. 'Bairnsdale ulcer'. A chronic inflammatory response in the skin to *Mycobacterium ulcerans* results in the formation of an irregular ulcer with widely undermined edges and pale and 'watery' granulation tissue in its base. Smears reveal many acid fast bacilli.

c. Syphilitic ulcer. Gummatous ulceration of tertiary syphilis is rare in developed places. It tends to occur on the outer side of the leg as the result of necrosis of a chronic granuloma of muscle and is typically a painless punched out ulcer vertical edges and a sloughing base.

NEUROPATHIC ULCERS

Ulcers occurring in association with diseases of the nervous system which result in sensory loss are called 'neuropathic', 'trophic' or 'penetrating' ulcers. The mechanism of their production is one of repeated injury or pressure which is allowed to occur because of loss of appreciation of pain in the area.

Conditions which underlie neuropathic ulceration include diabetic and alcoholic peripheral neuritis, tabes dorsalis and syringomyelia.

The ulcers commonly occur on the sole of the foot or the heel where they may penetrate to bone or joint levels.

(*Note.* Ulceration in association with *diabetes mellitus* may be precipitated by atherosclerosis, infection, peripheral neuritis or a combination of all these factors. The toes and feet are commonly affected.)

NEOPLASTIC ULCER

Metastases from a distant primary source can lodge in the skin and ulcerate but this is rare.

Primary tumour of the skin, e.g. squamous cell carcinoma or malignant melanoma, can also present as ulcers. Malignant change may occur in long-standing venous ulcers, in the scars of old ulcerated burns, or in chronically discharging osteomyelitic sinuses.

Neoplastic ulcers are usually recognized by their heaped up and proliferative edges.

CRYOPATHIC ULCER

Cryopathy is a term used to describe a condition resulting from cold.

a. Chilblains. These are probably the result of intense vasoconstriction of skin arterioles in areas exposed to cold and blisters and ulceration can occur, particularly on the feet.

b. Cold injury.
(i) Immersion of the foot in the wet at just above freezing temperatures can result in ischaemic changes in the skin and subcutaneous tissues which may result in superficial gangrene.
(ii) Exposure to freezing temperatures results in crystallization of tissues and probable denaturation of intracellular protein and destruction of enzyme systems. This causes gangrene of at least the full thickness of the skin.

IDIOPATHIC ULCER

a. Tropical ulcer. These ulcers occur on the legs and feet of people living in the tropics. There is no apparent arterial, venous, or infective process present but sometimes malnutrition appears to be a factor.

b. Martorell's ulcer. Patches of spontaneous skin necrosis of the legs may occur in patients with hypertension but without atherosclerotic peripheral arterial disease. These ulcers have also been described as 'hypertensive ulcers'.

SELF-INFLICTED ULCER

Injury to the skin by scratching, cutting or the injection of substances occurs most often in those who are psychologically abnormal or hope for some personal gain.

MISCELLANEOUS ULCERS

Ulceration of the leg may be associated with arteriovenous fistulae, poliomyelitis, ulcerative colitis, congenital haemolytic and allied anaemias, various collagen disorders and chronic lymphoedema.

Clinical features

These can be considered under the following headings:

THE ULCER

Any ulcer should be described according to its site, size, shape, floor, edge, base, exudate, and the nature of the lymph field draining the area. Whenever reasonable doubt exists as to the nature of the ulcer, a biopsy is required.

1. *Venous ulcer*—occurs typically over the lower and medial aspect of the leg
2. *Arterial ulcer*—occurs on the toes, dorsum of the foot or heel
3. *Traumatic ulcer*—occurs anywhere but when associated with plasters or prolonged bed rest they are closely related to bony prominences
4. *Neuropathic ulcer*—occurs on the sole or heel of the foot
5. *Syphilitic ulcer*—occurs classically on the lateral side of the leg and has a punched out appearance
6. *Bairnsdale ulcer*—has a widely undermined edge and watery granulation tissue
7. *Neoplastic ulcer*—has heaped-up edges
8. *Cryopathic ulcer*—follows a history of exposure to freezing or near freezing temperatures and the toes are commonly affected

THE CAUSE

1. *Arterial insufficiency.* This may be evident from the following:

a. History of intermittent claudication or rest pain
b. Presence of ischaemic changes in the limb, e.g., dry pale skin, loss of hair, fissuring of nails and absence of peripheral pulses

2. *Systemic manifestations* of any of the causes given above. Thorough clinical examination is mandatory.

In about 10% of cases no cause is apparent and special tests will be required.

SPECIAL TESTS

1. Urinalysis—particularly if diabetes is suspected
2. Full blood examination—if anaemias is suspected

3. Culture of ulcer discharge—for organisms including *Mycobacteria*
4. Biopsy of edge of ulcer—particularly if malignancy is suspected
5. Directional doppler ultrasound and venography—if suspicion of deep vein thrombosis persists
6. Arteriography—if there is suspicious of peripheral arterial disease
7. Plaster immobilization of affected part—if self-inflicted ulcer suspected

Treatment

ARTERIAL ULCER

The presence of an ulcer usually means that there is a severe degree of ischaemia. Thus, treatment of the causative disease (atherosclerosis, Buerger's disease) is not usually helpful; similarly, though correction of associated disorders such as diabetes and obesity is rational, the major therapy must be concentrated on the local lesion. The problem of arterial ulcer and arterial gangrene are the same and are therefore dealt with together here.

1. Relief of pain, which may be severe so that regular analgesics are required. A little alcohol may help and has also a vasodilatory effect. If a patient continues to smoke against strong advice, it is usually because he is not getting enough analgesic.
2. Simple dressings are used. A dry gangrenous part should be exposed. Obviously loose slough may have to be removed and pus drained.
3. Antibiotics are prescribed if there is spreading sepsis.
4. Restoration of circulation

   a. Lumbar sympathectomy dilates skin vessels and may possibly dilate collaterals around a major axial block. It is rarely effective in the severe problem of arterial ulcer or gangrene.
   b. Direct arterial surgery. Some idea of the likelihood of being able to restore flow by getting round a block in a major vessel may be gained clinically but arteriography is the best method. Every effort should be made to carry out direct arterial surgery or otherwise a major amputation is likely.

5. Establishment of skin closure by secondary intention healing or skin graft

NEUROPATHIC ULCER

Treatment of the cause, e.g., diabetes, alcoholism, tabes dorsalis.

Treatment of the limb. Clawing of the toes due to intrinsic muscle paralysis is treated with a well-fitted shoe and inner sole. When the toes become fixed then amputation may be necessary.

Treatment of the ulcer. Trophic ulcers are best treated

by rest and simple dry dressings and healing will occur unless infective or ischaemic factors are also present.

Soft shoes, thick socks and sponge rubber inner soles may retard the development of further ulcers.

Persistent trophic ulceration will require either amputation of an affected toe, or excision of a heel or sole ulcer together with underlying bony prominences. The defects are closed by primary suture or skin graft.

NEOPLASTIC ULCER

Wide excision and skin grafting will be indicated for epithelioma or malignant melanoma and the tumour is treated on its merits by supplementary management of the regional lymp nodes (see Chapter 37).

CRYOPATHIC ULCER

1. Protection from the cold is an essential prophylactic measure.
2. Vasodilator drugs may be helful with severe and recurrent chilblains.
3. Ulceration is treated conservatively. In severe cases of cold injury, in the absence of freezing, the gangrenous process may be superficial and amputation therefore unnecessary.

VENOUS THROMBOSIS AND PULMONARY EMBOLISM

Venous thrombosis most commonly affects the lower limbs; it may result in significant complications which include pulmonary embolism, perforator vein incompetence and varicose veins, or occasionally superficial gangrene.

CLASSIFICATION

Superficial vein thrombosis

1. Varicose veins
2. Veins used for intravenous therapy
3. Apparently normal veins:

   a. Hidden malignancy
   b. Buerger's disease (thrombo-angiitis obliterans)

Deep vein thrombosis

1. Upper limb:

   a. Superior vena cava
   b. Axillary vein

2. Lower limb:

   a. Soleal sinuses (calf vein thrombosis)
   b. Ilio-femoral (Phlegmasia alba dolens)
   c. Entire venous system (phlegmasia caerulea dolens)

SURGICAL PATHOLOGY

Predisposing factors

There are three commonly accepted predisposing factors to clot formation (Virchow's triad) all of which may interact in any single instance.

Stasis

Slowing of the circulation allows the central stream of platelets to become more peripheral and therefore able to become attached to the endothelial lining of the vessel.

Stasis is likely to occur in the following situations:

1. Heart failure
2. Confinement to bed which leads to reduced muscle pump activity and a slow rate of blood flow in the legs
3. Pelvic obstruction, for any reason, causing compression of iliac veins

Endothelial trauma

In arteries it is well known that intimal damage which occurs with artherosclerosis may predispose to clot formation. In veins endothelial trauma may occur in the following situations:

1. Rough handling of an unconscious patient
2. Pressure on unprotected calf muscles from unpadded operating tables or their fixtures
3. Intravenous therapy in association with trauma to the vein from a cannula, needle, or plastic tube
4. Nearby infection associated with inflammation of the vein wall

Altered constituents of the blood

1. Increased viscosity of the blood resulting from loss of water from the circulation, as in dehydration, or an increase in the cellular elements of the blood, as in polycythaemia, leukaemia and malignancy
2. Increased 'stickiness' of platelets after operation and parturition
3. Increased fibrinogen levels after operation
4. Reduced antithrombin levels after operation
5. Activated clotting factors IX, X and XI after operation
6. Other changes largely unknown associated with the contraceptive pill and malignancy

Thrombus formation

The features of thrombus formation are as follows:

Platelet deposition

A finely granular coral-like mass of platelets ('coraline clot' or 'white thrombus') is deposited on the endothelium and the proportion of white thrombus in any particular clot varies but it predominates in the arterial tree.

It is known that anticoagulants have little effect on platelet aggregations and results are disappointing when these drugs are used for arterial clots.

Deposition of other blood elements

Fibrin becomes interlaced between platelet clumps to strengthen and anchor them. Red and white cells are trapped in the mass and a complex structure develops which may occlude the vessel.

Wave of clotting

A red tail streams away from the head of the clot in the direction of the blood flow. This tail is smooth, slippery, non-adherent and particulary likely to break up to form emboli. This is the 'propagative' or 'consecutive clot' or 'red thrombus' of *phlebothrombosis* and there is little or no adherence to the vessel wall. The slower the blood flow the larger the clot. Anticoagulants are of considerable value in preventing the formation of this type of clot.

Chemical inflammation

This is probably the result of release of substances from disintegrating elements in the clot or more frequently of some extraneous substance, e.g. bacterial break-down products. An inflammatory reaction occurs in the wall of the vessel and the clot becomes adherent and therefore less dangerous. This is the stage of *thrombophlebitis* and is associated with symptoms and signs of inflammation. In a superficial vein a red, warm and painful cord is produced; in a deep vein, calf pain and an elevated temperature occur.

CLINICAL FEATURES

1. The predisposing cause

A history of varicose veins, Buerger's disease, or recent intravenous therapy, may indicate a cause for superficial vein thrombosis while a history of a recent operation, confinement to bed, heart failure, dehydration, or polycythaemia, may account for a deep vein thrombosis.

Massive deep vein thrombosis (phlegmasia caerulea dolens) and superficial thrombosis occurring in apparently normal veins must always raise suspicion of a hidden malignancy.

2. The stage of phlebothrombosis

Because the clot is propagative and not attached to the vein wall there are no local signs to indicate its presence. However if the patient has had one or more moderate or large pulmonary emboli then its existence will be known but its exact site of origin may be impossible to determine without special tests.

The inadequacy of clinical assessment has led to the development of objective tests to detect deep vein thrombosis before clinical features are manifest. These tests include the following:

a. Venography (phlebography) is probably the most accurate test and should be used if pulmonary embolism has occurred. The phlebographic diagnosis of deep vein thrombosis is based on the presence of well-defined filling defects in opacified veins and when correctly interpreted it probably displays all significant thrombi.

b. Labelled-fibrinogen uptake. Radioactive iodine-labelled fibrinogen is taken up and incorporated as fibrin into any new thrombus and this uptake can be detected with a scintillation counter. The test is performed by firstly blocking the uptake of iodine by the thyroid gland with sodium or potassium iodide and then giving $100\mu Ci$ of ^{125}I labelled fibrinogen intravenously and counting the radio activity at fixed points down the legs. If count rates show an unexpected and persistent elevation then deep vein thrombosis can be confidently diagnosed.

The test is reliable when compared with venography but it is of doubtful value in the upper thigh and of no value at levels above the inguinal ligament. There is also a delay of 24–48 hours after administering fibrinogen before the counts are of diagnostic value.

The test can be of practical value in all high risk patients (those over 40 years undergoing surgery or those with a previous history of deep vein thrombosis or pulmonary embolism).

c. Ultrasonics. Ultrasound is reflected off any interface between substances of different densities. An ultrasound wave reflected from a stationary interface is of the same frequency as that emitted. The two waves can be cancelled electronically. Ultrasound reflected from moving particles (e.g. red cells) is of slightly different frequency (Doppler shift) and the difference is in the audio range. It is heard with earphones or a loudspeaker and its pitch is proportional to the velocity of the blood. By listening over the femoral vein and manually compressing the calf an augmented signal can be heard if the axial vessels (popliteal, femoral, external iliac) are patent. Absence of augmentation implies occlusion.

3. The stage of thrombophlebitis.

a. Superficial vein. A tender, cord-like thickening is easily palpable over part of the course of the vein. The skin over the site may be reddened and elevation of temperature and pulse may be associated.

b. Deep vein. Calf tenderness, together with elevation of temperature, are constant features. Later swelling of the limb occurs with pitting oedema and, in the event of a massive deep vein thrombosis, severe shock may accompany oedema of the entire limb and the lower abdominal wall. In this situation pain may be agonizing and the limb can assume a dusky purple colour which persists on elevation, while subcutaneous veins are turgid and peripheral arterial pulses may be impalpable.

Clinicians often call the fully developed form of the disorder 'venous gangrene' but recovery of all but the most distal skin and subcutaneous tissue is likely with good treatment.

TREATMENT

Superficial vein thrombophlebitis

PROPHYLAXIS
This includes treatment of varicose veins and careful intravenous therapy techniques. Never use the lower limb for the latter.

CURATIVE TREATMENT
If the clot occurs in an apparently normal vein consideration must be given to hidden cancer or Buerger's disease. In the common situation however the clot has occurred in a varicose vein and there are two methods of treatment available:

Conservative
1. *Supportive bandaging.* This is prescribed for comfort and the patient is encouraged to remain ambulant.
2. *Elevation of foot end of bed* about 9 inches (24 cm) at night
3. *Anti-inflammatory agents* such as phenyl butazone may be prescribed for its analgesic and anti-inflammatory effects
4. *Antibiotics.* There is usually no place for antibiotics because the thrombotic process is basically one of chemical inflammation and not infection. However in the event of a thrombosis occurring in an arm or leg vein being used for intravenous therapy, the possibility of inoculation and bacterial infection cannot be dismissed; in this situatation a broad spectrum antibiotic is justifiable after blood culture has been taken.
5. *Anticoagulants.* It is doubtful whether anticoagulants have any place in the treatment of superficial vein thrombosis. However in the uncommon event of the phlebitic process rapidly extending to the region of the sapheno-femoral junction at which time there is a danger of propagation into the deep venous system, then anticoagulants may be advisable.

Operative
1. If the thrombotic process is seen early and is localized, and the patient has gross varicose veins, then the clot may be ignored and the varicosities treated on their merits.

2. Ligation of the sapheno-femoral junction should be considered in the unusual event of rapid propagation proximally of the thrombotic process.

Deep vein thrombosis

Superior vena caval thrombosis with its attendant chest wall collaterals is virtually always secondary to obstruction and is largely a problem of diagnosis of the cause rather than treatment and will not be discussed further. Similarly axillary vein thrombosis which occurs spontaneously, after excessive exertion in young adults or in association with the contraceptive pill and is attended with swelling and blueness of the upper limb, is an unusual condition which responds readily to general supportive and anticoagulant therapy.

Deep vein thrombotic episodes of the lower limb probably begin in the soleal sinuses in the majority of cases but primary iliofemoral thrombosis is responsible for about a third of postoperative cases.

PROPHYLAXIS

General measures
1. Pre-operative weight reduction if grossly overweight
2. Per-operative and post-operative graded stockings on the legs of all patients undergoing major surgery, particularly those with a past history of deep vein thrombosis, myocardial disease, or varicose veins with major perforator incompetence
3. Protection of leg veins during surgery with an adequately padded operating table and fittings in addition to stockings
4. Careful handling of a paralysed patient at completion of operation
5. Post-operative elevation of the foot of the bed 9 inches(24 cm)
6. Advising patient against sitting out of bed with legs dependent
7. Frequent leg exercises
8. Early ambulation after operation

Specific measures
1. Antithrombotic agents such as a small dose of subcutaneous heparin (5000 units every 12 hours for 7 to 10 days) or dextran 70 during and after operation
2. Per-operative mechanical prophylaxis such as intermittent electrical stimulation of the calf muscles or pneumatic calf compression are preferable when an extensive dissection is to be undertaken.

CURATIVE TREATMENT
1. *Support the limb with a one-way stretch elastic bandage*
2. *Elevate the foot end of the bed*
3. *Thrombolytic therapy*

There is no uniform agreement as to which schedule should be adopted. Available are:

a. Anticoagulant drugs. These will not unblock a vein totally occluded but they will reduce the extent of the consecutive thrombus and the incidence of pulmonary embolism. At present it appears that the best routine is to give 5000–10 000 units of heparin as a 'loading' dose by intravenous injection. This is followed by a continuous intravenous infusion of heparin in a dose of 20 000–40 000 units in each 24 hours delivered in 1000 ml of a 5% solution of dextrose. The dosage is adjusted to maintain the clotting time between 20 and 30 minutes. In the first 24 hours the clotting time is estimated on three occasions but thereafter it can be done daily. Some patients are heparin-sensitive while others may be resistant and therefore less or more of the drug may have to be given. The method is relatively safe even in the early post-operative period provided the treatment is carefully controlled. It is however probably best avoided in the presence of active peptic ulceration or late pregnancy while dosages may have to be reduced if liver or renal disease is present.

Bruising of the buttocks and haematuria may be the earliest signs of heparin overdosage and the urine must be tested daily and the buttocks inspected frequently while on treatment.

Heparin therapy should be continued for about 10 days but once local symptoms and signs in the leg have begun to improve the patient is allowed to be gradually ambulated with the legs bandaged. Near or at the end of heparin treatment, oral anticoagulants may be introduced and continued for about 6 months. Dosages are then adjusted so as to keep the prothrombin time between 2 and 22 times control.

All patients with major deep vein thrombosis should persevere with leg bandaging for 6 months.

b. Fibrinolytic drugs. Streptokinase, a plasminogen activator, may be considered, especially if the history of thrombosis is less than three days and in the absence of a recent (less than 10 days) wound. Many now consider it a more effective thrombolytic agent than heparin: 600 000 units can be given initially over 1 hour as an intravenous infusion with 5% dextrose solution; thereafter 600 000–900 000 units are given 6-hourly for about three days. Some recommend the addition of 100 mg hydrocortisone every 6 hours intravenously to control pyrexia and allergic reactions. If troublesome haemorrhage occurs the effect may be reversed with aminocaproic acid or aminomethyl-cyclohexane carboxylic acid and fresh blood or substitutes such as fresh frozen plasma or platelets.

4. Surgery

The place of surgery in deep vein thrombosis of the lower limbs remains controversial. Methods available include:

a. Caval plication. This should be considered if longstanding or recurrent pulmonary embolic episodes occur when anticoagulant therapy is ineffective or contraindicated. It may also be considered as an adjunct to pulmonary embolectomy for acute and massive pulmonary embolism.

Caval plication has, however, a significant mortality when performed on a very sick patient and about 30% of survivors subsequently experience trouble with chronic venous stasis.

b. Caval umbrella. An ingenious method for preventing recurrent embolic phenomena has been devised. Under local anaesthesia the internal jugular vein is exposed and a tiny umbrella attached to a flexible lead is threaded through it, the superior vena cava, the right heart and on into the inferior vena cava under X-ray control. Then the umbrella is opened out so that it impinges against the caval wall above the thrombotic process and the flexible lead is unscrewed and withdrawn out through the neck.

The early results with the use of the umbrella are encouraging but its place has yet to be established.

c. Thrombectomy. When thrombosis of the ilio-femoral segment is seen within the first 48 hours then through a groin incision the clot can be sucked out or pulled out with a balloon catheter. In addition venograms can be performed on the operating table to establish the completeness of the clot removal.

d. Outcome in deep vein thrombosis. When the clot is confined to the paraxial veins (principally the soleal sinuses) then little harm ensues. It is when an axial vein becomes blocked that long standing trouble is likely. The thrombotic process leads to either:

(i) Permanent occlusion of the vein, which is relatively uncommon, or
(ii) Damage to the valves both in the deep veins and at the communications between deep and superficial the perforating veins.

In either event there is venous hypertension distal to the site of thrombosis which commonly leads to venous ulceration

Pulmonary embolism

Lodgement of clots in the pulmonary artery tree from a peripheral phlebo-thrombosis of the leg or ilio-femoral veins may be a risk to life if the phenomenon is massive enough. Under these conditions emptying of the right heart is obstructed and circulatory failure occurs rapidly.

In the majority of cases pulmonary embolism occurs between the seventh and tenth post-operative days as a continuing process and not as a single and dramatic episode.

The lungs have a remarkable ability to dispose of emboli and even repeated emboli may be symptomless and/or completely lysed. However, massive emboli may cause instant or rapid death and repeated smaller emboli pulmonary hypertension as progressively more of the pulmonary vasculature is blocked off.

CLINICAL FEATURES

A large part of the pulmonary circulation can be occluded by emboli without any demonstrable alteration of pulse, blood pressure, chest X-rays, or electrocardiographic tracings.

In addition, more often than not, there are no features of a deep vein thrombosis present in a lower limb, indicating that the clot may have arisen in the iliofemoral segment.

Symptoms and signs
1. Massive and fatal—sudden collapse, severe dyspnoea and marked cyanosis before death
2. Less severe—retrosternal pain, circulatory collapse with lowered blood pressure, tachypnoea, tachycardia, cold blue extremities, elevation of central venous pressure and haemoptysis

SPECIAL TESTS
1. *Chest X-ray.* This may look normal; alternatively, there may be a paucity of vascular markings, a peripheral opacity or basal collapse.
2. *Electrocardiogram.* A useful test to exclude myocardial infarction. A normal ECG does not exclude pulmonary embolism. T-wave inversion in the right pre-cordial leads is the most common change, though it does not always occur immediately; evidence of right atrial enlargement or the development of right bundle branch block are helpful features. All the ECG changes are usually transient.
3. *Lung Scintiscan.* This test cannot be used in the massive and severe cases of pulmonary embolism because the patient is too ill to be moved and positioned in front of the gamma camera. However it is helpful both in diagnosis and in assessing progress in less massive instances. Intravenous ^{131}I or technetium labelled macro-aggregates of human serum albumin can be injected intravenously; scanning the lung fields will detect areas of poor perfusion as less radio dense portions of the scan. Underperfused areas on scan in the presence of a normal chest X-ray make the diagnosis highly probable. In some centres ventilation scans are also available using inhaled radionuclide so that ventilated but non-perfused areas can be delineated.
4. *Pulmonary angiography.* In suspected massive pulmonary embolism, pulmonary angiography is very useful in making the diagnosis and in determining the distribution and severity of obstruction before considering operative removal of the clot.
5. *Arterial blood gases.* Major pulmonary embolism is associated with arterial hypoxaemia and often severe metabolic acidosis.
6. Tests for the diagnosis of deep vein thrombosis (^{125}I-fibrinogen test, doppler ultrasound evaluation of venous flow and venography) are negative in 15–20% of patients with confirmed pulmonary embolism. The source of the thrombus may have been the internal iliac veins which are not well seen on venography. Therefore, in suspected pulmonary embolism, time should not be wasted on such tests.

TREATMENT
Prophylaxis—as for deep vein thrombosis.

CURATIVE TREATMENT
1. *General support*, which includes the use of analgesics for pain, the treatment of shock by inotropic agents and the administration of oxygen
2. *Anticoagulants.* Heparin therapy is begun whatever the final decision about surgery.
3. *Pulmonary embolectomy.* In the presence of a major embolism. Angiographic facilities are required to confirm the diagnosis and heart lung bypass is necessary to carry out the operation. The vena cava should be plicated at the end of the procedure.

SWELLING OF THE LOWER LIMB

Swelling of the lower limb is often due to medical conditions such as heart failure and renal disease but the surgeon is more concerned with peripheral causes, the majority of which are venous or lymphatic in origin.

CLASSIFICATION OF CAUSES

Central

1. Cardiac
a. Congestive cardiac failure
b. Constrictive pericarditis

2. Renal
a. Acute nephritis
b. Nephrotic syndrome

3. Hepatic

4. Nutritional
a. Protein lack or loss as in protein-loosing enteropathy
b. Thiamine lack

5. Hormonal
a. Cushing's syndrome
b. Myxoedema

Peripheral

1. Venous disease
a. Incompetent valves in the deep venous system
b. Calf vein thrombosis
c. Ilio-femoral thrombosis
d. Inferior vena cava thrombosis

2. Lymphoedema
a. Primary usually result of inadequate lymphatics
   (i) At birth (lymphoedema congenita and when familial, Milroy's disease)
   (ii) Adolescence (lymphoedema praecox)
   (iii) After 35 years (lymphoedema tarda)

b. Secondary usually the result of absent or inadequate lymph nodes

   (i) Previous excision
   (ii) Radiotherapy
   (iii) Malignant infiltration
   (iv) Inflammation
   (v) Parasitic infestation (filariasis)

3. Miscellaneous
a. Lipoedema
b. Erythrocyanosis frigida
c. Arteriovenous fistulae
d. Tight bandage or plaster
e. Injuries: fracture, and muscle contusion
f. Infection: cellulitis, abscess
g. Popliteal cyst rupture

SURGICAL PATHOLOGY

Venous disease

Engorgement of the venous system of the lower limb, due to deep venous incompetence or extensive thrombosis, allows the hydrostatic capillary pressure of blood to exceed its colloid osmotic pressure with the result that fluid of low protein content collects in the extravascular tissues causing pitting oedema of the limb.

Thrombosis of the inferior vena cava may occur as an extension from an ilio-femoral thrombosis; it may also occur in association with abdominal cancer, puerperal sepsis or other infective processes.

Oedema is seen in its most extensive form, involving the whole leg, after massive thrombosis throughout most of the deep venous system of the leg and the ilio-femoral veins (phlegmasia caerulea dolens).

Primary lymphoedema

The result of obstruction to lymphatic flow because of developmental subcutaneous lymphatic channel defects when the lymph vessels fail to remove protein molecules or larger particles adequately from the tissues. An increase in the tissue colloidal osmotic pressure takes place which increases filtration of fluid across the capillary membrane and decreases reabsorption with the result that fluid of a high protein content collects in the tissues and pitting oedema becomes evident.

Lymphangiographic studies have enabled primary lymphoedema to be subdivided into three groups:

1. Aplasia (13%), where there are no formed subcutaneous lymph channels; the defect is usually apparent at birth (lymphoedema congenita).
2. Hypoplasia (75%), where the lymph channels are too small or too few.
3. Varicose (12%), where the lymph channels are dilated, tortuous and incompetent. When these channels extend into the pelvic and para-aortic lymph trunks retrograde flow of intestinal chyle may occur into the groin and thigh allowing chyle-filled vesicles to appear beneath the skin.

Secondary lymphoedema

More common than primary lymphoedema

Whichever of the listed causes precipitates lymphoedema, as the condition becomes chronic the skin and subcutaneous tissues thicken and attacks of cellulitis, often caused by beta-haemolytic streptococci occur which accentuate the changes and pitting is lost. Later still the skin becomes hyperkeratotic or horny and vesicular eruptions appear which ulcerate and discharge clear lymph or milky lymph (chylous reflux).

Miscellaneous causes

1. Lipoedema is an abnormal and painful accumulation of fat, particularly around the thighs, buttocks, and ankles.

2. Erythrocyanosis frigida: exposure to cold combined with some constitutional susceptibility may cause the skin of the lower third of the legs of adolescent females to become cold, blotchy, blue and blistered (chilblains). The legs are fatter than normal and subcutaneous fat necrosis may result in the formation of hard, tender nodules. The condition presumably arises as the result of a hypoplastic micro-circulation through the skin.

3. Arteriovenous fistulae. Congenital arteriovenous fistulae in the lower limb may be localized or diffuse. The latter are often associated with a giant swollen limb, superficial angiomata, varicose veins and varicose lymphatics in the adolescent.

Traumatic arteriovenous fistulae follow penetrating injuries, when the limb gradually swells and becomes associated with varicose vein formation. Swelling is usually minor.

DIAGNOSIS

The cause of swelling of the lower limb can usually be established from a consideration of the following:

Is it central in origin?

Central causes for generalized oedema such as cardiac, renal, or hepatic disorders must be excluded by history and examination

Is it unilateral in distribution?

Unilateral swelling of the limb indicates that there must be a local cause, which is of venous or lymphatic origin in the majority of cases.

Is it venous or lymphatic in origin?

Venous
Most often some of the following features will be apparent:
1. History of deep vein thrombosis after pregnancy, operation, or confinemant to bed, with the subsequent development of a painful and swollen leg.

    Occasionally deep vein thrombosis may occur for no apparent reason; then hidden malignancy or the contraceptive pill may have to be considered as possible predisposing factors.
2. History of an acute episode of severe pain over most of the limb in association with marked shock, rapidly developing extensive oedema, cyanotic skin, turgid subcutaneous veins, and superficial skin ulceration, indicate a massive deep vein thrombosis (phlegmasia caerulea dolens).
3. The presence of varicose veins, perforator incompetence (blow outs, fascial pits, ankle flares), varicose dermatitis and varicose ulceration indicate chronic venous insufficiency.
4. The presence of oedema of the leg which may be pitting in the early phase, but non-pitting when chronic and associated with skin and subcutaneous thickening.

Lymphatic
Oedema of lymphatic origin, in contradistinction of that of venous origin, is rarely painful at any stage; in addition the skin of a lymphoedematous limb remains remarkably healthy for many years apart from recurrent attacks of cellulitis. Skin pigmentation and ulceration, which are typical of chronic venous stasis, are not apparent.

1. Primary lymphoedema (congenita, praecox, and tarda). There is a family history in 20% of cases; it is unilateral in 50% of cases and it is of gradual onset and apparently worse in warm weather. It is a soft pitting oedema in the early stages but, like chronic oedema of venous origin, it becomes non-pitting in the chronic phase when skin and subcutaneous thickening is present.

After many years hyperkeratotic, horny and vesicular changes may occur which lead to ulceration and discharge of lymph.

2. Secondary lymphoedema. This differs from primary lymphoedema in being of rapid onset and unilateral in distribution; most often there is an obvious cause for its occurrence.

Is it arteriovenous in origin?

On rare occasions when central and local causes are not apparent for the oedema, an arteriovenous abnormality will have to be considered.

Features suggestive of arteriovenous fistula formation vary according to whether it is localized or diffuse, congenital or traumatic.

Local
1. Gigantism of the limb occurs if the fistula is congenital or if it is acquired before completion of epiphyseal fusion of limb bones
2. Distended superficial veins
3. Superficial angiomata (congenital fistulae)
4. Warmth, thrill and bruit (machinery murmur) over a fistula are uncommon features except in the traumatic type
5. Coolness of the limb below the fistula
6. Muscle wasting below the fistula

Systemic
1. Elevated pulse pressure
2. Cardiac enlargement and later cardiac failure

Special tests

When the diagnosis is still in doubt the following special tests may be of value:

1. Venography (Phlebography). The injection of radio-opaque contrast medium into an ankle vein, femoral vein, or iliac crest intra-osseous vein (for suspected vena cava thrombosis) will outline the site and extent of a thrombotic process.

2. Lymphangiography. Dorsal foot lymphatics are visualized by an injection of a diffusible dye such as Patent Blue, then a suitable lymph trunk is injected with radio-opaque solution and X-rays are taken to outline the nature of the lower limb and abdominal lymphatics.

3. Arteriography. This a valuable test when arteriovenous fistula formation is suspected.

TREATMENT

Deep vein thrombosis

(see p. 269).

Lymphoedema

PRIMARY LYMPHOEDEMA

Conservative. This is indicated for mild oedema and includes:

1. Limb massage
2. Limb elevation at night
3. Application of well fitting elastic stockings or elastic bandages
4. Bed rest and antibiotics for attacks of cellulitis
5. Diuretics which may be beneficial in some cases

Operative. This is indicated for severe cases of oedema not responding to conservative measures, for chronic neglected cases with recurrent cellulitis, or for cosmetic reasons.

The operations none of which is dramatically successful are based on the principle of wide excision of the subcutaneous tissue because of the widespread nature of the lymphatic channel defects. The skin is regrafted onto the raw surface. Microsurgery with lympho-venous anastomosis has promising results.

Amputation may be necessary for severe and incapacitating lymphoedema, particularly when skin ulceration and leakage of lymph is present.

SECONDARY LYMPHOEDEMA

Conservative. Limb massage, elevation and bandaging, as above.

Operative. When the causative condition is inactive and lymphoedema is severe and incapacitating, a wide variety of operations has been considered, but results are not encouraging.

Arteriovenous fistulae

TRAUMATIC FISTULAE

Immediate operation and arterial and venous reconstruction, with or without arterial transplant or venous graft, will prevent limb swelling.

Alternatively a delayed operation and arterial and venous reconstruction or quadruple ligation may be performed when the collateral circulation is well established (three months).

CONGENITAL AND DIFFUSE FISTULAE

Treatment is of limited value.

1. Amputation will be necessary when gangrene occurs
2. Limb-shortening operations, such as bone resection or epiphyseal stapling, are not always satisfactory

36

Arterial surgery and amputations

ARTERIAL SURGERY

Surgeons have always been concerned with the management of severe limb ischaemia. Recently their role has extended to encompass the management of less severe conditions such as intermittent claudication.

SURGICAL PATHOLOGY

The causes of arterial disorders are:

1. Buerger's disease
2. Atheroma with or without diabetes
3. Embolism
4. Aneurysms
5. Systemic causes of small vessel disease—polyarteritis nodosa, systemic lupus erythematosis
6. Major vessel arteritis—seen most commonly in the tropics
7. Vasospastic conditions, e.g. Raynaud's syndrome
8. Injury (see Chapter 11)

Buerger's disease

The condition is a combination of inflammation and obliteration of arteries and their adjacent veins. It starts in the distal small vessels and spreads relentlessly proximally. A strong relationship with tobacco smoking is established but ethnic relations (Jews) are probably spurious. Buerger's disease is confined to young people and is rare though it continues to be seen in developing communities where 'raw' tobacco is widely used.

Atheroma

The major cause of vascular disease in Western countries. The process in the limbs which comes to the attention of the surgeon is part of a more general disorder involving cardiac, cerebral, extracerebral neck vessels and other sites to a bewildering and varying degree. The lesions may take the form of: atheromatous plaque with secondary thrombotic occlusions; ulceration and weak-

ening of the wall may occur leading to aneurysm; ulceration with thrombosis and distal embolization. Associated features are:

1. Heavy cigarette smoking
2. Hyperlipidaemia and hypercholesterolaemia
3. Diabetes mellitus
4. Obesity

The condition usually affects major vessels. In diabetes and more rarely without this disease, small vessels at digital level may be affected alone or in combination with larger vessel disease. The distinction is therapeutically important.

The classical sites for major arterial occlusion are:

1. The aorto-iliac region where there is most often diffuse involvement of the terminal aorta and common iliac arteries. Much less frequently the disease is localized at the aorta or common iliacs with relatively normal vessels above and below.
2. The superficial femoral artery in the thigh, particularly near the adductor hiatus
3. The popliteal artery
4. The bifurcation of the common carotid artery

Embolism

The major causes are:

1. Atrial fibrillation—usually the result of:

   a. Mitral valve disease
   b. Thyrotoxicosis
   c. Atheromatous coronary artery disease

2. Myocardial infarction and mural thrombus
3. Septic endocarditis in which case the embolus is also septic and a mycotic aneurysm may result
4. Detachment of thrombi from an atherosclerotic plaque—e.g. at the bifurcation of the aorta and of the common carotid artery

The effects of an embolus are principally related to the capability of blood getting round the point of obstruction and range from nil where the collateral circulation is adequate to death of tissue when the vessel involved is an end artery.

Aneurysms

These are classified into two types:

1. True aneurysms—where there is dilatation of the arterial wall. They are mainly due to arteriosclerotic degeneration of the media. Occasionally they may result from congenital defects in the media, e.g. Marfan's syndrome, 'berry' aneurysms of the circle of Willis (see p. 91).
2. False aneurysms—where the arterial wall is breached and the blood is contained by clot and surrounding tissues. They usually follow trauma, surgery or arteriography.

The common sites of aneurysms are:

1. The infrarenal aorta and at its bifurcation. Fortunately the disease usually spares the first 2 cm below the renal arteries, making reconstructive surgery possible.
2. The popliteal arteries—usually involved bilaterally and in association with abdominal aortic aneurysm.
3. The visceral arteries—splenic, renal and coeliac
4. The common femoral arteries—the commonest site of false aneurysm

Systemic disease

These conditions usually produce very distal (acral) disease which resembles that seen in diabetes.

Major arteritis

An ill-defined group of patients in which the abdominal aorta in particular is involved by a dense inflammatory process, sometimes with giant cells. Difficult to distinguish from Buerger's disease but probably pathologically separate.

Vasospastic condition

There is no specific disorder. The conditions associated with Raynaud's phenomen are discussed below.

CLINICAL FEATURES OF OCCLUSIVE VASCULAR DISEASE

Symptoms

PAIN

Pain is of two types:

1. Intermittent claudication
2. Continuous rest pain

Intermittent claudication

Intermittent claudication may in theory affect any muscle—angina is the same as claudication in the limb. However, claudication means literally limping (Latin claudicare—to limp) and is used to label pain experienced in the limb on exercise and which is relieved by rest. It is nearly always a lower limb symptom, though it can occur in the arms as a result of subclavian or innominate disease.

Surgical physiology of intermittent claudication. Pain produced in a limb on exercise is directly related to ischaemia of muscles in the region and is presumably caused by the liberation of pain-inducing metabolites.

The resting blood flow in both a normal and a limb with diseased vessels is usually about the same. On exercise the muscle bed dilates and blood flow is usually increased up to ten fold. When there is an arterial block this cannot happen beyond the obstruction. Indeed flow is often reduced and pulses previously present may disappear because of the dilated muscle bed proximal to the obstruction. The degree of distal deprivation relates to the amount of collateral circulation.

The pain of intermittent claudication is characteristically cramp like and varies from an ache to acute severe pain which arrests the patient's walking. The pain must be related to exercise to qualify for the description and must be relieved by rest. Useful information that may be sought relates to:

1. *Duration.*
2. *Progression or regression.* In many cases it is not possible to assess accurately the rate or direction of progression of the disease without observation over many months.
3. *Site.* The distribution of pain often provides an indication of the site of major vessel occlusion.
4. *Buttock pain* means internal iliac occlusion and calf pain is usually caused by a block of the superficial femoral artery in the thigh. Pain in the calves radiating up into the thighs is often due to aorto-iliac or generalized iliac artery disease. The patterns are, however, not constant.
5. *Type.* Intermittent claudication can be classified into three types.

    Type 1: This is the mildest type and the patient is able to continue walking after the onset of pain and provided he walks at the same speed the pain passes off.

    Type 2: This is the usual type. The pain persists with walking and the patient stops, not because the pain is unbearable, but because it is unpleasant.

    Type 3: The pain steadily worsens with walking and the patient is forced by the severity of the pain to stop.
6. *Claudication distance.* The distance travelled before

pain occurs is often an unreliable guide in that it is directly related to the amount of exercise performed and therefore depends on whether the patient is walking on flat ground or uphill. Patients usually state that pain occurs after they have walked a definite distance, 100 or 200 m, but the distance walked may vary from day to day. Also claudication in one leg may be so severe as to mask milder claudication in the other.

7. *Relief*. When pain in the leg is due to occlusive vascular disease it will always be relieved by rest. The relief is usually complete though some patients complain of an ache that continues after the cramp-like pain has abated.

Rest pain

Rest pain is characteristically boring, gnawing and severe, often worse at night and somewhat relieved by hanging the foot over the edge of the bed.

LOSS OF FUNCTION

The range is large. A patient with occlusive disease at the bifurcation of the aorta and some collateral circulation may have progressive weakness of his lower limb muscles and such specific functional loss as failure of erection (Leriche syndrome). At the other end of the scale a limb totally deprived of circulation will be flaccid and anaesthetic. Cold feet, numbness, bizarre tingling and burning are sometimes complained of, but are rare as presenting features of occlusive disease.

GENERAL SYMPTOMS OF ARTERIAL DISEASE

General symptoms of arterial disease are present in about 50% of patients with intermittent claudication. Cardiovascular disease may cause angina, shortness of breath and swelling of the ankles. Cerebral vascular disease may be associated with a past history of strokes or transient attacks of visual disturbance or limb weakness.

Signs

GENERAL

It is of particular importance to search for pulse irregularities, hypertension, evidence of cardiac failure, bronchitis and emphysema. The carotid, subclavian and renal vessels should be auscultated for bruits indicating stenotic disease. The abdominal aorta must be palpated for evidence of aneurysmal dilatation.

LOCAL

Inspection. Ischaemia of the lower limb may be associated with a dry pale skin, loss of hair, fissuring of nails, moist or infected interdigital clefts, ulceration and gangrene. Elevation of the affected limb will often cause pallor and blanching which may be accentuated by rapid ankle and toe movement. When the limb is lowered

below heart level it will regain its colour more slowly than on the healthy side and after a few minutes it may become blue and congested.

Palpation. 1. Palpation of the peripheral pulses is the most valuable clinial observation and in many instances the extent and position of the arterial disease can be estimated by this simple examination with a fair degree of accuracy. It is unusual for a patient with atherosclerosis to complain of symptoms before pulsation of one or more of the peripheral arteries has disappeared. If a pulse is absent at any point there must be a proximal block of the vessel concerned.

Thus if the common femoral pulse is not palpable in the groin, the occlusion will be in the aorta, common or external iliac arteries. If the femoral pulse is present, but the popliteal and ankle pulses are absent, then a portion of the superficial femoral or popliteal arteries will be occluded.

It must be remembered that the popliteal pulse may be difficult to detect and it should be sought with the knee flexed and with the patient face down on the bed. Also, the dorsalis pedis pulse is absent in about 10 per cent of normal individuals and the posterior tibial pulse in about 5 per cent.

2. Palpable collateral vessels may occasionally be detected when major vessels are occluded. A pulse over the medial side of the knee joint may indicate a wide open artery accompanying the long saphenous vein.

3. Palpation of the superficial veins of the leg may reveal the presence of thrombosis which accompanies thrombo-angiitis obliterans in 30% of patients.

4. Palpation for skin temperature change may show marked variation close to the site of a complete obstruction. Although patients with severe ischaemia will have a reduced skin temperature in the affected areas, the estimation of these temperatures is often unreliable, particularly if both limbs have not been equally exposed to the air. A warm knee may be found in patients with good collateral circulation.

Auscultation. A systolic bruit over a main vessel indicates the presence of a stenosis at that level or possibly higher up. Bruits from a stenotic aorta or iliac vessel may be heard anywhere from above the umbilicus to the groin.

Movements of joints. Reduced power of hip movements may be present with an aortic block. Similarly, weakened knee and ankle movements can occur with femoral and popliteal blocks.

The effects of exercise on the appearance of the limb and the distal pulses may be observed. In major vessel disease pallor ensues and weak or normal pulses can both disappear.

Special tests

1. Electrocardiography, chest X-rays and blood examination, together with an examination of the urine for glycosuria, are standard investigations in the general assessment of patients with occlusive disease.
2. The measurement of ankle pressure before and after a standard exercise using a sphygmomanometer and Doppler ultrasound blood velocity detector over the posterior tibial or dorsalis pedis arteries offers an objective quantitative measurement and a functional assessment of the severity of the disease. This test will save many patients with normal ankle pressures from unnecessary angiography because it demonstrates the anatomical extent of the disease and the feasibility of reconstruction.
3. Arteriography is by far the most important of all special tests. Trans-lumbar aortography or femoral arteriography will give information concerning the level and degree of obstruction, the condition of the collateral circulation and the state of vessels above and below the obstructed or stenotic site.

These procedures are safe only in experienced hands but they are still not without possible complications such as haemorrhage, damage to arterial wall and dissecting aneurysm formation. Therefore arteriography is not performed routinely and it is only carried out if clinical assessment indicates that reconstructive surgery is likely to be of benefit.

If symptoms are severe and incapacitating with signs of impending gangrene as indicated by rest pain, skin changes and ankle pressure measurements, then arteriography should be done urgently because arterial reconstruction is the only way of saving the limb.

Differential diagnosis in intermittent claudication

Sciatica. This may be confused with pain from arterial occlusive disease. The pain of intermittent claudication occurs after walking some distance, while sciatic pain is usually precipitated by stooping, straining or heavy lifting. The ankle pressure after exercise is increased or unchanged with absence of arterial disease.

Osteoarthritis of the hip. Degenerative disease of the hip joint may cause confusion, particularly as symptoms from it are most likely to occur after exercise and may be referred to the knee. However, the absence of local signs of peripheral arterial disease in the presence of restricted hip movements, should be enough to warrant an X-ray examination of the hip, after which the diagnosis should be apparent. Ankle pressure measurements will determine the presence or absence of significant haemodynamic disease.

MANAGEMENT OF OCCLUSIVE VASCULAR DISEASE

The underlying cause

1. Dietary manipulation. Only of use in patients with gross disturbance of cholesterol or lipids and not often very effective even then. May be supplemented by agents (e.g. Atromid) which lower serum cholesterol.
2. Weight reduction to reduce burden on the affected lower limbs
3. Cessation of smoking. Highly desirable in atheroma; mandatory in Buerger's disease if the condition is not to progress.
4. Control of diabetes.
5. Specific therapy for diseases such as polyarteritis or lupus erythematosis.

Management of the limb

General. Patients should be reminded that they have a limb or limbs that are at risk and that minor injury or infection may lead to gangrene. Specifically:

1. The feet must be kept clean and dry
2. The feet must be kept warm and overheating and possible blistering must be avoided
3. The toe-nails must be carefully trimmed
4. Corns, papillomata and fungal infection must be properly treated
5. Shoes should be soft and well fitting
6. Minor trauma such as having the toes trodden on in a crowd must be avoided

Vasodilators. Many have been tried and all are found wanting. When the problem is inflow it is of little use dilating the distal circulation.

Hypervolaemia. In patients with Buerger's disease who are having a wave of extension of the process, dextran 70 transfusion may temporarily increase perfusion and is used by some.

Specific

Claudication. Many patients with claudication can live within their distance. There is rarely any threat to the limb.

In the circumstance where claudication is incapacitating direct surgery should be considered (see below); sympathectomy is not helpful.

Major ischaemia from a proximal block with rest pain and impending or established gangrene.

1. Remove any remediable cause such as an embolus.
2. Try to restore blood flow by direct surgery. In aorto-

iliac disease this is usually by thrombo-endarterectomy (disobliteration) in which the clot and diseased intima and media are removed and the vessel reconstructed using only its adventitia. Below the inguinal ligament some form of bypass graft (reverse saphenous is the best) is used. Direct surgery can only be done if there are patent vessels distally as established by arteriography—what the vascular surgeon calls 'good run off'.

3. In the absence of run off, sympathectomy should be done but is unlikely to influence outcome.
4. Amputate dead tissue or occasionally allow this to separate. When the block is proximal and cannot be relieved major amputation is usual.

Ischaemia from distal block. By definition this is an end artery obstruction therefore sympathectomy or direct surgery are inapplicable. Conservatism should be practised; provided the dead tissue is dry it can often be left to separate spontaneously.

Local treatment of gangrene due to arterial disease. (*See* page 266)

SPECIAL CONSIDERATIONS

Diabetes

TYPES OF DISEASE
1. Major atheroma
2. Small vessel disease
3. Combinations of (1) and (2)
4. Neuropathy ±(1) or (2)

The first three have been dealt with. It is important that the fourth be recognized. Neuropathy is common in diabetes though its nature is largely unknown. When a patient presents with a septic/necrotic lesion on the foot it is vital to try and assess what proportion of neuropathy and vascular disease are separately responsible.

Vascular disease is characterized by:

1. System involvement—retina, kidney
2. Predominantly cutaneous and gangrenous lesions

Neuropathy typically has:

1. Sepsis
2. Perforating ulcers
3. Spreading sepsis in fascial plane involving necrosis of fascia and tendons in spite of what appears to be a good blood supply.
4. Clinical features of loss of sensation and of position sense

The septic/neuropathic foot can be treated by local surgery. Often this has to be radical, involving removal of digits which have been destroyed by infection and by the local arteritis that occurs. Wide excision of dead fascia may be required. However, major amputation can usually be avoided. Clearly advice on subsequent management for the patient must be rigorous.

Vasospastic diseases

Raynaud's phenomenon is characteristically attacks of pallor and pain in digits (nearly always the hand) followed by cyanosis and then rubor as the condition relents. The phenomenon is seen in.

1. Women without other cause when it can be styled Raynaud's disease
2. Both sexes, as a manifestation of some other disorder the most important of which are:

   a. Scleroderma or systemic sclerosis
   b. The prolonged use of vibrating tools
   c. Cold hypersensitivity associated with a positive Coomb's test when the lesion is probably 'sludging' of red cells in the capillaries.

Management is obviously related to cause.

1. *Raynaud's disease*. Opinion differs as to whether prolonged relief can be achieved by denervating the blood vessels. Proponents point to clinical success; opponents say that many patients relapse and that this is because by denervation the smooth muscle in the vessel wall is rendered more sensitive to whatever stimulus provokes a reaction.

2. *Raynaud's phenomenon*. The cause must be removed if this is possible, otherwise the patient must be encouraged to avoid cold stimulus.

Carotid arterial vascular disease

An aetiological advance in recent years has been the realization that stroke could result from the occlusion of major extracranial vessels. Two forms exist:

1. Occlusion of the carotid bifurcation when circle of Willis perfusion is inadequate (either anatomically or because of contralateral disease)
2. Emboli from an ulcerated plaque at the common carotid bifurcation

Both pathological situations may cause 'transient ischaemic attacks' (TIAs)—sudden loss of vision (amaurosis fugax), fleeting paraesthesiae in limbs, temporary paralysis and loss of cerebral function such as speech.

Patients who suffer TIAs should be investigated by auscultation of the carotid bifurcation and special noninvasive tests to ascertain carotid perfusion. The variety of such tests is currently bewildering but there is hope that a 'best buy' will soon emerge. If there is a suspicion on clinical examination or on non-invasive investigation that a carotid stenosis exists, then angiography is necessary.

Management. Opinion is equally divided amongst those who say that anticoagulant therapy will:

1. Prevent complete thrombotic occlusion
2. Avoid recurrent emboli from an ulcerating atherosclerotic plaque

and those who maintain that:

1. A completed stroke can be avoided by disobliteration of the carotid bifurcation
2. The same operation will 'rebore' the vessels and so prevent embolization

Both procedures carry a negligible morbidity.

Probably the answer rests on facilities. Where anticoagulant therapy is well controlled, patient compliance is adequate and the risks of operation high, non-operative treatment is appropriate. When any of the converse exist then surgery will give good results.

Aneurysms

The natural history can be:

1. Benign enlargement, possibly with spontaneous resolution by thrombosis
2. Thrombo-embolism, especially with popliteal aneurysms
3. Rupture. This is uncommon in aneurysms less than 5 cm in diameter. Beyond 5 cm the incidence of rupture increases progressively.

Symptoms can be due to:

1. Pressure on surrounding structures, e.g. duodenum, lumbar spine, iliac vein or ureter
2. Rupture. Sudden onset of pain and shock. Radiation of pain in rupture of an aortic aneurysm may be to the loin or groin, mimicking renal colic. Prompt diagnosis and urgent transfer to the operating theatre is vital.

Management. This applies to abdominal aortic aneurysms.

1. Asymptomatic and diameter less than 5 cm. Observe regularly, control hypertension if present and monitor size of aneurysm with annual ultrasound scan.
2. Symptomatic or diameter greater than 5 cm. Operative treatment is indicated. In the elective case, CT scan is helpful in defining the proximal extent.

The operation involves clamping the aorta below the renal arteries and the iliac arteries distal to the aneurysm. The aneurysm sac is opened longitudinally and the aortic segment is replaced with either a straight or bifurcation synthetic graft. The graft is laid inside the aneurysm which is then closed over it.

The operative mortality for ruptured aneurysms remains at about 50% whereas for elective resections it is about 5%.

AMPUTATIONS

In civilian surgical practice amputations are required most often for lower limb peripheral vascular disease.

INDICATIONS FOR AMPUTATION

A dead limb

The life of a limb (or part of it) may be destroyed by:

1. Trauma, when major blood vessels have been involved.
2. Atherosclerotic occlusive vascular disease of major vessels usually of the lower limb, when gangrene of the foot or digits has occurred. Then a midthigh or sometimes a below knee amputation will usually be indicated unless successful direct arterial surgery has been performed. In the latter event a major amputation may be avoided.
3. Diabetes mellitus, when gangrene of the foot is usually the result of a combination of factors (atherosclerosis, infection and peripheral neuritis). In these patients a limited amputation of toes or the foot is often successful when small vessel thrombosis only has occurred and major and more proximal limb vessels are unaffected.
4. Pyogenic infection, in the presence or absence of diabetes mellitus, when progression or gangrene of the foot or digits will require conservative amputation.

A lethal limb

The life of the patient may be threatened if the limb is retained under the following conditions:

1. An osteogenic sarcoma, when amputation of the whole of the affected bone is indicated if there remains no evidence of metastases after supervoltage radiotherapy.
2. A subungual malignant melanoma requires amputation of the digit. Amputation of a limb may be justified on some occasions to remove a foul fungating tumour which is not treatable by other means.

3. Gas gangrene, when amputation of whole or part of the affected limb will be required if all or most muscle groups are involved by spreading myonecrosis (*see also* Chapter 14).
4. An acutely ischaemic limb where restoration of the circulation may precipitate renal failure.

A useless limb

The affected limb may be considered inferior to an artificial limb or to no limb at all because it is:

1. Flail, as the result of poliomyelitis or some other nerve lesion.
2. Repeatedly infected, by osteomyelitis.
3. Intractably painful, when amputation is occasionally considered for such conditions as post-operative or post-radiotherapeutic brachial neuralgia which have failed to respond to less drastic measures; or for rest pain which cannot be controlled by reconstructive arterial surgery.

TYPE OF AMPUTATIONS

Provisional

This is performed when it is anticipated that primary healing is unlikely to occur because of infection or ischaemia. The amputation is performed at the lowest possible site so that if further amputation is necessary it will result in a stump of adequate length.

Technique. Skin and deep fascia flaps are raised as with definitive amputations but the wound is left open which allows delayed primary healing. This method is commonly used when the blood supply to the stump is doubtful or dead tissue and sepsis are present distally.

Definitive

Previously, these were classified according to whether or not the stump was weight-bearing. Now practically all amputations can be fitted with a non-end-bearing prosthesis.

1. End-bearing. As the weight is taken on the stump, a solid bony end is required with the scar situated anteriorly or posteriorly. The latter necessitates the cutting of unequal skin flaps.

Examples of end bearing stumps are:

a. Syme's amputation. This entails an initial disarticulation through the ankle joint; the tibia and fibula are then divided at the level of the joint and their ends are covered with a single flap of skin from the heel. The operation is performed most commonly for trauma but never for peripheral vascular disease.

b. Gritti-Stokes amputation. This is a supra-condylar amputation in which the femur is sawn across at the level of the adductor tubercle; the patella is then placed over the cut end to form a broad base for end bearing.

2. Non-end bearing (proximal bearing). In these amputations the weight of the body is transmitted by way of the artificial limb socket to structures other than the stump end.

Examples of non-end bearing stumps are:

a. Above knee amputation, where the weight is borne largely by the ischial tuberosity and the muscles of the thigh
b. Below knee amputation, where the weight is borne by the upper end of the tibia and the knee

Upper limb amputations are of course non-weight-bearing and the function of any prosthesis which may be used is to provide mobility for grasping objects. At the present time upper limb prostheses fail to provide the delicate movements of the forearms, wrist and fingers.

In the non-end bearing amputations the lengths of stumps considered to be ideal for maximum efficiency of fitted prosthesis are as follows:

For *above knee* amputations—25 to 30 cm (10 to 12 inches) from the greater trochanter
For *below knee* amputations—14 cm (5½ inches) from the knee joint
For *above elbow* amputations—20 cm (8 inches) from the acromium
For *below elbow* amputations—17 cm (7 inches) from the olecranon

OPERATIVE TECHNIQUE
1. Avoid a tourniquet if the amputation is for peripheral vascular disease
2. Measure the site of amputation
3. Cut equal skin flaps and raise them with some thickness of fascia and/or muscle
4. Divide soft tissue at the level of the proposed bone division
5. Secure vessels as they are encountered
6. Divide nerves above the level of the proposed bone division to avoid a painful neuroma
7. Avoid redundant skin flaps
8. Insert subcutaneous drain tubes to amputation site
9. Carefully apply a pressure dressing

Pre- and post-operative care

This entails a consideration of the patient, the amputation stump and the prosthesis.

THE PATIENT

1. Control pain until amputation can be undertaken.
2. Control other diseases but remember that diabetes is not likely to be stable until dead or infected tissue is removed.
3. Control spreading infection. Prevent operative contamination becoming a serious infection, particularly in bed-ridden or diabetic patients, by the use of perioperative antibiotics. The commonest cause of gas gangrene in civilian life is clostridial infection of a below knee amputation because of faecal contamination.
4. Maintain an optimistic outlook about rehabilitation.

THE STUMP

Management of the amputation stump must include the following:

1. Resting the stump on a pillow
2. Placing a bed cradle over the stump
3. Preventing flexion deformities of the hip and knee joints by using suitable splints
4. Avoiding major change of stump dressings for 5–7 days unless excessive oozing occurs or signs of infection are apparent

5. Removing drain tubes from the amputation site by 24 –48 hours
6. Removing skin sutures between 10 and 14 days
7. Encouraging stump muscle and joint exercise with the help of supervised physiotherapy
8. Using crepe bandages, elastic stump stockings or a plaster nylon to achieve a smooth conical stump

THE PROSTHESIS

This is fitted when the following situations prevail:

1. The stump is well healed and conical
2. The scar is stable
3. The patient's general and mental condition is optimal
4. In some major specialized centres immediate fitting is used but the technique has only limited application

SPECIAL COMPLICATIONS OF AMPUTATION

1. Haemorrhage—reactionary or secondary
2. Sloughing flaps
3. Skin eczema, callosites, ulceration, redundancy, adherent scar
4. Stump muscle wasting
5. Painful neuroma
6. Osteomyelitis and ring sequestrum
7. Phantom limb

37

Skin conditions

Numerous conditions of the skin are of surgical interest but only the commoner ones will be discussed.

CLASSIFICATION

Cysts

1. Epidermoid (sebaceous)
2. Dermoid

   a. Inclusion
   b. Implantation

3. Ganglion

Dermatofibroma
Kerato-acanthoma
Keloid
Lipoma
Dupuytren's contracture

Epidermoid tumours

1. Papilloma
2. Seborrhoeic keratosis
3. Senile keratosis
4. Bowen's disease
5. Basal cell carcinoma
6. Squamous cell carcinoma
7. Pigmented naevi
8. Malignant melanoma

Toe nails

CYSTS

Epidermoid (sebaceous) cyst

The term 'sebaceous' misrepresents this very common lesion, which actually consists of a cyst lined by epidermis and filled with keratinous debris—an offensive, creamy, 'toothpaste'-like material—not sebum. Epidermoid cysts are particularly common on the scalp, neck, scrotum and face but they can occur anywhere on the skin. The diagnosis is readily established from the typical features of a firm spherical swelling which is always in the epidermal layer of the skin and often associated with a punctum.

Treatment
Excision is recommended for cosmetic reasons and to prevent possible complications such as infection, ulceration, calcification or keratinous horn formation. Meticulous excision of all the epidermal lining will reduce the common tendency for recurrence.

Dermoid cysts

INCLUSION (SEQUESTRATION) DERMOID CYST
This occurs at sites of closure of embryonal fissures and may appear at the inner or outer angles of the orbit, the midline of the neck, abdomen or on the scalp.

There is a firm or tense unilocular cyst, not attached to skin; it differs from an implantation dermoid in that its wall contains hair, hair follicles, sweat and sebaceous glands.

Treatment
Excision is recommended to prevent infection or for cosmetic reasons.

IMPLANTATION DERMOID CYST
This occurs commonly in the palm of the hand or fingers as a subcutaneous cystic swelling which is sometimes associated with a scar from a precipitating injury. Gardeners who prune roses are one particularly prone group.

An implantation dermoid contains white greasy material which is surrounded by a wall of stratified squamous epithelium. Hair, hair follicles, sebaceous glands and sweat glands are absent.

The mode of development of an implantation dermoid is uncertain but explanations offered include:

a. Implantation of epidermal cells beneath the skin by a puncture injury
b. Epithelialization of a haematoma by cells from adjacent sweat glands, in the absence of a puncture wound

283

Treatment
Excision is recommended to prevent infection or for cosmetic reasons.

Infection of skin cysts

As has been implied, secondary infection is frequent in epidermoid or dermoid cysts. If the consequent abscess is merely drained, then recurrence is inevitable. It is better at the time of incision to curette the abscess under antibiotic cover so as to remove or destroy the lining of the cavity. Almost always such an approach is adequate.

Ganglion

Though not of cutaneous origin, ganglions are commonly mistaken for epidermoid cysts, but lie deep to skin and in the vicinity of joints. There is a tense unilocular cystic swelling lined by compressed fibrous tissue and containing gelatinous fluid which lies in close relation to or communicates with the synovial membrane of a joint or a tendon sheath. It occurs most frequently on the dorsum of the wrist or foot but occasionally is related to the long flexor tendons in the palm or the peroneal tendons at the ankle.

The pathogenesis of this lesion is uncertain; it may represent a herniation of a synovial membrane, myxomatous degeneration of connective tissue, or an extrasynovial benign synovioma.

Ganglia may cause pain or discomfort or interfere with the function of tendons.

Treatment
1. Immobilization of the affected joint if it is acutely painful
2. Excision under regional or general anaesthetic and bloodless field. This is the most certain method of treatment but recurrence is still common, perhaps because the condition is not taken seriously.

DERMATOFIBROMA (HISTIOCYTOMA)

This presents as a firm nodule, 0.5–2 cm in diameter, fixed to the epidermis but freely mobile. The lesion is usually found on the lower leg, is often singular and is thought to result from minor trauma such as an insect bite which causes a reactive proliferation of histiocytes leading to fibrosis and scarring.

Treatment is excision for cosmetic reasons.

KERATO-ACANTHOMA (MOLLUSCUM SEBACEUM)

An affliction of adults who are usually over the age of 50,

it occurs exclusively on hair-bearing areas, particularly those exposed to sunlight, such as the face, neck and dorsal surfaces of the hands and forearms.

The lesion grows rapidly over 1 or 2 months to appear as an elevated dome-shaped swelling with smooth sides and central umbilication containing a keratotic plug which can be peeled off with difficulty to reveal a bleeding granular floor.

Untreated, the lesion gradually regresses over 6–9 months to leave finally an irregular depressed scar.

The aetiology is unknown but it probably arises from hyperplasia of hair follicle epithelium and metaplasia of sebaceous glands.

Treatment
Excision is usually recommended as it is often difficult to distinguish a molluscum sebaceum from an epithelioma.

When the diagnosis is certain, curettage of the central keratin plug and the floor of the lesion will hasten regression; the alternative is to do nothing and allow it to disappear spontaneously.

KELOID

This is an irregular hypertrophy of vascularized collagen forming a raised ridge on the site or scar of previous injury. Individual and racial predisposition is an important factor in keloid formation but in ordinary circumstances the condition occurs more in burns and wounds that heal by secondary intention. Spontaneous keloid may occur over the sternum.

Ridges of keloid often form 'claw-like' projections invading the surrounding skin *outside* the borders of the original scar, thus differentiating it from a hypertrophied scar.

Treatment
Inevitable recurrence follows excision; however, repeated monthly injections of triamcinolone acetonide into the lesion for 6 months generally give satisfactory results.

LIPOMA

This is the commonest of all benign tumours, occurring in any situation where there is fat but particularly in the subcutaneous tissue of the trunk and limbs. Lipomata also occur in sub-periosteal, sub-peritoneal (rectroperitoneal), sub-fascial and sub-synovial planes and in the submucosa of the bowel.

They usually appear in adult life as soft lobulated, fluctuant tumours and have definite and definable edges when subcutaneous in position.

Calcification is an occasional occurrence in a lipoma but it is rare for liposarcomatous changes to occur.

Adiposis dolorosa of Dercum is a term applied to diffuse or nodular painful deposits of fat in women. Sclerosis — loss of blood supply — can make a lipoma painful but may be followed by shrinkage or even disappearance.

Treatment
Excision is recommended if lipomata are large, unsightly, or troublesome.

Sub-fascial lipomata may extend through intermuscular planes and create difficulties if the operation is performed under local anaesthetic.

DUYPUYTREN'S CONTRACTURE

This condition is not strictly of cutaneous origin but is included here for convenience. There is thickening of the palmar fascia resulting in flexion contractures of the fingers of the hand with particular involvement of the ring and little fingers. The cause is unknown but it is thought to be familial and the incidence is increased in those of Celtic origin, alcoholics, diabetics and epileptics treated with phenytoin. The condition is more common in males. Some patients have similar contractures of the penis, associated with bowing of the penis (Peyronie's disease), or involvement of the plantar fascia of the feet. There is no known association with trauma. Microscopically there is a fibroblastic proliferation without special features.

Clinical features
The first signs are nodules in the palm at the base of the affected finger, followed by a thick palpable cord with subsequent contraction leading to flexion of the digit.

Treatment
Surgical treatment is the only effective form of therapy. Local excision of the affected palmar fascia is most commonly practised, allowing sufficient opening of the hand but minimizing the risk of complications such as the cutting of digital nerves or skin necrosis.
Post-operatively, the hand is immobilized in a firm wool and crepe dressing with gentle mobilization commencing after the first week.

EPIDERMAL TUMOURS
Papilloma

A common benign, sessile or pedunculated and sometimes pigmented tumour composed of squamous epithelium.

The common wart (verruca vulgaris) is a papilloma which probably arises from a virus infection. It may be single or multiple, and may disappear spontaneously. When the lesion occurs on the sole of the foot it may be difficult to differentiate from a corn which is a localized horny plug of epithelial cells in the epidermis. However if it is pared down until tiny haemorrhagic spots emanating from the finger-like projections of hyperplastic prickle cells of the papilloma are seen, the distinction will be made.

Treatment
Papillomata are usually excised for cosmetic reasons. However plantar warts often demand removal because of pain; they may be treated with silver nitrate, curettage, or excision.

Seborrhoeic wart (seborrhoeic keratosis)

A common benign and sessile condition of the elderly which appears as a dark brown raised area on the face, limbs, or trunk. It is a hyperplastic condition of the basal cell layer of the skin with laminated pearls of keratinized material or dendritic melanin forming cells. The lesion is typically 'greasy' to touch but may occasionally be impossible to distinguish from a melanoma.

Treatment
Excision is indicated when melanoma cannot be excluded.

Senile keratosis

A hard scaly condition of the elderly occurring particularly on the exposed parts of the skin. It is composed of hyperkeratotic areas with mitotic figures in the basal layers of the epidermis.

Treatment
Malignant change to squamous cell carcinoma occurs in about 25% of cases and excision is therefore recommended as a prophylactic measure.

Bowen's disease

A slowly growing premalignant reddish-brown lesion with well-defined margins affecting the middle-aged and elderly. It tends to form crusts and ulcerate; multiple lesions, which tend to coalesce, are common.

Microscopically there is hyperkeratosis with mitotic acitivty in the basal layers, where multinucleated giant cells and large clear cells are seen.

Treatment
Malignant change to squamous cell carcinoma may occur after many years and excision is therefore recommended.

Basal cell carcinoma (rodent ulcer)

This is particularly liable to occur in fair and dry skinned people constantly exposed to sunlight. Elderly subjects are usually affected and the majority of lesions occur on the face above the line joining the angle of the mouth and the lobe of the ear but no part of the skin is exempt.

Macroscopically the tumour begins as a pearly nodule with tiny venules coursing across the surface; it later proceeds to central ulceration with a raised, rolled, or beaded edge.

Microscopically the typical features are densely packed islands of uniform cells continuous superficially with the basal layer of the epidermis. The cells of the periphery of the islands are more deeply staining and have a palisade arrangement; prickle cells and cell nests (keratinized cores) are absent.

Direct spread superficially or deeply to involve other structures is the rule but rarely lymphatic and blood spread may occur.

Occasionally a basal cell tumour arises from the basal cells of hair follicles or sweat glands of the scalp of adolescents and enlarges to involve the entire scalp and face and neck (epithelioma adenoides cysticum or 'turban tumour').

Treatment

Radiotherapy. Superficial radiotherapy will cure over 90% of lesions.

Surgery. Wide excision and skin grafting is indicated in the following circumstances:

1. Recurrence after radiotherapy.
2. Involvement of muscle, cartilage, or bone.
3. Occurrence close to cartilage or the eye

Squamous cell carcinoma (epithelioma)

Like basal cell carcinoma, this lesion occurs particularly in elderly fair skinned people exposed to sunlight.

Prediposing factors

1. Senile keratosis
2. Bowen's disease
3. Lupus vulgaris (tuberculosis of the skin)
4. Xeroderma pigmentosum
5. Exposure to sunlight or irradiation
6. Chronic irritation

   a. Leukoplakia (see Chapter 17)
   b. Burn scar, varicose ulcer, osteomyelitis sinus (Marjolin's ulcer)
   c. Charcoal burner on abdominal wall (Kangri cancer of Kashmir)
   d. Sleeping on oven bed (Kang cancer of buttocks, heels and elbows of Tibetans)

Macroscopic features. The lesion may appear as a warty growth or as a malignant ulcer with raised and everted edges.

Microscopic features. There are solid clumps of epithelial cells extending into the dermis with finger-like projections. Cell nests or epithelial pearls with central keratinized cores and surrounding cells arranged in 'onion skin' fashion are characteristic, while intercellular bridges and small round cell infiltration of the dermis are usually present.

Direct spread to surrounding structures is slow and while lymphatic involvement is usually late it is an ever present danger.

Treatment

Radiotherapy. Superficial radiotherapy will cure over 80% of early lesions.

Surgery. Wide excision is indicated for the same reasons as those pertaining to basal cell carcinoma. Lesions on the hands, feet, perineum and vulva are ideally treated by surgery.

Lymph nodes. If the regional lymph nodes are clinically involved, a block dissection is indicated and when the primary lesion and the nodes are closely approximated, a dissection in continuity is preferable.

Pigmented naevi

SURGICAL PATHOLOGY

Pigmented naevi (moles) are composed of proliferations of melanocytes at different layers of the skin. Melanocytes are probably derived embryologically from neural crest elements of ectoderm that migrate into the skin and are capable of forming melanin from dioxyphenylalanine (DOPA). Melanin may be transfered from melanocytes to other cells. Melanocytes reside mainly in the basal layer of the epidermis and numerically are in constant ratio with the prickle cells of the basal layer but may migrate into the dermis or less often the epidermis. The deeper the collection of melanocytes the bluer the naevus.

Pigmented naevi of benign nature are of five types.

1. Junctional naevus. This is a smooth, flat or elevated naevus of all shades of brown, which can occur anywhere on the body from birth to later life.

When naevi occur on the palm, soles, digits, or genitalia, they are always junctional in type.

Microscopically there is a proliferation of melanocytes

at the epidermo-dermal junction. The cells have clear cytoplasm, dark nuclei, and varying amounts of melanin.

Junctional naevi rarely become malignant but nevertheless it is from this group that 90% of malignant melanomas occur.

Increased 'activity' of a junctional naevus, which indicates malignant change, is evidenced by:

a. Increase in size
b. Increase in pigmentation
c. Ulceration, crusting, or haemorrhage
d. Satellite pigmented spots
e. Microscopic evidence of hyperchromasia, anaplasia, mitotic figures and sub-epithelial spread

2. Intradermal naevus (common mole). When junctional activity ceases the naevus cells lie within the dermis and form a mature pigmented lesion which is rare in children but commoner with increasing age. It is a light or dark brown in colour and may be papillary, flat, or warty; it is often raised and hairy and occurs anywhere on the body except the palms, soles, and genitalia; it never becomes malignant.

Microscopically the overlying epidermis appears normal and the dermal naevus cells are arranged in characteristic alveoli or ribbons. The cells have lost the typical features of clear cells but some of them coalesce to form giant cells.

3. Compound naevus. Junctional cells migrate into the dermis so that both junctional and intradermal components are present. The later is inactive and incapable of multiplication or pigment production but the junctional component is responsible for this lesion being potentially malignant.

4. Blue naevus. This is a flat hairless bluish lesion devoid of surface elevation which is seen on the face, dorsum of the hands and feet, and the buttocks of babies (Mongolian spot).

The blue neavus is not premalignant and when occurring in babies it usually disappears before the age of 5 years.

Microscopically there are spindle-shaped and melanin-containing melanocytes in ribbon-shaped masses or whorls in the dermis.

5. Juvenile melanoma. Malignant melanoma is a very unusual occurrence before puberty but a pigmented hairless and warty melanoma occurring at this time and pursuing a benign course may have all the microscopic features of malignant melanoma. This is the juvenile melanoma in which junctional activity is marked with prominent mitotic figures and segregation of bizarre-looking multinucleate giant cells. There is however no dermal invasion and the outcome is always favourable.

TREATMENT OF NAEVI

Naevi appearing at birth are innocent tumours and are removed only for cosmetic reasons.

Naevi appearing before puberty are mainly flat junctional naevi and, since malignant melanoma does not occur in this age group, their removal is again indicated for cosmetic reasons only.

Naevi appearing after puberty should be removed if they are;

1. Situated in potentially dangerous areas (soles of feet, palms of hands, and genitalia).
2. Subjected to repeated trauma from clothes, braces, belts and razors.
3. Showing signs of malignancy.

Naevi appearing at birth or before puberty can be excised close to their margins; all other naevi must be widely excised if malignancy is suspected.

Any excised naevus must be subjected to careful histological study.

Malignant melanoma (melanoma)

This forms about 2–3% of all skin malignancies, and in Australia the incidence has increased fourfold in the last 30 years. 90% of melanomas arise from junctional elements of pre-existing naevi and in ten percent of cases the lesion arises *de novo*.

Females are affected more often than males, particularly in the age group 20–40 years. A melanoma is more likely in the lower extremity of a female and the trunk or arm of a male; Celtic ancestry and exposure to the sun are well documented pre-disposing factors. Black-skinned people are relatively resistant to melanomas, although these may occur on their palms, soles or mucous membranes.

Melanoma is one of the most malignant and dangerous forms of cancer and although occurring most often on the skin it can arise in any part of the body, especially the eye, beneath the nail (subungual melanoma), the intestine or meninges. Occasionally, widespread metastases present without the primary site being discovered.

SURGICAL PATHOLOGY

Macroscopic features. Malignant change in a pre-existing innocent mole will manifest itself by an increase in size with elevation above the surface, an increase in pigmentation, nodularity, haemorrhage, ulceration, or satellite pigmentations.

Microscopic features. There is marked junctional activity and invasion of the dermis and deeper structures. The cell structure and arrangement varies considerably; it may appear like a carcinoma in which cells are epithelial in character and arranged in alveoli, or it may appear like a sarcoma in which spindle cells predominate.

Spread. There may be lymphatic spread by emboli, to regional lymph nodes, or by permeation, to produce secondary nodules in the vicinity of the primary lesion.

Dissemination by the blood stream to any part of the body is usually a late development.

Special features. There is no doubt that malignant melanoma incites an immune response and that this may account at least in part for the remarkable variation of the clinical course.

CLASSIFICATION AND PROGNOSIS

Histological grading

The depth or level of invasion of the skin and the thickness of the lesion are two factors that indicate the invasiveness of the tumour and are useful for grading, determining appropriate treatment and indicating prognosis.

1. Level of invasion. Clark divides the skin into five levels for purposes of staging melanoma, the deeper the invasion the worse the prognosis:

Level I   Intra-epidermal (in-situ, premalignant)
Level II   Invasion into the papillary layer of the
              dermis
Level III   Invasion into the junction of the papillary
              and reticular dermis
Level IV   Invasion of the reticular dermis
Level V   Invasion of the subcutaneous fat

The 5-year survival for Level II is greater than 90% whereas for Level V it is less than 50%.

2. Tumour thickness. Breslow expresses invasiveness in terms of thickness in millimetres as measured histologically and this scheme correlates well with prognosis. Tumours less than 0.75 mm rarely metastasize, whereas approximately 30% of those between 0.76 and 1.5 mm will metastasize and for lesions greater than 3.0 mm in thickness more than 80% will metastasize.

General prognostic features

Other pathological features indicating a poor prognosis are:

1. Ulceration
2. Amelanosis
3. Poor lymphocytic reaction
4. Satellitosis—tiny deposits away from the main growth
5. High mitotic index

Lesions of the extremities have a good prognosis compared with those of the trunk. Subungual lesions have a particularly favourable outcome. Melanomas in females have an overall better prognosis than those in males, partly related to the different distributions in site.

Education programmes aimed at the public and the medical profession result in greater awareness, earlier presentation and better overall outcome, as illustrated in Queensland, Australia.

CLINICAL PATTERNS

Three typical patterns of melanoma are recognised.

1. Lentigo maligna (Hutchinson's freckle). This presents on the malar region of the face in middle-aged women and is the least malignant type. The lesion is flat, rounded in shape with an irregular edge and uneven pigmentation. Melanocytes invade the dermis but the tumour is not very thick (usually less than 0.75 mm). Treatment is local excision with a narrow margin and prognosis is excellent.

2. Superficial spreading (Pagetoid melanoma). The commonest form of melanoma this occurs in any area exposed to the sun. The lesion is raised, has an irregular edge and a variegated colouration. All levels of invasion exist but epidermal invasion predominates and lymphatic infiltration is prominent.

3. Nodular melanoma. The melanoma is elevated, convex or even pedunculated, occuring at sites not exposed to the sun and is often amelanotic. This is the most ominous form of melanoma with: extensive dermal invasion; rapid growth; and early metastases.

TREATMENT

Co-operation between the pathologist and surgeon is vital for the diagnosis and treatment of melanoma. Although paraffin sections are the safest means of making a histological diagnosis and grading the tumour, advances in interpretation of frozen sections of melanomas enables excision biopsy and definitive surgery to be performed at the one operation.

Early cases

1. Primary lesion. A wide local excision of the melanoma and a margin of at least 2.5 cm in width, and as deep as the deep fascia, is performed. Wider margins and excision of the deep fascia are now considered unnecessary. The defect is replaced by a split-skin graft taken from the contralateral limb, to avoid lymphatic seeding in the proximal ipsilateral limb.

2. Regional lymph nodes. There is no universal agreement on the treatment of the regional lymph nodes.

1. Regional nodes not clinically involved
    a. *Immediate 'prophylactic' block dissection.* All agree
       that if a block dissection is to be performed it

should be in the form of an en bloc excision of the primary lesion, the intervening lymphatics, and the first echelon of lymph nodes, whenever this is anatomically possible. A lesion of the thigh can be removed in continuity with the ilio-inguinal lymph nodes, but for a lesion below the knee, there is no advantage in removing the subcutaneous tissue and deep fascia between the primary lesion and the groin as many intervening lymph plexuses and potential metastatic deposits must necessarily be missed by such a dissection.

Many surgeons consider that when melanoma is distant from the regional lymph nodes, a lymph node dissection may provoke dissemination of the malignancy to unpredictable areas by operative trauma and by removing immunological control.

b. *Delayed 'prophylactic' dissection.* A block dissection of the regional lymph nodes may be performed 2–3 weeks after adequate excision of the primary. A possible benefit of the delay is to allow time for any malignant cells in lymphatics to travel to regional lymph nodes.

Block dissection, whether immediate or delayed is associated with a significant morbidity (swollen limb and flap necrosis)

c. *Regional perfusion combined with surgery.* The rationale of this method is that tumour cells are constantly en route to the regional nodes and must be destroyed by a high local concentration of cytotoxic agent. This can be achieved by isolating the circulation of the limb and perfusing, using a pump oxygenator. The lesion is then excised. The 5-year survival in lower limb melanoma is improved by this approach but unfortunately its use is limited to special centres.

d. *Observe closely.* It is considered by some surgeons that the results of immediate or delayed 'prophylactic' node dissection do not justify its use and that nothing more than continued observation is required.

Block dissection is performed if nodes becomes clinically involved.

e. *Treatment based on histological grading.* A somewhat more rational approach may be used based on histological grading. Melanomas of Level I or II and less than 0.75 mm require excision only, because metastases are rare. Lesions of Level IV or V and greater than 3.0 mm in thickness have a poor prognosis and may benefit from a combination of prophylactic lymph node dissection and limb perfusion. The best choice of treatment for the intermediate group Level III or IV and thickness 0.76–1.5 mm has not yet been established but the combination of excision and limb perfusion has gained in popularity.

2. *Regional nodes clinically involved.* Once the regional nodes are involved with malignant melanoma, the prognosis is very poor and only 5% of these patients survive 5 years.

The methods of treatment available are as follows:

a. *Immediate block dissection*
b. *Endolymphatic therapy plus block dissection.* The block dissection should be performed about 4 weeks after the intralymphatic injection, when the isotope has had time to decay to safe level. The operation can however be technically more difficult if more than 4 weeks have been allowed to elapse. The disadvantages of the treatment is that it can only be performed in a specialized radiosotopic unit.
c. *Perfusion and block dissection*

Advanced cases

When the lesion is locally irremovable or when metastases are present then systemic combination chemotherapy, including imidazole carboxamide (DTIC), may be employed but response is not universal. B.C.G. vaccination, either intra-lesionally for recurrent melanoma or by multiple intradermal injection, has been used to stimulate an immunological response but the results have been disappointing.

Amputation of a limb may occasionally be justified on some occasions to remove a foul, fungating tumour.

TOENAILS

These may be the site of various surgical conditions. Apart from paronychia and glomus tumour, which usually occur on fingers, most nail abnormalities are found on the great toe.

Classification of toenail disorders

1. *'Ingrown' toenail* (onychocryptosis)
2. *'Overgrown' toenail* (onychogryphosis)
3. *Nail bed lesions*

   a. Subungual haematoma
   b. Subungual exostosis
   c. Melanoma
   d. Glomus tumour

Surgical pathology

1. 'INGROWN' TOENAIL

The basic defect is a pressure necrosis of the nail wall and nail sulcus due to persistent contact with the edge of the nail plate. Subsequent ulceration, inflammation and suppuration cause the nail wall and nail sulcus to swell and develop exuberant granulation tissue which in turn exaggerates the contact with the nail plate.

Factors which predispose to abnormal pressure between the nail plate and the nail wall and sulcus are as follows:

Soft tissue abnormalities
a. A toenail cut short and curved allows the unsupported pulp of the toe to roll over the nail edge when upward pressure is exerted on walking (Fig. 37.1)
b. A soft and lax pulp, which may result from debilitating diseases and hyperhidrosis, rolls easily over the nail plate edges.
c. A crowded foot in an ill-fitting or pointed shoe may cause pressure to be exerted between the nail wall and nail plate of the first or second toe.

Nail abnormalities
A congenitally hypercurved nail or a secondarily hypercurved nail. The latter may result from peripheral arterial disease, pulmonary disease or ageing.

Bone abnormalities
a. Subungual exostosis
b. Upward tilt of the tip of the distal phalanx

These defects may cause the nail plate to become domed and allow abnormal pressures to be exerted between the nail-plate edge and the nail wall.

2. 'OVERGROWN' TOENAIL
Excessive growth of the nail plate occurs by proliferation of the cells in the germinal matrix. This causes the nail to thicken, lengthen, and pile up to form a nail which is said to resemble a ram's horn.

3. NAIL BED LESIONS

Subungual haematoma. This is a tense and painful haematoma beneath a nail as the result of a crushing injury.

Subungual exostosis. This is a small overgrowth of bone on the dorsal surface of the distal phalanx which may enlarge and deform the nail and destroy the nail bed.

Melanoma. Malignant melanoma not uncommonly occurs in a nail bed.

Glomus tumour. This is an extremely painful and well encapsulated tiny bluish tumour. It is benign and arises from the neural tissue of specialized subcutaneous arteriovenous anastomoses which are concerned with heat regulation. Most of these tumours occur in the upper extremities and about 30% are subungual but the subungual regions of the lower extremities are not excluded.

Microscopically there is a tangled mass of blood vessels surrounded by a musculo-endothelial or neuromatous stroma.

Treatment

1. 'INGROWN' TOENAIL

Conservative
This should be adopted initially in all cases, and includes:

a. Correct trimming of the nail so that pulp is unable to roll over the nail plate edge (Fig. 37.1)
b. The wearing of clean socks and the use of foot baths when excessive sweating is present
c. The careful application of dusting powder to the toe and web spaces, making sure that the nail sulcus is not 'caked'
d. The placing of cotton wool beneath the nail plate edge and along the sulcus to facilitate the separation of these structures
e. Thinning of the central portion of the nail with a razor blade, sandpaper, or file, to make it more pliable and able to give way more readily to the forces applied during walking
f. Control of exuberant granulation tissue on the nail wall with silver nitrate
g. Advice regarding correctly fitting shoes

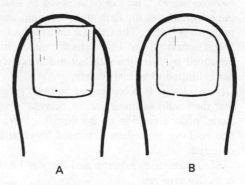

Fig. 37.1 Toenail trimming *A.* Correct *B.* Incorrect

Operative
This is indicated when pain or discomfort persists despite conservative treatment or when drainage of pus is necessary.

The operations available are:

1. Nail plate operations. Simple avulsion of the nail is indicated when it is essential to establish free drainage of pus. Wedge excision of portions of the nail only serves no permanently useful function.

2. Nail wall operations. Excision of most of the soft tissue from the side of the toe with or without pedicle grafts is not popular, but can be justified when pulp migration is considered the initiating factor.

3. Nail bed operations. Excision of whole or part of the nail bed concerned with nail growth (germinal matrix) is the most popular operation because by preventing regrowth of the nail recurrence is uncommon.

Any of three operations may be employed and all can be performed using a digital nerve block and tourniquet assuming circulation to the toe is normal.

a. Wedge resection (Watson-Cheyne operation). A V-shaped portion of the affected nail together with the underlying portion of the matrix is performed. It is not recommended, as the matrix removal is often incomplete.

b. Winograd's operation. This is most satisfactory when peripheral arterial disease or diabetes precludes a more radical procedure, and in such circumstances is best performed with general anaesthesia without tourniquet.

Good exposure of the matrix, by a longitudinal incision in the nail fold, allows excision under vision of the half of the nail involved and the related matrix (Fig. 37.2).

c. Zadik's operation. This operation produces excellent and long-lasting results.

The incisions are planned to contain adequately any swollen or granulating nail wall and two proximal extensions are made from the edges of the nail fold towards the distal interphalangeal joint, so that a wide flap of skin

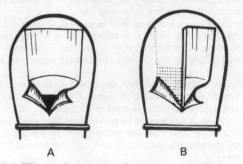

Fig. 37.2 Winograd's operation for ingrown toenail *A*. V-shaped cut to display half of germinal matrix *B*. Half nail and germinal matrix excised

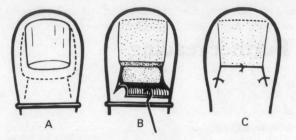

Fig. 37.3 Zadik's operation for ingrown toenail *A*. Line of incision *B*. Nail removed, flap raised, germinal matrix excised and phalanx exposed *C*. Flap replaced and sutured to non-germinal matrix

can be raised to allow access to the nail root and the matrix. The nail is removed, the limits of the matrix are dissected out, and a block of tissue containing the matrix is excised to leave bare phalanx. The flap is then replaced and sutured to the proximal edge of the remaining nail bed (Fig. 37.3)

2. 'OVERGROWN' TOE-NAIL ONYCHOGRYPHOSIS

Conservative
Repeated trimming with heavy cutters may keep the condition under control.

OPERATIVE
A nail bed ablative procedure is the only permanently effective cure.

3. NAIL BED LESIONS

Subungual haematoma. Relief of pain is obatined by evacuating the clot through a hole made in the nail with a trephine or the red-hot end of a paper clip.

Subungual exostosis. The nail is avulsed and the exostosis excised through the nail bed.

Melanoma. Excisional biopsy and histological confirmation is essential before amputation of the digit and either block dissection of the ilio-inguinal lymph nodes or perfusion therapy.

Glomus tumour. Excision is associated with dramatic and lasting relief of pain.

Further reading

This book is a guide and though it endeavours to give the average undergraduate what he needs to know, it does not claim to be wholly comprehensive. Indeed, individual clinical courses vary so much that it would never be possible to write a book or set of notes to encompass them all. The best one can do is use one's own teaching and that of one's colleagues to create a book which expresses the course in your School but has some generality. This book combines Melbourne, Adelaide and London. Some other books of a similar nature are:

Browse N L 1978 An introduction to the symptoms and signs of surgical disease. Edward Arnold, London
Clain A 1982 Demonstration of physical signs in clinical surgery (Hamilton Bailey), 16th edn. Wright, Bristol
Ellis H, Calne R Y 1977 Lecture notes on general surgery, 5th edn. Blackwell, Oxford
Macfarlane D, Thomas L P 1984 Textbook of surgery, 5th edn. Churchill Livingstone, Edinburgh

Large textbooks are aimed more at the technical side of surgery and at postgraduates but may be useful to the student for reference. Anyone who has made up his or her mind to go into surgery should be perusing them and owning one. Examples are:

Dunphy J E, Way L (eds) 1981 Current surgical diagnosis and treatment, 5th edn. Lange, Los Altos, Cal
Harding Rains A J, Ritchie H D (eds) 1981 Bailey and Love's short practice of surgery, 18th edn. Lewis, London

For help in the immediate period after qualification during pre-registration training the following may be useful:

Fraenkel G, Ludbrook J, Dudley H, Hill G, Marshall V 1982 Guide for house surgeons in the surgical unit, 7th edn. Heinemann, London
Kyle J (ed) 1984 Pye's surgical handicraft, 21st edn. Wright, Bristol

Many texts dealing with operative or specialized aspects of surgery are available. Among these are:

Adams, J C 1983 Outline of fractures, 7th edn. Churchill Livingstone, Edinburgh
Adams, J C 1983 Outline of orthopaedics, 9th edn. Churchill Livingstone, Edinburgh
Jennett W B 1977 An introduction to neurosurgery, 3rd edn. Heinemann, London
Kirk R M (ed) 1978 General surgical operations. Churchill Livingstone, Edinburgh
Rintoul R F (ed) 1984 Farquharson's textbook of operative surgery, 7th edn. Churchill Livingstone, Edinburgh

Reading the literature

This is the hardest thing to do. If you want to know about surgery there is no substitute for scanning the journals.

The *British Journal of Surgery* is a definitive, middle of the road, *important* journal for surgical documentation and advance.

The American journals such as *Surgery, Surgery, Gynecology & Obstetrics, Archives of Surgery, Annals of Surgery*, and the *American Journal of Surgery* are usually more technically orientated but well worth skimming over.

Specialist journals such as the *Journal of Bone and Joint Surgery, Journal of Urology, British Journal of Urology*, etc. are on the whole not student fodder. However, if you want to pursue a subject in depth these journals are where you will find it.

General journals: *The Lancet*, the *British Medical Journal* and the *New England Journal of Medicine*. Unfortunately too little of major surgical interest appears in such general places. Nevertheless, if you want to be part of medicine (which is a life-long study) and whatever specialty you may profess, the general journals are essential, if now rather neglected, reading.

Index

Abdomen,
  burst, 25
Abdominal
  injuries, 51 *et seq*
  paracentesis, 52
  pain, 3 *et seq*
  wall, infections, 75
Abdomino-perineal excision of rectum, 211, 213
Abscess,
  abdominal, 24
  amoebic, 198
  appendiceal, 202, 204, 209
  breast, 123
  cerebral, 85, 90 *et seq*
  cold, 73, 81, 101
  crypt, 192
  extradural, 91
  hand, 79 *et seq*
  intracranial, 90 *et seq*
  ischio-rectal, 216, 218, 220
  liver, 166
  mediastinal, 78
  metastatic, 66, 78
  pelvic, 24
  pelvi-rectal, 217
  peri-anal, 216, 218, 220
  pericaecal, 209
  pericolic, 190, 191, 192, 209, 210
  perinephric, 203, 249
  pilonidal, 217, 218, 221
  residual, after abdominal surgery, 23 *et seq*
  spinal, 105
  subaponeurotic, 85
  submucous, 217, 218, 220
  subphrenic, 24
Achalasia of oesophagus, 141 *et seq*
Achlorhydria, 157
Acid secretion studies, *see* Gastric acid studies
Acidophilic cell carcinoma, 104
Acinic carcinoma, 104
Acoustic neuroma, 90
Actinomycosis, 74, 105
Adenocystic carcinoma, 104
Adenoma,
  acidophilic cell, 104
  chromophobe, 90
  colon, 206 *et seq*

eosinophilic, 90
  multiple endocrine, syndrome, 156
  parathyroid, 119
  pleomorphic, 104
  salivary, 104
  tubular, 206
  tubulo-villous, 206
  villous, 206
Adenitis,
  cervical, 101
  mesenteric, 202
Adenosarcoma, kidney, 250
Adenosis, breast, 122
ADH, 8, 9
  secretion in injury, 12
Adhesions, in bowel obstruction, 187
Adiposis dolorosa of Dercum, 285
Adjuvant therapy in breast cancer, 127
Adrenalectomy, in breast cancer, 129, 130
Adrenocorticoid insufficiency, 19
Adrenocorticoid secretion in injury, 12
Adson manoeuvre, 132
Adult respiratory distress syndrome, 17, 20
Alcohol, in acute pancreatitis, 171
Air encephalogram (AEG), 87
Airway,
  in chest injuries, 45
  obstruction, 48
  in tracheostomy, 49
  in unconscious patient, 40, 48
Aldosterone secretion in injury, 12
Allergy,
  in Crohn's disease, 195
  in ulcerative colitis, 192
Allison repair, 147
Alpha fetoprotein, tumour marker, 245
Amaurosis fugax, 279
Amelanosis, 288
Amnesia, in head injuries, 42
Aminocaproic acid, 92, 270
Amoebiasis, 198 *et seq*
Amoeboma, 199
Ampulla of Vater, 171, 175, 180
Ampullary carcinoma, 175
Amputations, 280 *et seq*
  above knee, 281
  below knee, 281
  complications, 282
  end-bearing, 281

Gritti-Stokes, 281
  in lymphoedema, 274
  in melanoma, 289
  in osteogenic sarcoma, 280
  indications, 280
  non-end bearing, 281
  prostheses, 282
  stump care, 282
  Syme, 281
Amylase, serum, 164, 173
Amyloid disease, 101
Anaemia,
  after gastric surgery, 152
  haemolytic, 179
  in large bowel cancer, 209, 210
  pernicious, and gastric cancer, 157
Anal
  fissure, 215, 217, 219, 228
  fistulae, 217, 220
  glands, 216
  papilla, hypertrophied, 215
  papilloma, 217
  sphincter, 215
  stretch, 219
  warts, 217
Anal canal and anus,
  anatomy, 213
  carcinoma, 213 *et seq*
Anaplastic carcinoma, thyroid, 119
Anastomosis, extracranial-intracranial, 92
Anastomotic ulcer, 152
Anchovy sauce pus, 199
Aneurysms, 276 *et seq*
  aortic, abdominal, 229, 280
  cerebral, 91
  dissecting, 137, 138
  false, 57, 276
  femoral, 236
  neck, 105
  saccular, 91
  subclavian, 102
Angina
  pectoris, 136, 138
  Vincent's, 95
Angiography, *see* Arteriography
Aniline dyes and bladder cancer, 250
Ankle flare, 262
Ano-rectal suppuration, 216 *et seq*
  abscess, 216, 218, 220
  fistulae, 217, 220

Ano-rectal suppuration (cont'd)
  in Crohn's disease, 196
  in ulcerative colitis, 193
  sites of, 216
  treatment, 220
Ano-rectal examination, 228
Anthrax, 73
Antibiotic resistance, 67
Anticoagulants,
  in peripheral vascular disease, 280
  in pulmonary embolism, 271
  in venous thrombosis, 268, 269, 270
Antigens, milk, in ulcerative colitis, 192
Antioestrogen therapy, see Oestrogen
    antagonists
Antithrombotic agents, 269
Antithyroid drugs, 113
Antitoxin,
  gas gangrene, 72
  tetanus, 70
Anus, see Anal canal and anus
Aorta,
  coarctation, 136
  rupture of thoracic, 47
Aorto-enteric fistula, 229
Aortography,
  in chest injuries, 44
  in dissection aneurysm, 138
  translumbar, 278
Aphthous ulcer, 95
Appendicectomy, 204
Appendicitis, acute, 200 et seq
  classification, 200
  differential diagnosis, 201–204
  generalised peritonitis, with, 203
  inflammatory mass, with, 202
  treatment, 204
Apudoma, 156
Arterial injuries, 35, 56
  spasm, 56
  surgery, 275 et seq
Arteriography,
  carotid, 87, 92
  in abdominal injuries, 52
  in coronary artery disease, 137
  in ischaemic colitis, 198
  in liver injuries, 53
  in pancreatic disease, 175, 177
  in peripheral vascular disease, 278
  in pulmonary embolism, 271
  in rectal bleeding, 229
  in renal trauma, 54
  in thoracic outlet syndrome, 132
  vertebral, 92
Arteriovenous,
  fistulae, 57, 293
  malformations,
    bowel, 230
    intracranial, 92
Arteritis, 276
Arthritis, septic, 81, 82
Astrocytoma, 89
Atheroma, 275
Auerbach, plexus of, 141
Auto-antibodies,
  in Crohn's disease, 195
  in ulcerative colitis, 192

primary biliary cirrhosis,
    antimitochondrial, 181
  thyroid, 110
    antimicrosomal, 111, 118
    antithyroglobulin, 111, 118
Autonephrectomy, 249
Axillo-bifemoral graft, 230
Azathioprine, in colitis, 194

Bacillus anthracis, 73
Bacteraemia, 65, 66
Bacteria, antibiotic-resistant, 67
Bacterial toxins, 18
Bacteroides infections, 73, 78
Bairnsdale ulcer, 265
Ballance's sign, 53
Balloon tamponade intra-aortic, 18
Barbiturate-induced coma, 42
Barium
  enema, 190, 191, 193, 198, 210
  meal, 142, 146, 150, 159, 210
  meal and follow-through, 210
  swallow, 142, 146
Barrett's oesophagus, 140
Basal cell carcinoma, 286
Basal metabolic rate (BMR), 114
Bassini operation, 237
BCG vaccination, 73
  in melanoma, 289
Bed sores, 21, 265, 266
Belsey repair, 147
Beta-adrenergic receptor antagonists, in
    thyrotoxicosis, 113, 114
Bezoar, 161
Biliary,
  calculi, 162 et seq
  colic, 163
  fistula, external, 169
  peritonitis, 169
  sepsis, 63
  surgery, complications, 168
Bilirubin, metabolism and disorders,
    178 et seq
Billroth I gastrectomy, 151, 152, 160,
    225
Biofeedback therapy, in incontinence,
    258
Biopsy,
  aspiration, prostate, 255
  excision, breast, 122
  incision, pancreas, 177
  needle, breast, 126
    pancreas, 177
    prostate, 255
Bile,
  diversion of, 176
  leakage, 169
  lipid composition, 162
  lithogenic, 162
  pigment, metabolism and disorders,
    179
  salts, 162
Bile duct,
  anatomy, 168, 169
  abnormalities, 163, 168
  axial, 163
  exploration, 167

injury, 167, 168
  obstruction, 163, 175
  paraxial, 163
  residual and reformed stones, 170
  stricture, 168
  T-tubes, 167, 169, 170
Bladder, see also Incontinence
  atonic, 258
  injuries, 35
  neck, stenosis, 256
  perforation, 256
  training, 258
  tumours, 250 et seq
    staging, 251
    treatment, 254
  unstable, 258
Bleeding, see Haemorrhage
Bleeding diatheses, 29
Block dissection,
  inguinal, in melanoma, 289
    in prostatic cancer, 255
  neck, 98
  prophylactic, in melanoma, 288 et seq
    in testicular tumours, 244
Blood,
  flow, peripheral, 15
  loss, 15 et seq
  transfusion, 32, 224, 225
  volume, circulating, 15
Blumberg's sign, 201
Bochdalek, foramen hernia, 144
Body composition, table, 9
Body water, 7, 9
  disorders, 9, 12
  turnover, 8
Borrelia Vincenti, 95
Bowel,
  inflammatory disease, 189 et seq
  ischaemic disease, 229
  intussusception, 229
  injuries, 51
  large, bleeding, surgery in, 230
    cancer, 207 et seq
      complications, 209
      Dukes classification, 209
      pre-operative preparation, 212
      treatment, 211
    polyps, 206 et seq
  obstruction, 184 et seq
    adhesions, 187
    closed loop, 184
    management, 185
    mechanical, 184
    paralytic, 184
    post-operative, 187
    simple occlusion, 184
    strangulation, 184, 185
  preparation, 212
  pseudo-obstruction, 188
  small, bleeding, surgery in, 230
Bowen's disease, 285
Brachial plexus injuries, 56
Brain,
  compression, 38, 40, 85
  death, 42
  herniation, 87
  injuries, 37

Brain, injuries (cont'd)
  complications, 41
  lesions, 86 *et seq*
  oedema, 85
  shift, 87
  tumours, 88 *et seq*
  vascular disorders, 91
  volume, 85
Branchial
  cyst, 102, 104, 106
  fistula, 105
Breast, 121 *et seq*
  abscess, 123
  anatomy, 121
  biopsy, needle, 126
  cancer, 124 *et seq*
    advanced, 128
    diagnosis, 128
    dissemination, 126, 127, 128
    hormone dependent, 128
      manipulation, 128
    oestrogen receptor assay, 126
    prognosis, 128
    screening, 125
    staging, TNM classification, 127
    treatment, 127
      local, 127
      advanced, 128
  cysts, 122, 123
    aspiration, 122
    galactocele, 123
    retention, 122
  duct, ectasia, 123
    papilloma, 123
  examination, 125
  fat necrosis, 123
  fibroadenoma, 122
  fibroadenosis, 122
  fistula, 122
  lumpy, 122
  mass, 122
  Paget's disease, 124
  pigeon, 131
  sarcoma, 130
Breslow, tumour thickness in
  melanoma, 288
Bronchopneumonia, post-operative, 20
Bronchoscopy, 106, 133, 134
Bronchus, rupture, 46
Bubonocele, 234
Buerger's disease, 265, 266, 267, 275
  et seq
Burns, 59 *et seq*
  aftermath, 64
  antibiotic therapy, 62
  chemical, 64
  chest problems, 63
  depth, 60
    method of assessment, 60
  haemoglobinuria, 61
  myoglobinuria, 61
  infection, 63
  irradiation, 64
  local management, 62
  nutrition, 63
  pain relief, 62
  prevention, 64

  pruritis, 64
  rehabilitation, 64
  scars, management, 62
  shock, 61
  sweating, 64
  thermo-regulation, 64
Burr holes, 41
  aspiration, 91
  biopsy, 89
  exploratory, 41, 88
Bursa, subhyoid, 100, 102

C-cells, 119
Caecostomy, 212
Caecum, carcinoma, 202
Calciferol (Vitamin D), 117
Calcitonin, 119
Calculus,
  biliary, 162 *et seq*
    residual, reformed, 170
  pancreatic, 175
  renal, 253
  salivary, 102, 104, 106
  ureteric, 202, 253
  urinary, 248, 256
  vesical, 251, 256
Calf vein thrombosis, 267, 272
Campylobacter sp., 202
Cannon ball lesion, lung, 135
Caput medusa, 181
Carbimazole, 113, 114
Carbuncle,
  face, 94
  neck, 99
Carcino-embryonic antigen (CEA), 211
Carcinoma, *see* Organs affected
Carcinoma-in-situ,
  bladder, 150
  skin, 285
Cardiac
  catheter studies, 137
  injuries, 47
  tamponade, 18
Cardiomyotomy, 143
Cardioplegia, 138
Cardiopulmonary bypass, 138
Carotid
  angiography, 87, 92
  arterial vascular disease, 279
  body tumour, 102, 105, 106
Castration, *see* Oophorectomy,
  Orchiectomy
Cat scratch disease, 101
Catecholamine secretion,
  in injury, 12
  in shock, 18
Catheterization, *see also* Central venous
  urethral, 257
Causalgia, 56
Caval, *see* Vena cava
Cavernous sinus,
  syndrome, 86, 91
  thrombosis, 94
Cellulitis, 66
  clostridial, 71
Cephalohaematoma, 84
Central venous,

catheterization (cannula), 61
  pressure, 61, 76, 174
Cerebral oedema, 42
Cerebrospinal fluid (CSF)
  circulation, 85
  leak, 42
  otorrhoea, 42
  rhinorrhoea, 42
  volume, 85
Chain of lakes, in chronic pancreatitis,
  175
Charcot's triad, 166
Cheilosis, 95
Chemotherapy in cancer, *see* Cytotoxic
  therapy
Chest,
  flail, 46
  infections, 77
  injuries, 44 *et seq*
    management, 45 *et seq*
  tunnel, 131
Chest wall
  disorders, 131 *et seq*
  tumours, metastatic, 131
Chilblains, 265, 267, 272
Child's grading, in portal hypertension,
  226
Cholangiohepatitis, oriental, 162
Cholangitis, 166
  malignant, 168
  sclerosing, 168
Cholangiogram, *see* Cholegrams
Cholecystectomy, 165, 169
  complications, 168 *et seq*
Cholecystitis
  acalculous acute, 167
  acute, 164 *et seq*
  anaerobic, 167
  emphysematous, 167
  treatment, 165
Cholecyst-jejunostomy, 177
Cholecystokinin, 167
Cholecystostomy, 165
Choledochoduodenostomy, 167, 176
Choledochography, *see* Cholegrams
Choledochojejunostomy, 177
Choledocholithiasis, 166 *et seq*
Choledochoscope, 165
Cholegrams
  E.R.C.P., 167, 175, 182
  intravenous, 164, 166, 175
  operative, 165, 182
  oral, 166, 175
  P.T.C., 167
  post-operative T-tube, 166, 167
Cholestasis
  extra-hepatic, 179, 180
  intra-hepatic, 179
Cholesterol, in bile, 162
Choriocarcinoma, 244
Chromium (Cr^{51}), red cell labelled, 229
Chvostek-Weiss sign, 116
Chylothorax, 47, 132, 133
Chylous reflux, 272
Cimetidine, 64, 143, 149, 150
Cirrhosis, primary biliary, 180, 181
Clark's levels of invasion, melanoma, 288

Claudication, intermittent, 276, 278
Clavicle, tumours, 103
Clear cell carcinoma, kidney, 249
Cleft lip, 93
Cleft palate, 93
Clonorchis senensis, 162
Cloquet's
    hernia, 238
    node, 237
Cock's peculiar tumour, 85
Clostridium
    difficile, 22, 199
    oedematiens, 71
    septicum, 71
    sporogenes, 71
    tetani, 69
    welchii, 71
Coeliac plexus, injection, 177
Coin lesion, 135
Cold injury, 265, 267
Colectomy, *see also* Hemi-colectomy
    sigmoid, 213
    total, with mucosal proctectomy, 195,
        197
        with ileo-rectal anastomosis, 195,
            197, 230
        with ileostomy, 195, 197
    transverse, 212, 213
Colitis
    amoebic, 198
    chemical, 199
    Crohn's, 196
    ischaemic, 197, 229
    pseudomembranous, 22, 199
    ulcerative, 192
Collagen, in wound healing, 28 *et seq*
Colon
    carcinoma, 207 *et seq*
        treatment, 211 *et seq*
    diverticula, *see* Diverticular disease
    inflammation, *see* Inflammatory
        bowel disease
    obstruction, *see* Bowel obstruction
    polyps, *see* Polyps
Colonoscopy, 207, 229
Colostomy,
    in diverticular disease, 191
    in large bowel obstruction, 186, 192
    loop transverse, 213
Commando operation, 97
Common bile duct, *see* Bile ducts
Complications, post-operative, 20 *et seq*
Condyloma accuminata, 217
Coning, *see* Herniation, brain
Contact bleeding, in colitis, 193
Contraction, contractures, *see* Wound
Cooper, ligament of Astley, 233, 237
Coomb's test, in haemolysis, 181
Cope's sign, 201
Coraline clot, 267
Coronary artery, autogenous vein graft,
    138
Coronary endarterectomy, 138
Corticosteroids, in ulcerative colitis, 194
Cortisol secretion, in injury, 12
Costoclavicular syndrome, 131

Courvoisier's law, 177, 181
Craniectomy, 41
    posterior fossa, 89, 90
Craniopharyngioma, 90
Craniotomy, 41, 88
Crigler-Najjar's disease, 178
Crohn's disease, 195 *et seq*
    of colon, 196
    of oesophagus, 142
    regional enteritis, 196
Cross-infection, 22
Cruveilhier's sign, 236
CT scan, for,
    dissecting aneurysm, 138
    head injuries, 38
    intracranial lesions, 87
    lung disorders, 135
    jaundice, 182
    pancreatic lesions, 177
    subphrenic abscess, 25
    testicular tumours, 245
Cullen's sign, 172
Cupid's bow, 94
Curling's ulcer, 148, 223
Cushing's syndrome, 272
    ulcer, 223
Cylindroma, 85
Cyst
    branchial, 102, 104, 106
    breast, 122, 123
    dermoid,
        inclusion, 283
        implantation, 283
        large bowel, 206
        sublingual, 95, 100
    epidermoid (sebaceous), 85, 90, 283
    epididymal, 246
    retention, of buccal mucous gland, 95
    suprasellar, 90
    thyroglossal, 100, 102, 106
    vitello-intestinal, 205
Cystectomy, total with urinary
    diversion, 254
Cyst-gastrostomy, in pseudocyst, 174
Cystic artery, anatomical variants, 169
Cystic duct
    anatomical variants, 168
    obstruction, 163, 165, 166
    stump syndrome, 170
Cystic hygroma, 102, 105
Cyst-jejunostomy, Roux-en-Y, 174
Cystogram, 257, 258
Cystometrogram, 257, 258
Cystosarcoma phylloides, 130
Cystoscopy, 252, 253, 254
Cysto-urethrogram, in pelvic fractures,
    35
Cytotoxic therapy
    in breast cancer, 127, 129, 130
    in large bowel cancer, 212
    in testicular tumours, 245

Dactylitis, tuberculous, 81, 82
Debridement, *see* Wound excision
Decompression, intestinal, 77
Delphian node, 108, 119

Denonvillier's fascia, 251
De Quervain's disease
    tenosynovitis, 81
    thyroiditis, 118
Dercum's disease, 285
Dermatofibroma, 284
Dermoid cysts, skin, 283
    sublingual, 100
Detrusor instability, 257
Dexamethasone, 42, 88
Diabetes, in injury, 13
    in peripheral vascular disease, 275,
        279, 280
Diabetic gangrene, *see* Ulcer,
    neuropathic
Diaphragm
    eventration, 144
    hernia, 144
    hiatal hernia, 144
    rupture, 47, 144
Diazoxide, in insulinoma, 178
Dioxyphenylalanine (DOPA), 286
Disobliteration, 279
Diverticular disease and diverticulitis,
    189 *et seq*
Diverticulum, colonic, 189
    Meckel's, 205, 229
Dohle bodies, neutrophils, 18
Doppler
    shift, 268
    ultrasound
        in arterial disease, 278
        in venous disease, 262, 268, 271
Douglas, semilunar fold of, 240
Dubin-Johnson disease, 179
Ductus arteriosus, patent, 136
Dukes, classification of large bowel
    cancer, 209
Dumping syndrome, 152
Duodenal
    carcinoma, 176
    ulcer, *see* Peptic ulcer
Dupuytren's contracture, 285
Dysphagia, 139 *et seq*
    lusoria, 141
    post-vagotomy, 141
    sideropenic, 141

Echo-cardiography, 137
Echo-encephalography, 41
Ectasia, vascular, of bowel, 229
Ehlers-Danlos, syndrome, 222
Electro-encephalography (EEG), 41, 87
Elemental diets, 14
Embolectomy, pulmonary, 271
Embolism
    air, 115
    arterial, 275
    pulmonary, 18, 267, 271, 272
Embryoma, 250
Embryonal carcinoma, testis, 244
Emphysema
    surgical, 44
    mediastinal, 44
Empyema, 77
Encephalitis, 42

Encephaloid carcinoma, breast, 124
Encephalopathy, porto-systemic, 225
Endolymphatic therapy, in melanoma, 289
Endorphin system, 2
Endoscopic retrograde pancreatico-cholangiography (ERCP), 167, 175, 182
Endotoxins, 18
Energy, expenditure in injury, 13
Enkephalins, 2
Entamoeba histolytica, 198
Enteral feeding, 14, 63
Enteritis, regional *see* Crohn's disease
Entero-colitis, pseudo-membranous, 22
Ependymoma, 89
Epidermal tumours, 285
Epidermoid
  carcinoma, 104
  cyst, 283
Epididymectomy, 243
Epididymis, 241 *et seq*
  cysts, 246
Epididymo-orchidectomy, 243
Epididymo-orchitis, 242 *et seq*
  acute, 242
  chronic, 243
  tuberculous, 243
Epitheliosis, breast, 122, 124
Erb's palsy, 56
Erythema nodosum, 193
Erythrocyanosis frigida, 272
Ethanolamine oleate, sclerosing agent, 262
Exomphalos, 239
Exophthalmos, 114, 117
Exostosis, subungual, 290
Exotoxins, 18
Exteriorization operation, colonic, 191
Extra-cellular fluid (ECF) and extra-cellular water (ECW), 7 *et seq*
  acute deficiency, 9
  excess, 16
  loss, 16

Face, 93 *et seq*
Factor VIII, 29
Faecal impaction, 21
Fainting, 14
Fallot's tetrology, 137
Falx cerebri, 85
Fasciitis, necrotizing, 72
Fasciotomy
  in fractures, 33
  in vascular injuries, 57
Fat necrosis, breast, 123
Feeding
  intravenous, 14
    in burns, 64
    infection in, 67
  tube (enteral), 14
    in burns, 14
    in unconscious patient, 40

Feet
  care in peripheral vascular disease, 278
  neuropathic, 279
  ulcers, 265
Felon, 79
Femoral
  hernia, 236 *et seq*
  sheath, 237
Fiberoptic endoscopy, *see* Colonoscopy; Gastroscopy; Sigmoidoscopy
Fibre diet, high, 219
Fibrinogen
  level, in pancreatitis, 272
  radio-active iodine labelled in venous thrombosis, 268
Fibrinolysis, 29
Fibrinolytic therapy, 270
Fibroadenoma, 122
Fibroadenosis, 122
Filariasis, 272
Finger, infections, 79 *et seq*
Fissure-in-ano, *see* Anal fissure
Fissurectomy, 219
Fistula
  ano-rectal, 193, 217
  aorto-enteric, 229
  arterio-venous, 57, 273
  biliary, external, 168
  breast, 122
  bronchial, 78
  broncho-pleural, 78
  chylous, 98
  colo-cutaneous, 190
  diverticular, 190
  duodenal, 170
  enteric, post-operative, 26
  entero-colic, 196, 209
  faecal, 192
  gastro-intestinal, nutrition in, 13
  gastro-jejuno-colic, 152
  ileo-colic, 209
  mammillary, 122
  peri-anal, *see* Anorectal fistula
  recto-vaginal, 209
  thyroglossal, 100
  tubal, 190
  uterine, 190
  vaginal, 190
  vesico-colic, 190, 191, 192, 209, 210
Flail chest, 46
Fluoride excess, 109
Follicular carcinoma, thyroid, 119
Foramen
  caecum, 100
  incisive, 93
  of Bochdalek, 144
  of Lushka, 85
  of Magendie, 85
  of Monro, 85
  of Morgagni, 144
Foreign bodies
  hand, 83
  in appendicitis, 200
  oesophagus, 140, 141, 142
  stomach, 161

Fractures, 32 *et seq*
  complications, 33
  healing, 32
  immobilization, 33
  pelvic, 35
  reduction, 33
  rib, 44
  skull, 42
Fraenum linguae, 94
Free thyroxine index (FTI), III
Friedrichsen-Waterhouse, syndrome, 19
Froment's sign, 55
Frusemide, 11, 182
Fundoplication, stomach, 147
Fusiformis fusiformis, 95

Galactocele, 123
Galea, 84
Gall bladder
  dyskinesia, 167
  empyema, 203
  mucocele, 163
  surgery, 165, 167
    complications, 168–170
Gall-stone ileus, 164
Gall-stones, 163 *et seq*
  in pancreatitis, 171
Gamma camera, 271
Ganglion, 284
Ganglioneuroblastoma, 136
Gangrene, 63
  amputation for, 281
  arterial, 266
  dry, 66
  in appendicitis, 200
  in bowel obstruction, 185
  in hernia, 238, 239
  in infection, 65
  in ischaemic colitis, 197
  in peripheral vascular disease, 278
  skin, 265, 266
  synergistic, 72
  venous, 269
Gardner's syndrome, 208
Gas gangrene, 71 *et seq*
  amputation for, 281
Gastrectomy
  Billroth I, 151, 152, 160, 225
  cancer following, 157
  complications, 151 *et seq*
  Polya, 151, 152, 154, 160, 225
  radical subtotal, 160
  radical total, 160
  radical upper partial, 160
  total, for Zollinger-Ellison syndrome, 156
Gastric
  acid studies, 146, 150, 156, 159
  cancer, 157 *et seq*
  cytology, 159
  mucosa, heterotopic, 205
Gastrin, 156
Gastritis
  atrophic, 153
  bile reflux, 153
  chronic, 157

Gastro-enteritis, 202
Gastro-enterostomy, 151, 225
Gastrografin contrast examination
  in bowel obstruction, 185
  in oesophageal rupture, 47
Gastro-intestinal haemorrhage, 222
    et seq
  classification, 222
  investigation, 223
  per-rectum, 226–230
  upper, 222–226
Gastroscopy, 150, 159, 224
Gastrostomy
  feeding, 14
  for gastric decompression, 21, 77, 186
Genetic defects
  in jaundice, 178
  in thyroid disease, 109
Germ cells, testes, 243
Gigantism, 273
Gilbert's disease, 179
Gimbernat's ligament, 233, 237, 238, 239
Giraldes, organ of (paradidymis), 246
Glasgow coma scale, 39
Glioblastoma multiforme, 89
Glioma, 89
Globus hystericus, 141
Glomerular filtration rate (GFR), 12
Glomus tumour, 290
Glossitis, 94 *et seq*
Glottic oedema, 115
Gluconeogenesis, 13
Goitre, 102, 103, 108 *et seq*
Goitrogens, 109
Gonadotrophin
  in testicular maldescent, 242
  in testicular tumours, 243
Grafts
  arterial, synthetic, 280
  split skin, 62, 266
  vein, reversed saphenous, 279
Granulomas, in Crohn's disease, 195
Grave's disease, 110
Grawitz tumour, kidney, 249
Grey Turner's sign, 172
Gritti – Stokes amputation, 281
Gumma, 74
Gynaecological conditions, mimicking
    appendicitis, 202
Gynaecomastia, 244
Gynandroblastoma (orchioblastoma), 244

Haematemesis, 222 *et seq*
Haematocele, 247
Haematoma
  expanding, 57
  intracranial, 37, 38, 41
  peri-anal, 216, 218, 220
  pulsating, 57
  scalp, 84
  subungual, 290, 291
Haematuria, 248 *et seq*
  investigation of, 252 *et seq*
Haemobilia, 54
Haemodialysis, 11

Haemodilution, in shock, 16
Haemoglobinuria, in burns, 61
Haemoperitoneum, 47
Haemoptysis, 222
Haemorrhage
  diverticular, 190
  extradural, 38
  gastro-intestinal, 222–230
    per rectum, 226–230
    upper, 222–226
  in shock, 16
  in ulcerative colitis, 193
  intracranial, 38
  scalp, 39
  subarachnoid, 38, 91
  subdural, 38
Haemorrhoids, 215 *et seq*
  bleeding, 226, 227
  degrees of, internal, 216
  injection, 219
  operations for, 219
  position of, primary, 216
  recurrent, 220
Haemothorax, 46, 47
Hamartoma, 92, 206
Hand
  foreign bodies, 83
  infections, 78 *et seq*
Hartmann's
  pouch, 163
  solution, 11, 17, 61, 76, 186
Hashimoto's disease, 111, 117, *et seq*
Hasselbach's
  hernia, 238
  ligament, 234
  triangle, 234
Head injuries, 37 *et seq*
  complications, 41
  management, 38
Heart disease, 136 *et seq*
Heller's cardiomyotomy, 143
Hemicolectomy
  extended right, 212
  left, 212
  right, 212
Henry's incision, 238
Hepatectomy, 53
Hepatic
  coma, 225
  injury, 53
Heparin, in venous thrombosis, 270
Hepatitis
  amoebic, 198
  primary biliary, 179
  viral, 179
Hernia, 231 *et seq*
  Bochdalek, foramen of, 144, 145
  Cloquet's (pectineal), 238
  diaphragmatic, 144 *et seq*
    congenital, 144, 145, 146
    traumatic, 47, 144, 145, 146
  dual, 234
  epigastric, 240
  external, 231 *et seq*
  femoral, 236, 237–240
  gluteal, 240
  Hasselbach's 238

hiatus, 144 *et seq*
  haemorrhage and, 223
  para-oesphageal (rolling), 145
  sliding, 141, 142, 144, 146, 223
  incarcerated, 232
  incisional, 25
  inguinal, 233 *et seq*
    complicated, 236
    treatment, 237
    types of, 234
  internal, 186
  Langier's (lacunar), 238
  Littre's, 232
  lumbar, 240
  Maydl's, 232
  Narath's (external femoral), 238
  obturator, 240
  Ogilvie's, 234
  pantaloon, 234
  para-umbilical, 239
  pectineal, 238
  prevascular, 238
  recurrent, 233, 237
  Richter's, 232, 238
  saddlebag, 234
  sciatic, 240
  scrotal, 236
  Spigelian, 240
  treatment of, principles, 232
  umbilical, 239
Hernia-en-glissade, 144
Herniation
  brain, 87
  foraminal, 87
  stomach, 47
  tentorial, 87
Hernioplasty, 232, 237
Herniorrhaphy, 232, 237, 238
  Bassini operation, 237
  Shouldice operation, 237
  Tanner's slide, 237
Herniotomy, 232, 237
Herpes simplex, 94
Hiatus hernia, 144 *et seq*
  see also Dysphagia
  treatment, 146–147
HIDA isotope secretion scan, 164
Hill repair, 147
Hip, osteoarthritis, 278
Hippocratic facies, 203
Histamine H_2 antagonists, 64, 143, 149, 150
Histiocytoma, 284
Hodgkin's disease, 101, 102, 103
Hofmeister valve, 151
Homeostasis
  kidney, 8
  potassium, 11
  water, 8
Horner's syndrome, 102, 116, 134
Human chorionic gonadotrophin
    (HCG), tumour marker, 244, 245
Hutchinson's freckle, 288
Hydatid disease, 180, 182
Hydatid of Morgagni, 246
Hydrocele, 246 *et seq*
  aspiration, 247

Hydrocele (cont'd)
  canal of Nuck, 236, 246
  encysted of cord, 236, 246
  operative treatment, 247
Hydrocephalus, obstructive, 90
Hydrocortisone, in shock, 19
Hydroxyproline, urinary in breast
      cancer, 126
Hygroma
  cystic, 102, 105
  subdural, 38
Hyperabduction syndrome, 131
Hyperbaric oxygen, 72
Hyperbilirubinaemia, familial, 179, 180
Hyperchlorhydria, 148
Hypercholesterolaemia, 275
Hyperlipidaemia, 171, 275
Hypernephroma, 249
Hyperparathyroidism, 171
Hyperpyrexia, in head injuries, 40
Hypertension, portal, 223, 226
Hyperthyroidism, see Thyrotoxicosis
Hyperventilation, in cerebral oedema,
      42
Hypoglycaemia, insulin induced, 19
Hypokalaemia, 11
Hyponatraemia, in prostatic surgery,
      256
Hypoparathyroidism, 113
  post-thyroidectomy, 116
Hypophysectomy
  in breast cancer, 130
  transethmoidal, 90
Hypopituitarism, 90
Hypothyroidism, 111
  post-thyroidectomy, 117

Ileitis, 202
  acute regional, 196
Ileo-colitis, 195
Ileo-cystoplasty, 255
Ileo-rectal anastomosis, 195, 230
Ileostomy, 195, 197
  split loop, 195
Ileus
  gall stone, 164
  paralytic, 76, 77, 172, 184, 185, 190
  management, 187
Image intensifier, 83
Imidazole carboxamide (DTIC), in
      melanoma, 289
Impacted faeces, 186
Incisions
  burr holes, 41
  hand infections, 81, 82
  Henry's, 238
  McEvedy's, 238
Incontinence
  urinary, 257 et seq
  overflow, 258
  stress, 257
  total, 258
  urge, 258
Infections
  abdominal wall, 75
  acute, 65 et seq
    chemotherapy, 66

cross-infection, 22
  facial, 94
  hand, 78
  hospital-acquired, 67
  management, 66
  opportunistic, 67
  palmar-space, 79
  prevention, 66
  pulp-space, 79
  specific sites, 75 et seq
  specific species, 69 et seq
  spread, 65
  thenar-space, 79
  web-space, 79
  wound, see Wound infection
Inflammatory bowel disease, see Bowel
Infra-tentorial
  exploration, 88
  lesions, 86
Ingrown toe nails, see Toe nails
Inguinal
  canal anatomy, 233
  hernia, 233 et seq
  lymph nodes, see Lymph nodes and
      Block dissection
Injection, of haemorrhoids, 219
Injuries, see also organs affected
  blast, 44
  general management, 31 et seq
  high velocity, 29, 51
  low velocity, 29, 51
Injury
  metabolic response, 12 et seq
  neuro-endocrine response, 12
Insensible losses, 8
Insulinoma, 178
Intermittent claudication, see
      Claudication
Intermittent positive pressure
      ventilation (IPPV)
  in brain death, 43
  in respiratory support, 48
  in shock lung, 21,
  in tetanus, 70
Interstitial cell tumours, 244
Intestinal obstruction, see Bowel
      obstruction
Intestine, see Bowel
Intimal tear, 57
Intracellular fluid, 7, 9
Intracranial
  abscess, 90
  aneurysms, 91
  blood volume, 85
  calcification, 87
  pressure, 85
  tumours, 88 et seq
Intrathoracic conditions, 131 et seq
Intravenous urogram (IVU), 252, 253,
      255
  in kidney trauma, 54
  in large bowel cancer, 211
  in pelvic fractures, 35
Intubation, endotracheal, 48
Intussusception, 229
Inverted 3 sign, in pancreatic mass, 176
Iodine

deficiency, 109
I^{131}, 111
  Lugol's, 114
  radio-active, 113, 119, 120
Ion exchange resins, 11
Ionic concentration, body fluids, 9
Ischaemia, 57
  of bowel, 197, 229
  of lower limb, 277, 278, 279
Ischaemic colitis, 197
  heart disease, 136, 138
  transient attacks, 92, 279
  vascular disease, 278, 281
Ischio-rectal abscess, 216, 218, 220
Isotope scan, see Radioactive isotope
      scan
Isotopes, see Chromium, Iodine,
      Technetium.

Jaboulay's operation, 247
Jaundice, 178 et seq
  acholuric, 178
  classification, 178
  diagnosis, 180
  haemolytic, 178
  in bile duct stricture, 168
  in choledocholithiasis, 166
  in pancreatic carcinoma, 177
  in pancreatitis, 172, 174, 175
  obstructive (surgical), 178
  pre-operative preparation, 182
  surgical treatment, 182
Jejunostomy, feeding, 14
Joint stiffness, after fracture, 34
Junctional naevus, 286
Juvenile melanoma, 287

Kallikrein inhibitor, see Trasylol
Kangri cancer of Kashmir, 286
Kehr's sign, 53
Keloid, 29, 284
Keratitis, 88
Kerato-acanthoma, 284
Keratosis
  seborrhoeic, 285
  senile, 285
Kidney
  injuries, 54
  stones, 253
  tuberculosis, 249
  tumours, 249 et seq
Killian, dehiscence of, 100
Kissing ulcer, duodenal, 149
Klumpke's palsy, 56
Koch pouch, 195
Krukenberg tumour, 158

L.A.T.S., 110
Langhans layer, 244
Langier's hernia, 238
Lannier's triangle, 100
Laparoscopy, 202
Large cell carcinoma, lung, 134
Laryngeal nerve injury, after
      thyroidectomy, 116
Laryngocele, 100, 102, 106
Laryngoscopy, 106
  indirect, 114

Laryngostomy, emergency, 49
Larynx, carcinoma, 101
Laser photocoagulation, endoscopic, 225
Leather-bottle stomach, 157
Leg
  amputation, 280 et seq
  arterial disease, 275 et seq
  swelling of, 271 et seq
  ulceration, 263 et seq
Lentigo maligna, 288
Leriche syndrome, 277
Leukoplakia, 94, 96
Leydig cell, 243
  tumour, 244
Lid, lag and retraction, 110
Lieberkühn, crypts of, 192
Ligament
  inguinal, 233
  interfoveal (Hasselbach), 234
  lacunar (Gimbernat), 233
  pectineal (Astley Cooper), 233
Limb, lower, swelling, 271 et seq
Limb shortening operations, 274
Linea alba hernia, 240
Linitis plastica, 157
Lip
  carcinoma, 95 et seq
    treatment, 98
  cleft, 93
  cysts, 95
Lipoedema, 272
Lipoma
  large bowel, 206
  neck, 99, 103, 106
  skin, 284
  spermatic cord, 236
Littré's hernia, 232
Liver, see also Hepatic
  biopsy, 181
  failure, 180
  in portal hypertension, 226
  injuries, 53
Lobectomy, pulmonary, 89
Lockwood operation, 239
Lotheissen operation, 239
Ludwig's angina, 95
Lugol's iodine, 114
Lumbar hernia, 240
Lumbar puncture, 87
Lumbar sympathectomy, 366
Lumbar triangle of Petit, 240
Lung
  biopsy, 134
  carcinoma, 135 et seq
  contusion, 46
  disorders, 133 et seq
  laceration, 46
Lupus vulgaris, 286
Lushka, foramen of, 85
Lymph node biopsy, 106
Lymph node dissection, see Block dissection
Lymph nodes and lymphatics
  axillary 121
  breast, 121
  cervical, 97

Cloquet's, 237
Delphian, 108, 119
  hilar, 135
  inguinal, 214
  internal mammary, 121
  jugulo-digastric, 97
  jugulo-omohyoid, 97
  para-aortic, 244
  posterior intercostal, 121
  scalene, 134
  stomach, 158
  supraclavicular, 98
  swellings, 101 et seq
Lymphadenectomy, see also Block dissection
  in testicular tumours, 245
Lymphadenitis, 66, 101, 102
Lymphangiitis, 66
Lymphangiography, 245, 274
Lymphoedema, 272 et seq
Lymphoma, 136   see also Hodgkin's disease
Lympho-venous anastomosis, 274

McBurney's point, 201
McCutcheon's theory, in pancreatitis, 171
McEvedy's incision, 238
Macronutrients, 13
Magendie, foramen of, 85
Malignant pustule, 73
Mallory-Weiss syndrome, 141, 223
Mammary duct ectasia, 123
Mammillary fistula, 122
Mammography, 106, 125
Mannitol
  in head injuries, 42
  in jaundice, 182
  in neurosurgery, 88
Mantoux test, 95
Marfan's syndrome, 137
Marjolin's ulcer, 286
Marseilles symposium on pancreatitis, 174
Martorell's ulcer, 265
Mask (danger) area, face, 94
Mastectomy, 127
Mastitis, 123
Maydl's hernia, 232
Mayo repair, 239
Medulloblastoma, 89
Meckel's diverticulum, 205, 229, 232
Mediastinoscopy, 134
Mediastinum
  disorders, 135 et seq
  emphysema, 44
Medullary carcinoma
  breast, 134
  thyroid, 119
Megacolon, toxic, 193
Meig's syndrome, 132
Melaena, 222 et seq
Meleney's synergistic gangrene, 72
Melanin, 286
Melanocyte, 286
Melanoma (malignant), 287 et seq
  histological grading, 288

  juvenile, 287
  nodular, 288
  Pagetoid, 288
  subungual, 280, 287
  superficial spreading, 288
    treatment, 288 et seq
Mendelson's syndrome, 21
Menetrière's disease, 161
Meningioma, 90
Meningitis, in head injuries, 42
Meningococcal septicaemia, 18
6-Mercaptopurine, in ulcerative colitis, 194
Mesenteric
  adenitis, 202
  occlusion, 203
  tears, 51
Mesothelioma, 132
Metastases in cancer, see organs affected
Metaplasia, intestinal, 157
Metabolic response to injury, 12 et seq
Methaemalbumin in pancreatitis, 173
Metronidazole, 73, 77
  in amoebiasis, 199
  in appendicitis, 205
Micronutrients, 13, 29
Mid-inguinal point, 234
Mikulicz disease, 104
Millard's operation, 94
Milroy's disease, 272
Moles, 286 et seq   see also Naevus
Molluscum sebaceum, 284
Mongolian spot, 287
Monro, foramen of, 85
Morgagni
  foramen of, hernia, 144
  hydatid of, 246
Mouth, 93 et seq
  carcinoma, floor of, 95 et seq
    treatment, 98
  congenital disorders, 93
  cysts, 95
  inflammatory disorders, 94
Mucocele of gall bladder, 163
Muco-epidermoid carcinoma, 104
Mucoid carcinoma, breast, 124
Multiple antibiotic-resistant bacteria, 67
Multiple endocrine adenoma (MEA) syndrome, 156
Mumps, 104, 242
Murphy's sign, 164
Muscle tumours, 105
Myasthenia gravis, 136
Mycobacterium ulcerans, 265
Myoglobinuria, see Burns
Myonecrosis, clostridial, 71
Myxoedema, 272 et seq
Myxoma, atrial, 137, 138

Naevus
  pigmented, 286 et seq
    treatment, 287
  blue, 287
  compound, 287
  intradermal, 287
  junctional, 286
Nail disorders, 289 et seq

Nail operations, 290
Narath's hernia, 238
Narcotics, in head injuries, 40
Nasogastric drainage, 77, 186
Natal cleft, 221
Neck
  anatomy, 99
  lymph nodes, 97 *et seq*
    block dissection, 98, 106
  swellings, 99 *et seq*
  triangles, 99
  wry, 105
Neoplastic polyps, colon, 206 *et seq*
Nephrectomy
  auto, 249
  for calculus, 253
  for carcinoma, 254
  partial, 253
Nephroblastoma, 250, 254
Nephrolithiasis, *see* Renal calculi
Nephrolithotomy, 253
Nephro-ureterectomy, 254
Nerve
  cervical sympathetic, 116
  conduction test, 132
  femoral, 56
  funiculi, 56
  injury, 55 *et seq*
    in fractures, 34
  intercosto-brachial, 121
  laryngeal, recurrent, 113, 116, 135
    superior, 116
  median, 55
  radial, 55
  sciatic, 35, 56
  ulnar, 55
Neurilemmoma, 136
Neuroblastoma, 136
Neurofibroma, 99, 136
Neuroglia, tumours, 89
Neuroleptanalgesia, in neurosurgery, 88
Neuroma
  acoustic, 90
  of amputation stump, 282
Neuropathy, in vascular disease, 279
Neuropathic ulcer, 265
Neuropraxia, 55
Neurotmesis, 55
Nines, rule of, in burns, 59
Nipple
  discharge, 123
  Paget's disease, 124
Nissen fundoplication, 147
Nitrogen, excretion in injury, 13
Nocturnal proctalgia, 217
Nodule
  thyroid, 112, 119
  pulmonary, 135
Nück
  canal of, 231
  hydrocele of, 236
Nutrition, *see also* Feeding
  enteral, 14, 63
  in burns, 63
  in head injuries, 40
  in injury (surgery), 13

in tetanus, 70
parenteral, 14

Oat cell carcinoma, 134
Obstruction, *see* Bowel obstruction
Occult blood, faecal, 160, 210
Octapressin, 225
Oddi, sphincter of, 170, 171, 173, 180
  stenosis of, 176
Oedema
  cerebral, 42
  lymphatic, 272
  venous, 272
Oesophageal varices, 225
Oesophageal web, 141
Oesophagectomy, 143
Oesophagitis, reflux (peptic), 141 *et seq*, 223
Oesophagoscopy, 106, 143, 146
Oesophagus, 139 *et seq*
  achalasia, 141
  anatomy, 139
  Barrett's, 140
  carcinoma, 140
  Crohn's disease of, 140, 142
  cytology, 143
  lacerations, 141
  manometry, 143, 146
  motility, 139
  perforation, 141
  rupture, 47
  stricture, corrosive, 143
    peptic, 143
Oestrogen
  antagonists, 129, 127
  receptors, in breast cancer, 126
  therapy, in prostatic cancer, 255
Ogilvie's hernia, 234
Oligodendroglioma, 89
Omphalitis, 75
Onkocytes, 104
Onychocryptosis, 289
Onychogryposis, 289
Oophorectomy, in breast cancer, 127
Ophthalmoplegia, in thyrotoxicosis, 110
Opiate receptors, 2
Opisthotonus, 70
Orchidopexy, 242
Orchiectomy
  in prostatic cancer, 255
  in testicular tumour, 245
Orchioblastoma, 244
Osteoarthritis, hip, 278
Osteogenic sarcoma, amputation in, 280
Osteomyelitis
  acute, 65
  chest wall, 131
  hand, 81, 82
  ribs, 78, 131
  skull, 85
Overgrown toe nail, *see* Toe nail
Oxygen carrying capacity, 17, 31

Paget's disease of nipple, 124
Pagetoid melanoma, 288
Pain, 1 *et seq*
Palate, cleft, 93

Palmar space infection, 79 *et seq*
Pampiniform plexus, 246
Pancoast syndrome, 134
Paneth cells, 157
Pancreas, 170 *et seq*
  biopsy, 175, 177
  carcinoma, 176 *et seq*
    surgery in, 177
  cytology, 177
  enzymes, 173
  fat necrosis, 171
  function tests, 175
  injuries, 54
  pseudo-cyst, 54, 171, 172, 174
  scan, 175
Pancreatectomy, 176, 177
Pancreatic divisum, 175
Pancreatic duct obstruction, 171, 176
Pancreatico-gastrostomy, 176
Pancreatitis
  acute, 170 *et seq*
    peritoneal lavage, 174
    prognostic signs, 172
  chronic and relapsing, 174 *et seq*
  classification, Marseilles, 174
  haemorrhagic, 171
Pancreatogram, operative, 176, 183
Pancreozymin, 175
Papillary carcinoma, thyroid, 118
Papilloedema, 86
Papilloma
  anal, 217, 220, 228
  bladder, 250
  cutaneous, 285
  duct, breast, 123
Paradidymis, cyst of, 246
Paradoxical respiration, 47, 49
Parafollicular cells, 119
Parathormone, 117
Park's pouch, 195
Parenteral nutrition, 14, 63, 186
Paronychia, 79 *et seq*
Parotid gland, tumours, 104 *et seq*
Parotitis
  acute, 104
  mumps, 104
Patent blue, in lymphangiography, 274
Patent ductus arteriosis, 136
Paterson-Kelly syndrome, 141
Paul's tube (latex rubber), drain, 220
Peau d'orange, 124
Pectus carinatum, 131
Pectus excavatum, 131
Pelvic fractures, 35
Pelvic inflammatory disease, 202
Peptic oesophagitis, *see* Oesophagitis
Peptic ulcer, 148 *et seq*
  bleeding, 222
    surgery in, 224
  complicated, 149, 153 *et seq*
  perforated, 153
    definitive surgery in, 154
  pyloric stenosis, 154
  treatment, 150 *et seq*
Percutaneous transhepatic
  cholangiogram (PTC), 182

Perfusion, limb, in melanoma, 289
Periampullary carcinoma, 177
Perianal, see also Anal canal
  haematoma, 216, 218, 220
Perichondritis, thyroid cartilage, 101
Pericolic abscess, 190, 209
Perineal hernia, 240
Peritoneal lavage
  in pancreatitis, 174
  in trauma, 52, 77
Peritoneal toilet, 77, 187
Peritonitis, 51 et seq, 75 et seq
  biliary, 169
  in appendicitis, 201 et seq
  in diverticular disease, 190
  in herniae, 236
  in large bowel cancer, 209
  in ulcerative colitis, 193
Pernicious anaemia, in gastric cancer,
  157
Perspiration, sensible, 8
Petit's triangle, 240
Peutz-Jeghers syndrome, 206
Peyronie's disease, 285
Phaeochromocytoma, 119
Phantom limb, 282
Pharyngeal carcinoma 98
Pharyngeal pouch, 100, 142
Pharyngitis, 105
Phenyl alanine mustard, in breast
  cancer, 127
Phlebography, see Venography
Phlebothrombosis, 268
Phlegmasia alba dolens, 267
Phlegmasia caerulea dolens, 267, 272
Photo-coagulation, endoscopic laser,
  225
Pigmented naevi, see Naevus
Pile
  sentinel, 215
  thrombosed external, 216
Piles, see Haemorrhoids
Pilonidal sinus, 217, 218, 220
Pituitary fossa tumours, 90
Plasma loss, 16
Plasmids, 66
Plaster sores, 265, 266
Pleural
  aspiration (thoracentesis), 133
  biopsy, 133
  effusion, 132
Pleural cavity, disorders, 132 et seq
Plummer-Vinson syndrome, 141
Pneumo-encephalography, 41
Pneumo-peritoneum 52
Pneumonectomy, 135
Pneumothorax, 46
  after thyroidectomy, 115
Polya gastrectomy, 151, 152, 154, 160,
  225
Polyposis
  familial (polyposis coli), 206 et seq
  Gardner's syndrome, 208
  juvenile, 206
Polyps
  gastric, 157

hamartomatous, 206
inflammatory, 192
large bowel, 206 et seq
neoplastic, 206
pseudo-polyps, 192
Portal
  hypertension, 223, 226
  pyaemia, 75
  vein thrombosis, 75
Porto-azygos disconnection, 226
Porto-systemic
  encephalopathy, 225
  shunts, 226
Positive end expiratory pressure
  (PEEP), 21
Post-cholecystectomy syndrome, 170
Post-concussion syndrome, 42
Post-cricoid carcinoma, 143
Post-traumatic
  epilepsy, 42
  pulmonary insufficiency, 20
Potassium, 8, 11, 12
Pott's puffy tumour, 85
Pre-auricular sinus, 94
Prednisolone, in breast cancer, 130
Pregnancy,
  abdominal pain in, 202
  in thyroid disease, 114
  ruptured ectopic, 203
Prendred's syndrome, 109
Processus vaginalis, 247
Proctalgia fugax, 217
Proctitis, 192 et seq
Procto-colectomy, 195, 197
Proctoscopy, 228
Propranolol, in thyrotoxicosis, 113, 114
Proptosis, 110
Prostate
  benign hypertrophy, 251, 252, 255
  carcinoma, 251 et seq
    staging, 255
    treatment, 255
  surgery, complications, 256
Prostatectomy, 255, 256, 257
Prostatomegaly, retention in, 256, 257
Prostheses, after amputation, 282
Prothrombin time, in jaundice, 181
Pruritis ani, 217
  in burns, 64
  in jaundice, 180
Pseudocyst, see Pancreas
Pseudo-membranous colitis, 22, 199
Pseudo-obstruction, bowel, 188
Pseudopolyps, 192, 196
Pseudoxanthoma elasticum, 222
Psoas sign, 201
Puestow's operation, 175, 176
Pulmonary arterial wedge pressure, 61
Pulmonary
  embolectomy, 271
  embolism, 18, 271 et seq
  metastases, 135
Pulp space infection, 79 et seq
Pump failure, 17
Pyaemia, 65, 66
  portal, 75

Pyelitis, 202
Pyelogram, see also Intravenous
    urogram
  retrograde, 54
Pyelolithotomy, 253
Pyloric stenosis, 154 et seq
Pyloric channel ulcer, 150
Pyloroplasty, 151, 225
Pyoderma gangrenosum, 193

R-factors, in antibiotic resistance, 67
R-regimen
  in pancreatitis, 173
  in ulcerative colitis, 193
Radiation burns, 64
Radio-active iodine, in thyrotoxicosis,
  113
Radio-active isotope scan, see also
    Technetium
  bone, in breast cancer, 126
  brain, 87
  HIDA, 164
  in bleeding Meckel's diverticulum,
    205
  in bleeding per rectum, 229
  iodine-labelled fibrinogen, 268
  leukocyte-labelled, 25
  liver, 53, 126, 181
  liver-lung, in subphrenic
    abscess, 25
  lung, in pulmonary embolism, 271
    ventilation perfusion, 271
  thyroid, 111
Radio-immuno-assay (RIA), in thyroid
  disease, 111
Radiotherapy in cancer, see Organs
    affected
Ranson, prognostic signs in pancreatitis,
  172
Ranula, 95
  plunging, 101, 102, 106
Rathke's pouch, 90
Raynaud's disease, 279
Raynaud's phenomenon, 102, 132, 279
Rectum
  bleeding per, 226 et seq
    causes, 227
    diagnosis, 227
    management of massive, 230
    specific syndromes, 229
  carcinoma, 208 et seq, 228
    treatment, 211 et seq
  polyps, 206, 207
  prolapse, 227
Red-currant-jelly stool, in
    intussusception, 229
Reflux, duodeno-gastric, 148
Reflux oesophagitis, 141 et seq
Regional enteritis, see Crohn's disease
Renal
  calculi, 253
  failure in pancreatitis, 172
  trauma, 54
  tumours, 249 et seq
Respiratory
  distress syndrome, adult, 17, 20

Respiratory (cont'd)
  failure in pancreatitis, 172
  management in surgery, 48 *et seq*
  quotient, 13
Rest pain, 277
Retention of urine, 256 *et seq*
Reticulo-endothelial system (RES), 18, 178
Rhinorrhoea, CSF, 42
Rib
  cervical, 102 *et seq*, 131
  fracture, 45, 46
  osteomyelitis, 131
Richter's hernia, 232, 238
Riedel's thyroiditis, 118
Roux-en-Y reconstruction
  choledocho-jejunostomy, 168
  cysto-jejunostomy, 174
  oesophago-jejunal, 160
Rovsing's sign, 201
Ryle's ten questions, in pain, 2

Saegesser's sign, 53
Salazopyrine, in colitis, 194
Salivary gland, 104 *et seq*
  calculi, 102, 104, 106
  swelling, 104
  tumours, 104
Santorini, pancreatic duct of, 175
Saphena varix, 236
Sarcoid foci, *see* Granulomas
Sarcoma
  breast, 130
  gastric, 161
Satellitosis, in melanoma, 288
Scalds, 64
Scalene node biopsy, 134
Scalenus anticus syndrome, 131
Scalp, 84 *et seq*
Scan, *see* CT, Radio-isotope, Ultrasound
Scarpa's fascia, 238
Schatzki ring, 141
Schistosoma haematobium, 250
Sciatica, 278
Scintiscan, *see* Radio-isotope scan
Scirrhous carcinoma, breast, 124
Scleroderma, 279
Sclerotherapy, injection
  in haemorrhoids, 219
  in oesophageal varices, 226
  in varicose veins, 262
  in venous ulcers, 264
Sebaceous cyst, *see* Epidermoid cyst
Seborrhoeic keratosis, 285
Secretin, 175
Seminoma, 243–245
Senile keratosis, 285
Sengstaken-Blakemore tube, 226
Sentinel loop, in pancreatitis, 173
Sentinel pile, 215
Sepsis, massive, 18
Septicaemia, 18, 66
Sequestrum, of bone, 23, 65
Sertoli cell, 243
    tumour (sertolioma), 244
Shock, 15 *et seq*

anaphylactic, 19
bacteraemic (bacterial), 18
burn, 61
cardiogenic, 17
neurogenic, 15
septic, 18
spinal, 15, 34
toxic, 18
Shock lung, *see* Adult respiratory distress syndrome
Shouldice operation, 236, 237
Shunt
  porto-systemic, 226
  Warren, 226
  ventriculo-atrial, 88
  ventriculo-peritoneal, 88
Sialangiectasis, 104
Sialolithiasis, 104
Sideropenic dysphagia, 141
Sigmoidoscopy
  fiberoptic, 210, 229
  rigid, technique, 228
Sign
  Ballance's, 53
  Blumberg's, 201
  Chvostek-Weiss, 116
  Cope's, 201
  Cruveilhier's, 236
  Cullen's, 172
  Froment's, 55
  Grey Turner's, 172
  Kehr's, 53
  Murphy's, 164
  psoas, 201
  Rovsing's, 201
  Saegesser's, 53
  Troisier's, 101, 158
  Trousseau's, 116, 177
Silver sulphadiazine in burns, 63
Sinus
  cavernous, thrombosis of, 94
  pilonidal, 217, 218, 220
  pre-auricular, 94
  umbilical, 205
  wound, 27
Sistrunk's operation, 100
Sjögren's syndrome, 104
Skin, 283 *et seq*
  closure in fractures, 33
  cysts, 283
  grafts, 30, 62, 266
  tumours, 265, 284 *et seq*
Skull
  fracture, 41, 42, 84
  osteomyelitis, 42
Slough, definition, 65
Smoking, in vascular disease, 275
Sodium, 8, 12
Space blanket, in burns, 63
Space-occupying lesions, intracranial, 85 *et seq*
Spermatic cord, 246 *et seq*
  encysted hydrocele of, 236
  lipoma of, 236
Spermatocele, 246
Spermatogenesis, 241, 246

Spherocytosis, hereditary, 179, 181
Sphincteroplasty, transduodenal, 167, 176
Sphincterotomy, endoscopic, 170
Spigelian hernia, 240
Spinal cord, injury, 34
Spinal fractures, 34
Spinal shock, 15, 34
Splanchnicectomy, in pancreatitis, 176
Spleen, rupture, 53
Splenectomy, vaccination after, 53
Spleno-renal shunt, distal, 226
Sputum retention, 48
Squamous cell carcinoma
  breast, 124
  head and neck, 95
  lung, 134
  oesophagus, 140
  renal pelvis, 250
  skin, 286
Staghorn calculus, 253
Staging in cancer, *see* Organs affected
Staplers, intraluminal, circular, 211
Starvation, 11
Stercobilinogen, 178
Sternomastoid tumour, 102, 105
Sternum, osteomyelitis, 131
Stilboestrol, in prostatic cancer, 255
Still's disease, 101
Stomach, *see also* Gastric,
  carcinoma, 157 *et seq*
    complications, 158
    haemorrhage, 223
    prognosis, 158
    spread, 158
    treatment, 160
  sarcoma, 161
  lymphoma, 161
Stomatitis, 95
Stones, *see* Calculi
Streptokinase, 270
Stress ulcer, 13, 64
Stroke, 279
Stricture
  biliary duct, 167
  ischaemic, colonic, 197
  oesophageal, 141, 143
  urethral, 256
Strychnine poisoning, 70
Stuart's transport medium, 73
Subarachnoid haemorrhage, 38, 91
Subdural
  haemorrhage, 38
  hygroma, 38
Subhyoid bursa, 100
Sublingual dermoid, 100
Submucous abscess, anal, 217, 218, 220
Subphrenic abscess, 24
Subungual
  exostosis, 290
  glomus tumour, 290
  haematoma, 290
  melanoma, 280, 287, 290
  paronychia, 79
Succussion splash, 155
Sulphur granules, in actinomycosis, 105

Suprapubic cystostomy, 257
Supratentorial, lesions, 86
Surgery, complications of, 20 *et seq*
Surgical emphysema, 44
Sutures
  in hernia repair, 232
  monofilament nylon, 77
  PGA, 33
  polypropylene, 77
Swan Ganz catheter, 61
Sweating, in burns, 64
Swellings in neck, 99 *et seq*
Swollen leg, surgical aspects, 271 *et seq*
Sylvius, aqueduct of, 85
Sympathectomy
  in pancreatitis, 176
  in vascular disease, 279
  lumbar, 266
Syndrome
  adult respiratory distress, 17, 20
  cavernous sinus, 86, 91
  costo-clavicular, 131
  Cushing's, 272
  cystic duct, 170
  dumping, 152
  Ehlers-Danlos, 222
  Friedrichsen-Waterhouse, 19
  Gardner's, 208
  Horner's 102, 116, 134
  hyperabduction, 131
  Leriche, 277
  Mallory-Weiss, 141, 223, 225
  Marfan's, 137, 276
  Meig's, 133
  Mendelson's, 21
  multiple endocrine adenoma, 156
  Pancoast, 134
  Paterson-Kelly, 141, 142, 143
  Peutz-Jeghers, 206, 207
  Plummer-Vinson, 141
  post-cholecystectomy, 170
  post-concussion, 42
  Prendred's, 109
  scalenus anticus, 131, 132
  Sjögren's, 104
  thoracic outlet, 131, 132
  Tietze's, 131
  toxic shock, 18
  Zollinger-Ellison, 148, 149, 152, 156
Syphilis, 74

T₃, 108, 111
T₃ resin uptake, 111
T₃ suppression test, 111
T₄, 108, 111
T-tube
  after exploration common bile duct, 167
  cholegram, post-operative, 167, 170
  problems, 169
  track, removal of stones, 170
Tamoxifen, 127, 129, 130
Tanner's slide, 237
Tarsorrhaphy, lateral, 88
Technetium (⁹⁹ᵐTc)
  scan, 111, 205, 229, 271
  sulphur colloid, 229

labelled macro-aggregates of albumin, 271
Temperature
  in burns, 64
  in head injuries, 40
Tenosynovitis, 80 *et seq*
Tenovaginitis, 81
Tentorial hiatus, 37
Tentorium cerebelli, 37, 86
Teratodermoids, 136
Teratoma, 136, 244
Tertiary waves, oesophageal, 139
Testis, 241 *et seq*
  anatomy, 241
  ectopic, 236, 241
  horizontal, 245
  imperfect descent, 241
  retractile, 242
  torsion, 242, 245
  tumours, 243 *et seq*
  undescended, 236, 241
Tetanus, 69 *et seq*
  prophylaxis, 55, 62, 70
  treatment, 70
Thenar space infection, 79, 80, 82
Thermography, breast, 125
Thermoregulation, 64 *see also* Temperature
Third space phenomenon, 16, 171
Thoracentesis, 133
Thoracic duct, rupture, 47
Thoracic outlet syndrome, 131, 132
Thoracotomy, 45, 46, 47
Thorax, *see* Intrathoracic conditions
Thrombectomy, 270
Thrombo-angiitis obliterans, *see* Buerger's disease
Thrombo-embolism, 280
Thrombo-endarterectomy, 279
Thrombophlebitis, 263, 268, 269
  migrans, 116, 177
Thrombosis
  arterial, post-operative, 20
  venous, 267 *et seq*
Thrombus formation, 267
Thumb printing, in ischaemic colitis, 197
Thymoma, 136
Thyrocardiacs, 113
Thyroglossal
  cyst, 100
  tract, 100
Thyroid
  binding globulin (TBG), 108, 111
  binding pre-albumin, 108
  carcinoma, 118 *et seq*
  crisis, 117
  function tests, 111
  gland, 107 *et seq*
    blood supply, 107
    disorders, 108 *et seq*
    physiology, 108
  hormones, 108
  lateral alberrant, 101
  lobectomy, 112
  nodules, 112
  releasing hormone (TRH), 111
  stimulating hormone (TSH), 108, 111

Thyroidectomy, 109, 112, 114 *et seq*
  complications, 114 *et seq*
  subtotal, 114
  total, 112
Thyroiditis, 117 *et seq*
Thyrotoxicosis, 113
  recurrent, 117
Thyroxine, 111, 113 *see also* T₃, T₄
Tietze's syndrome, 131
TNM classification, in breast cancer, 127
Toe nail, abnormalities, 289 *et seq*
  trimming, 290
Tongue, 93 *et seq*
  carcinoma, 95 *et seq*
    surgery in, 98
  congenital furrowing, 94
  fissuring, 94
  furring, 94
  geographical, 94
  inflammation, 94
  lymph drainage, 96, 97
  tie, 94
  ulcers, 95
Tonsillitis, 105
Tourniquet tests, in varicose veins, 262
Toxic goitre, *see* Goitre
Toxic granulations, neutrophils, 18
Toxic megacolon, 139, 199
Toxic shock syndrome, 18
Tracheal
  carcinoma, 101
  collapse, after thyroid surgery, 116
  rupture, 46
  stenosis, 50
Tracheitis, after thyroidectomy, 115
Tracheo-bronchitis, post-operative, 20
Tracheo-oesophageal fistula, 47, 50
Tracheostomy 48 *et seq*
  in anaphylactic shock, 19
  in burns, 63
  in chest injuries, 45, 46, 47
  in head injuries, 40
  in recurrent laryngeal nerve injury, 116
  in respiratory support, 48 *et seq*
  in tetanus, 70
Transcellular water, 7, 9, 16
Transethmoidal pituitary ablation, 90
Transient ischaemic attacks (TIAs), 92, 279
Transitional cell carcinoma, 250
Transpiration, water of, 8
Transurethral resection prostate, 255
Trasylol, 173
Triamcinolone, in Keloid, 284
Troisier's sign, 101, 158
Trousseau's sign, 177
Truss, 232
Tryptophane metabolism, 250
Tuberculosis, 73–74
  epididymis, 243
  hand, 81, 82
  neck swellings in, 101, 102–103
  urinary, 249, 253
Tuberculous dactylitis, 81

Tumours
  carotid body, 105
  chest wall, metastatic, 131
  Cock's peculiar, 85
  glomus, 290
  intracranial, 88 et seq
  Krukenberg, 158
  large bowel, 206 et seq
  neurogenic, 136
  pituitary fossa, 90
  Pott's puffy, 85
  salivary, 104
  testicular, 243 et seq
  turban, 85
  Warthin's, 104
  Wilm's, 250
Tunica vaginalis, 241
  hydrocele of, 246

Ulcer
  anastomotic, 152
  aphthous, 95
  arterial, 265, 277
  Bairnsdale, 265
  cryopathic, 265
  Curling's, 148, 223
  Cushing's, 223
  duodenal, 149 et seq, 223
    surgery in, 151 et seq, 225
  gastric, 149 et seq, 223
    surgery in, 151 et seq, 225
  hypertensive, 265
  infective, 265
  kissing, duodenal, 149
  leg, 263 et seq
  Marjolin's, 286
  Martorell's, 265
  neoplastic, 265
  neuropathic, 265
  peptic, 148 et seq, 222–226
  pyloric channel, 150, 155
  pyogenic, 265
  rodent, 286
  self-inflicted, 266
  syphilitic, 265
  traumatic, 265
  trophic, 265
  tropical, 265
  venous, 263
Ulceration of leg, 263 et seq
Ulcerative colitis, 192 et seq
  carcinoma, and, 208
  pre-operative preparation, 195
  surgery in, 194
Ulcerative procto-colitis, see Ulcerative
  colitis
Ultrasound scan, see also Doppler
  in arterial disease, 278
  in breast cancer, screening, 125
  in cholecystitis, 164, 166, 167
  in jaundice, 181
  in pancreatic disorders, 177
  in thyroid disorders, 110, 112
  in venous disease, 262, 268, 271
Umbilical hernia, 239
Umbilicus, infection, 75
Unconscious patient, management,

38 et seq
Uraemia, 76
Ureter
  calculus, 202, 253
  tumours, 254
Ureteric colic, 202
Ureterolithotomy, 253
Urethral
  catheterization, 36, 257
  injury, 35
  stricture, 256
Urinary
  calculi, 248–249, 253
  diversion, after cystectomy, 254
    for total incontinence, 259
  incontinence, 257 et seq
  retention, 256
  tuberculosis, 249, 253
Urine
  examination, 252
  exfoliative cytology, 252
Urobilinogen, 166, 178, 181
Urography, see Intravenous urogram

Vaccination
  anti-pneumococcal, 53
  for anal warts, 220
Vagotomy, 147, 151, 225
  highly selective, 151, 154, 225
  selective, 151
  truncal, 151, 225
    and gastroenterostomy, 225
    and pyloroplasty, 225
Valsalva effect, 15
Valve replacement, cardiac, 137
Valvotomy, cardiac, 137
Vancomycin, in pseudo-membranous
  colitis, 22
Varices, oesophageal, 225
Varicocele, 246
Varicose
  ulcer, see Venous ulceration
  veins, 260–263, 267–269, 273
Vascular
  disease, occlusive, 276 et seq
    peripheral, 276 et seq
  injuries, 56 et seq
  surgery, see Arterial surgery
Vasopressin, in bleeding oesophageal
  varices, 225
Vasospastic disease, 276, 279
Vaso-vagal attack, 15
Vater, ampulla of, 171, 175, 180
Vein
  diploid, 84
  emissary, 84
  femoral 261
  gluteal, 261
  graft, 57
  injury to, 57
  internal iliac, 261
  long saphenous, 260
  perforator (communicating), 260
  popliteal, 261
  of round ligament, 261
  short saphenous, 260
  thrombosis, 267

ulceration, 263 et seq, 271
Vena cava
  plication, 270, 271
  thrombosis, 273
  umbrella, 270
Venography
  in swollen limbs, 273
  in varicose veins, 262
  in venous thrombosis, 268
Venous
  gangrene, 269
  pressures, ambulatory, 262
  thrombosis, 267 et seq
    deep, prophylaxis, 269
  ulceration, 263 et seq
Ventriculography, 87
Verruca vulgaris, 285
Vesical calculi, see Bladder calculi
Vesico-colic fistula, see Fistula
Villous adenoma, rectum, 206
Vincent's angina, 95
Virchow's triad, 20, 267
Vitamin D, in post-operative tetany,
  117
Vitamin deficiencies, 75
Vitamin K, in jaundice, 182
Volkmann's ischaemic contracture, 34
Volume obligatoire, 8, 12
Volvulus, of sigmoid colon, 186
Vomiting
  bilious, 153
  post-operative, 21
Vomitus, aspiration of, 21
Von Willebrand's disease, 29

Waldeyer's ring, 98
Warren shunt, 226
Wart
  anal, 217, 220
  common, 285
  plantar, 285
  seborrhoeic, 285
Warthin's tumour, 104
Water
  body, 7 et seq
  extracellular, 7, 9
  interstitial, 719
  intoxication, 9
  intracellular, 7, 9
  lack, acute, 9
  loss of, 16
  transcellular, 7, 9
  transpiration of, 8
Water and electrolytes
  disorders, 9
  organization in body, 7
Watson-Cheyne operation, 291
Web space infections, 79 et seq
Wedge resection, toe nail, 291
Wen, 85
Whipple's triad, in insulinoma, 178
Willis, circle of, 88, 91
Wilm's tumour, 250
Winograd's operation, 291
Wirsung, pancreatic duct of, 171,
  176
Wolffian duct system, 246

Wound
  burn, 59
  chemotherapy, 30
  closure, 23
    delayed primary, 29, 77
    primary, 29
  contraction, 28
  contractures, 28
  debridement, *see* Wound excision
  disruption, 25

  dressings, 23
  excision, 29, 32, 71
  exclusion, 23
  gas-gangrene prone, 71
  healing, 23 *et seq*
  infection, 22, 29, 30, 66, 80
  management, 28 *et seq*
  sinus, 27
  tensile strength, 28
  tetanus prone, 69

Xeroderma pigmentosum, 286

Yersinia sp., in gastroenteritis, 202

Z-plasty, in pilonidal sinus, 221
Zadik's operation, 291
Ziehl-Nielsen stain, 73
Zollinger-Ellison syndrome, 148, 156